ISCCM Manual of Noninvasive Ventilation

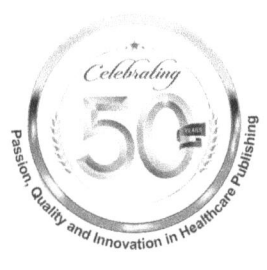

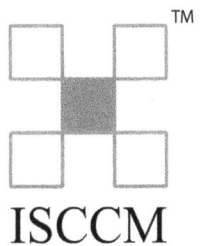

ISCCM

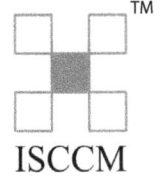

ISCCM Manual of Noninvasive Ventilation

Editors

Subhal Bhalchandra Dixit
MD IDCCM FICCM FICP FCCM
Consultant Critical Care and Director ICU
Department of Critical Care, Sanjeevan and MJM Hospitals
Pune, Maharashtra, India

Dhruva Chaudhry
MD (Med) DNB (Med) DM (PCCM)
Senior Professor and Head
Department of Pulmonary and Critical Care Medicine
Pandit Bhagwat Dayal Sharma Postgraduate Institute of Medical Sciences
Rohtak, Haryana, India

Yatin Mehta
MD MNAMS FRCA FAMS FIACTA FICCM FTEE
Chairman
Institute of Critical Care and Anesthesia
Medanta—The Medicity
Gurugram, Haryana, India

Kapil Zirpe MD FICCM FCCM
Director
Neuro Trauma Unit
Ruby Hall Clinic
Pune, Maharashtra, India

Foreword
Shirish Prayag

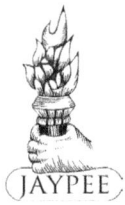

JAYPEE BROTHERS MEDICAL PUBLISHERS
The Health Sciences Publisher
New Delhi | London

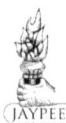 **Jaypee Brothers Medical Publishers (P) Ltd**

Headquarters
Jaypee Brothers Medical Publishers (P) Ltd
4838/24, Ansari Road, Daryaganj
New Delhi 110 002, India
Phone: +91-11-43574357
Fax: +91-11-43574314
Email: jaypee@jaypeebrothers.com

Overseas Office
J.P. Medical Ltd
83 Victoria Street, London
SW1H 0HW (UK)
Phone: +44 20 3170 8910
Fax: +44 (0)20 3008 6180
Email: info@jpmedpub.com

Website: www.jaypeebrothers.com
Website: www.jaypeedigital.com

© 2020, Jaypee Brothers Medical Publishers

The views and opinions expressed in this book are solely those of the original contributor(s)/author(s) and do not necessarily represent those of editor(s) of the book.

All rights reserved. No part of this publication may be reproduced, stored or transmitted in any form or by any means, electronic, mechanical, photocopying, recording or otherwise, without the prior permission in writing of the publishers.

All brand names and product names used in this book are trade names, service marks, trademarks or registered trademarks of their respective owners. The publisher is not associated with any product or vendor mentioned in this book.

Medical knowledge and practice change constantly. This book is designed to provide accurate, authoritative information about the subject matter in question. However, readers are advised to check the most current information available on procedures included and check information from the manufacturer of each product to be administered, to verify the recommended dose, formula, method and duration of administration, adverse effects and contraindications. It is the responsibility of the practitioner to take all appropriate safety precautions. Neither the publisher nor the author(s)/editor(s) assume any liability for any injury and/or damage to persons or property arising from or related to use of material in this book.

This book is sold on the understanding that the publisher is not engaged in providing professional medical services. If such advice or services are required, the services of a competent medical professional should be sought.

Every effort has been made where necessary to contact holders of copyright to obtain permission to reproduce copyright material. If any have been inadvertently overlooked, the publisher will be pleased to make the necessary arrangements at the first opportunity. The **CD/DVD-ROM** (if any) provided in the sealed envelope with this book is complimentary and free of cost. **Not meant for sale.**

Inquiries for bulk sales may be solicited at: jaypee@jaypeebrothers.com

ISCCM Manual of Noninvasive Ventilation

First Edition: **2020**

ISBN: 978-93-89776-42-3

Printed at:

Editors

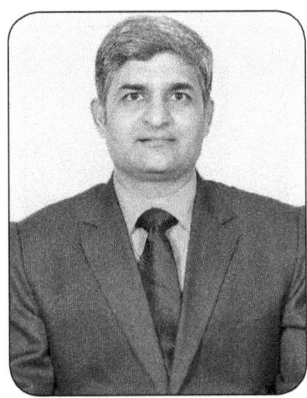

Subhal Bhalchandra Dixit
MD IDCCM FICCM FICP FCCM
Consultant Critical Care and Director ICU
Department of Critical Care
Sanjeevan and MJM Hospitals
Pune, Maharashtra, India

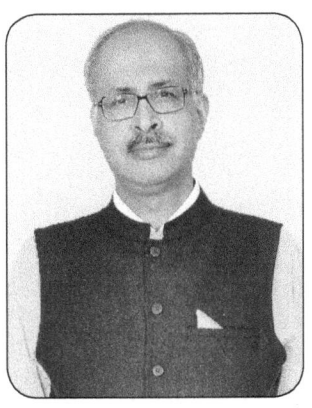

Dhruva Chaudhry
MD (Med) DNB (Med) DM (PCCM)
Senior Professor and Head
Department of Pulmonary and
Critical Care Medicine
Pandit Bhagwat Dayal Sharma Postgraduate
Institute of Medical Sciences
Rohtak, Haryana, India

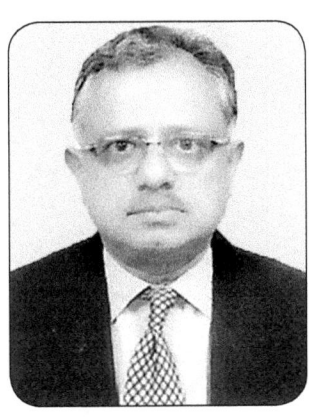

Yatin Mehta
MD MNAMS FRCA FAMS FIACTA FICCM FTEE
Chairman
Institute of Critical Care and Anesthesia
Medanta—The Medicity
Gurugram, Haryana, India

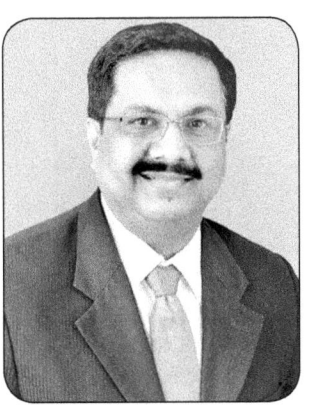

Kapil Zirpe MD FICCM FCCM
Director
Neuro Trauma Unit
Ruby Hall Clinic
Pune, Maharashtra, India

Section Editors

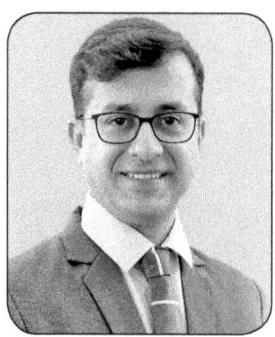

Bharat Jagiasi MD IDCCM
Head
Department of Critical Care
Su'asth Healthcare India Ltd
Mumbai, Maharashtra, India

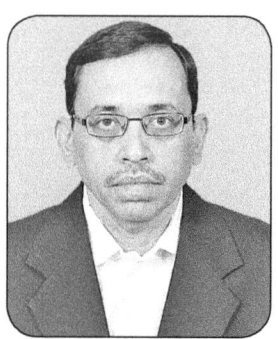

Khalid Ismail Khatib MD FICCM
Professor
Department of Medicine
Smt Kashibai Navale Medical College
Pune, Maharashtra, India

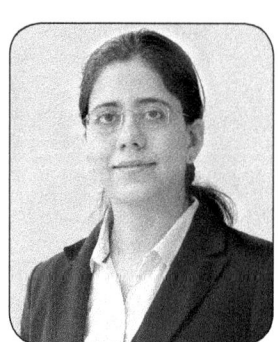

Gunjan Chanchalani MD FNB IFCCM EDIC
Chief Intensivist
Department of Critical Care Medicine
Bhatia Hospital
Mumbai, Maharashtra, India

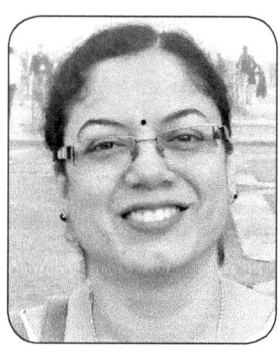

Banani Poddar MD (Pediatrics) DNB (Pediatrics)
Professor
Department of Critical Care Medicine
Sanjay Gandhi Postgraduate Institute of
Medical Sciences
Lucknow, Uttar Pradesh, India
Neonatology and Pediatrics Section

Contributors

Aakanksha Chawla MD IDCCM
Attending Consultant
Department of Respiratory, Critical Care and Sleep Medicine
Indraprastha Apollo Hospitals
New Delhi, India

Aanchal Singh MBBS DNB
General Practitioner
NMC Specialty Hospital
Al Nahada, Dubai, UAE

Abha Mahashur DNB IDCCM
Junior Consultant Chest Physician
Department of Respiratory, Critical Care and Sleep Medicine
Lilavati Hospital
Mumbai, Maharashtra, India

Akshaykumar Chhallani DNB FNB MNAMS
Consultant Honorary Intensivist
Departmentt of Critical Care Medicine
BARC Hospital
Mumbai, Maharashtra, India

Amit Goel DNB PDCC (Critical Care Medicine) EDIC
Senior Consultant
Department of Critical Care Medicine
Max Superspecialty Hospital
New Delhi, India

Amit Singh Vasan MD
Graded Specialist (Resp Medicine)
Department of Pulmonary Critical Care and Sleep Medicine
Command Hospital
Panchkula, Haryana, India

Anand Srivastava MD IDCCM
Consultant Intensivist
Department of Critical Care
Su'asth Healthcare India Ltd
Mumbai, Maharashtra, India

Anish Gupta MD FNB EDIC
Consultant
Department of Critical Care Medicine
Max Superspecialty Hospital
New Delhi, India

Anita Singh MD DNB
Associate Professor
Department of Pediatrics
Sanjay Gandhi Postgraduate Institute of Medical Sciences
Lucknow, Uttar Pradesh, India

Anjali Mishra MD
Fellow
Department of Critical Care Medicine
Max Superspecialty Hospital
New Delhi, India

Ansuman Mukhopadhyay DTCD MD (Respiratory Medicine) DNB (Respiratory Medicine)
Consultant
Department of Pulmonology
AMRI Hospitals
Kolkata, West Bengal, India

Archana Suraj Thakur MBBS DA IDCCM IFCCM EDIC
Head
Department of Critical Care
MGM New Bombay Hospital
Mumbai, Maharashtra, India

Ashish Shukla MD
Consultant
Department of Critical Care
Sir HN Reliance Foundation Hospital
Mumbai, Maharashtra, India

Atul Prabhakar Kulkarni MD FISCCM PGDHHM FICCM
Professor and Head
Department of Anesthesiology
Critical Care Medicine and Pain
Tata Memorial Hospital
Mumbai, Maharashtra, India

Babu Abraham MD MRCP (UK) FICCM
Senior Consultant
Department of Critical Care Medicine
Apollo Hospitals
Chennai, Tamil Nadu, India

Banani Poddar MD (Pediatrics) DNB (Pediatrics)
Professor
Department of Critical Care Medicine
Sanjay Gandhi Postgraduate Institute of Medical Sciences
Lucknow, Uttar Pradesh, India

Bharat Jagiasi MD IDCCM
Head
Department of Critical Care
Su'asth Healthcare India Ltd
Mumbai, Maharashtra, India

Carol D'silva MD FNB EDIC
Assistant Professor
Department of Critical Care Medicine
St Johns Medical College Hospital
Bengaluru, Karnataka, India

Deeksha Tomar DA IDCCM IFCCM EDIC
Consultant, Critical Care
Narayana Superspecialty Hospital
Gurugram, Haryana, India

Deepak Govil MD EDIC FCCM
Director
Department of Critical Care Medicine
Medanta – The Medicity
Gurugram, Haryana, India

Deven Juneja DNB FNB EDIC FCCP IFCCM FCCM
Associate Director
Department of Critical Care Medicine
Max Superspecialty Hospital
New Delhi, India

Dhruva Chaudhry MD (Med) DNB (Med) DM (PCCM)
Senior Professor and Head
Department of Pulmonary and Critical Care Medicine
Pandit Bhagwat Dayal Sharma Postgraduate Institute of Medical Sciences
Rohtak, Haryana, India

Divija Sannapareddy MD IDCCM
Consultant
Department of Critical Care
Maxcure Hospital
Hyderabad, Telangana, India

GC Khilnani MD FCCP (USA) FAMS FICCM FICP FNCCP FISDA FICS
Chairman
PSRI Institute of Pulmonary
Critical Care and Sleep Medicine
Pushpawati Singhania Hospital and Research Institute
New Delhi, India

Ganshyam Jagathkar MD FNB (Critical Care)
Director
Department of Critical Care
Maxcure Hospital
Hyderabad, Telangana, India

Gopal Raval MD DNB (Resp Med) DTCD MNAMS FSM IBSM
Consultant Pulmonologist
Critical Care and Sleep Disorders Specialist
Department of Critical Care Medicine
Sterling Hospital and Sparsh Chest Diseases Center
Ahmedabad, Gujarat, India

Gunjan Chanchalani MD FNB IFCCM EDIC
Chief Intensivist
Department of Critical Care Medicine
Bhatia Hospital
Mumbai, Maharashtra, India

Jacob George Pulinilkunnathil MD IDCCM EDIC FCCP
Senior Resident
Department of Anesthesia, Critical Care and Pain
Tata Memorial Hospital
Mumbai, Maharashtra, India

Jaikumar D Mulchandani DNB (Gen Med) MRCP IDCCM
Intensivist
Department of Critical Care
Inlaks and Budhrani Hospital
Pune, Maharashtra, India

Contributors

Jayeshkumar Dobariya MD IDCCM
Director
Department of Pulmonary and
Critical Care Medicine
Synergy Superspecialty Hospital
Rajkot, Gujarat, India

Jhuma Sankar MD IAP-ISCCM Fellowship in
Pediatric Critical Care
Assistant Professor
Department of Pediatrics
All India Institute of Medical Sciences
New Delhi, India

Jigar Padalia MBBS CTCCM IDCCM
Consultant
Department of Critical Care Medicine
Synergy Superspecialty Hospital
Rajkot, Gujarat, India

Jigeeshu Divatia MD FICCM FCCM
Professor and Head
Department of Anesthesia
Critical Care and Pain
Tata Memorial Hospital
Mumbai, Maharashtra, India

K Swarna Deepak MD (Internal Medicine) MRCP
(UK) EDIC IDCCM IFCCM
Consultant
Department of Critical Care Medicine
Apollo Health City
Hyderabad, Telangana, India

Kana Ram Jat MD FCCP
Associate Professor
Department of Pediatrics
All India Institute of Medical Sciences
New Delhi, India

Kapil S Borawake DNB IDCCM
Consultant
Department of Intensive Care Medicine
Vishwaraj Hospital
Pune, Maharashtra, India

Kapil Zirpe MD FICCM FCCM
Director
Neuro Trauma Unit
Ruby Hall Clinic
Pune, Maharashtra, India

Khalid Ismail Khatib MD FICCM
Professor
Department of Medicine
Smt Kashibai Navale Medical College
Pune, Maharashtra, India

Khusrav Beji Bajan MD EDIC
Consultant Critical Care
Head, Department of Emergency
Medicine, PD Hinduja National Hospital and
Medical Research Center
Mumbai, Maharashtra, India

Kirti M Naranje MD
Associate Professor
Department of Pediatrics
Sanjay Gandhi Postgraduate Institute of
Medical Sciences
Lucknow, Uttar Pradesh, India

Lakshmi Sasidhar Puvvula MD
Fellow
Department of Critical Care
Continental Hospitals
Hyderabad, Telangana, India

Leena Patil DNB (Anesthesia), IDCCM
Consultant Intensivist and Anesthesiologist
Secretary SCCM Jalgaon Branch, BCLS Trainer
Department of Critical Care
Dr KD Patil Multispecialty Hospital
Jalgaon, Maharashtra, India

Maitree Pandey MD
Director and Professor
Department of Anesthesiology and Critical Care
Lady Hardinge Medical College
New Delhi, India

Milap Mashru MD (Internal Medicine) FNB
(Critical Care) EDIC
Director
Department of Internal Medicine and Critical
Care Medicine
Synergy Superspecialty hospital
Rajkot, Gujarat, India

Minal Jariwala MD IFCCM EDICM
Chief Intensivist
Critical Care department
Nanavati Superspecialty Hospital
Mumbai, Maharashtra, India

Neetu Jain DNB FCCP FICCM
Consultant
Department of Pulmonary Critical Care and Sleep Medicine
Pushpawati Singhania Hospital and Research Institute
New Delhi, India

Niranjan Thomas MD (Pediatrics) DNB (Pediatrics) Fellowship in Neonatal Perinatal Medicine (Toronto)
Professor and Unit Head
Department of Neonatology
Christian Medical College
Vellore, Tamil Nadu, India

Nirmalyo Lodh MD
Fellow
Department of Anesthesia, Critical Care and Pain
Tata Memorial Hospital
Mumbai, Maharashtra, India

Nishanth Baliga MD
Fellow
Department of Anesthesia, Critical Care and Pain
Tata Memorial Hospital
Mumbai, Maharashtra, India

Nitin Dhochak MD DM
Senior Resident
Department of Pediatric Pulmonology and Intensive Care
All India Institute of Medical Sciences
New Delhi, India

Palepu B Gopal MD FRCA FCCM FICCM
Head
Department of Critical Care Medicine
Continental Hospitals
Hyderabad, Telangana, India

Prasad Padwal MD (Pulmonary Medicine) FNB (Critical Care Medicine)
Associate Consultant
Department of Critical Care
Fortis Hospital
Mumbai, Maharashtra, India

Prashant Nasa MD FNB (Critical Care Medicine) EDICM CIC
Specialist and Head, Critical Care Medicine
Chairman Prevention and Control of Infection
NMC Specialty Hospital
Al Nahada, Dubai, UAE

Prashant Singh DNB IDCCM
Associate Consultant
Department of Critical Care Medicine
Max Superspecialty Hospital
New Delhi, India

Pratheema Ramachandran DNB IDCCM IFCCM EDIC
Consultant
Department of Critical Care Medicine
Apollo Hospitals
Chennai, Tamil Nadu, India

Praveen Kumar G MD FNB EDIC
Associate Consultant
Department of Critical Care Medicine
Medanta – The Medicity
Gurugram, Haryana, India

Priyanka Singh MD DNB
Graded Specialist (Resp Medicine)
Department of Pulmonary Critical Care and Sleep Medicine
Army Hospital Research and Referral
New Delhi, India

Rahul Agrawal MD
Consultant Internist
Department of Critical Care
Maxcure Hospital
Hyderabad, Telangana, India

Rahul Pandit FCICM FJFICM EDICM FCCP FICCM MD DA
Director
Intensive Care Unit
Fortis Hospital
Mumbai, Maharashtra, India

Rajeev Kumar Thapar MD (Pediatrics) Post Doctoral Fellowship in Neonatology
Professor
Department of Pediatrics
Command Hospital (Central Command)
Lucknow, Uttar Pradesh, India

Rajesh Chandra Mishra MBBS MD (Medicine) FNB EDIC FCCM FCCP FICP
Consultant Intensivist and Internist
General Secretary ISCCM 2019-20
Ahmedabad, Gujarat, India

Contributors

Rajesh Chawla MD FCCM FCCP
Senior Consultant
Department of Respiratory
Critical Care and Sleep Medicine
Indraprastha Apollo Hospitals
New Delhi, India

Rajesh Pande MD PDCC FICCM FCCM
Director
BLK Center of Excellence for Critical Care
BLK Superspecialty Hospital
New Delhi, India

Raymond Dominic Savio MD DM EDIC FISCCM
Consultant
Department of Critical Care Medicine
Apollo Hospitals
Chennai, Tamil Nadu, India

Ripenmeet Salhotra MD (Anesthesiology) IDCCM
IFCCM EDIC
Director and Head
Department of Critical Care Medicine
Fortis-Escorts Hospital
Faridabad, Haryana, India

Rohit Yadav Diploma in Anesthesia IDCCM
Senior Consultant
Department of critical care
Nayati Medicity
Mathura, Uttar Pradesh, India

Roseleen Kaur Bali DNB IDCCM
Consultant
Department of Respiratory, Critical Care and
Sleep Medicine
Indraprastha Apollo Hospitals
New Delhi, India

Ruchi Gupta Singla MD FNB
Associate Consultant
Department of Critical Care Medicine
Medanta – The Medicity
Gurugram, Haryana, India

Sachin Gupta MD IDCCM IFCCM EDIC FCCM FICCM
Head
Department of Critical Care
Narayana Superspecialty Hospital
Gurugram, Haryana, India

Safal Muhammed MK MD (Pediatrics)
Assistant Professor
Department of Pediatrics
Command Hospital (Central Command)
Lucknow, Uttar Pradesh, India

Sameer Jog MD EDIC IDCCM
Consultant Intensivist
Department of Intensive Care Medicine
Deenanath Mangeshkar Hospital and
Research Center
Pune, Maharashtra, India

Samriti Gupta MD DM
Senior Resident
Department of Pediatrics
All India Institute of Medical Sciences
New Delhi, India

Sandesh Kumar MD FNB EDIC
Consultant Intensivist
Department of critical care
Cloud Physician Healthcare
Bengaluru, Karnataka, India

Sateesh A MD
Fellow
Department of Pulmonary and Critical Care Medicine
Pandit Bhagwat Dayal Sharma Postgraduate
Institute of Medical Sciences
Rohtak, Haryana, India

Satya Ranjan Sahu DNB IDCCM MNAMS
Associate Consultant
Department of Pulmonary Critical Care and
Sleep Medicine
Pushpawati Singhania Hospital and
Research Institute
New Delhi, India

Sharmili Sinha MD DNB EDIC
Senior Consultant
Department of Critical Care Medicine
Apollo hospitals
Bhubaneswar, Odisha, India

Sheila Nainan Myatra MD FICCM FCCM
Professor
Department of Anesthesia, Critical Care and Pain
Tata Memorial Hospital
Mumbai, Maharashtra, India

Shivangi Khanna MD
Fellow National Board
Department of Critical Care
Artemis Hospital
Gurugram, Haryana, India

Simran Singh MD EDIC FRCP (London) IDCC FICCM
Consultant Intensivist and Physician
Hinduja Hospital
Mumbai, Maharashtra, India

Sonali Ghosh DCH MRCPCH IDPCCM
Consultant
Department of Pediatrics
QRG Health City
Faridabad, Haryana, India

Subhal Bhalchandra Dixit MD IDCCM FICCM FICP FCCM
Consultant Critical Care and Director ICU
Department of Critical Care
Sanjeevan and MJM Hospitals
Pune, Maharashtra, India

Sumit Ray MD FICCM
Chairperson
Department of Critical Care
Artemis Hospital
Gurugram, Haryana, India

Suneel Kumar Garg MD FNB IFCCM EDIC FICCM FCCP FCCM
Senior Consultant
Department of Critical Care Medicine
Max Superspecialty Hospital
New Delhi, India

Supradip Ghosh DNB (Internal Medicine) EDIC FICCM
Director and Head
Department of Critical Care Medicine
Fortis-Escorts Hospital
Faridabad, Haryana, India

Suresh Ramasubban AB (Internal Medicine, Pulmonary and Critical Care)
Senior Consultant
Department of Respiratory, Critical Care and Sleep Medicine
Apollo Gleneagles Hospital
Kolkata, West Bengal, India

Susruta Bandyopadhyay MD Dip Card
Director
Department of Critical Care
AMRI Hospitals
Kolkata, West Bengal, India

Swapna Chitra Vijaykumaran MD
Resident
Department of Anesthesiology
Pain and Critical Care
Tata Memorial Hospital
Mumbai, Maharashtra, India

Tushar Sontakke MD (Medicine) IDCCM
Intensivist
Department of Critical Care
MGM New Bombay Hospital
Mumbai, Maharashtra, India

Vikas Marwah MD (Pulmonary Medicine)
SCE (Resp Med) RCP (UK)
Senior Advisor (Resp Medicine), Trained in Pulmonary Critical Care
Professor (AFMC)
Department of Pulmonary Critical Care and Sleep Medicine
Military Hospital (CTC)
Pune, Maharashtra, India

Vivek Kumar MD DNB IFCCM EDIC FICCM FICP FACP MNAMS
Chief Intensivist
Department of Respiratory, Critical Care and Sleep Medicine
Sir HN Reliance Foundation Hospital
Mumbai, Maharashtra, India

Yash Javeri DA IDDCM FICCM
Director
Apex Healthcare Consortium
New Delhi, India

Foreword

It gives me a great pleasure to write this foreword for the *ISCCM Manual of Noninvasive Ventilation (NIV)*.

We are all aware of the great strides taken by the science of mechanical ventilation of the critically ill patients. From just being a machine being used to support failing respiratory system in 1950s, the science of this field has come a long way. Among the important strides being taken have been the ones associated with noninvasive ventilation.

The evolution of noninvasive positive pressure ventilation over the last 20 years has been quite enormous and interesting. It has started from the need to reduce the chances of ventilator associated pneumonitis with reducing the tracheal invasion during mechanical ventilation. It started with attempted use during various situations requiring mechanical ventilation for a short period of time. It has now evolved into two distinct categories of uses: one in the ICU or hospital as a substitute for invasive ventilation for conditions which are not so severe. The second category is the use at home for chronic long-term support.

Both these uses need their own detailed discussion in terms of conditions and stages in which to use, equipment, monitoring, complications and many other aspects.

This is the basic need for a workbook like this one being brought out by ISCCM.

The readers will be very attracted to the long list of topics included in this book and their curiosity and appetite will be whetted by this interesting list of contents.

I sincerely hope that the book meets the reader's expectations and adds laurels to the long list of achievements of ISCCM. I also hope that the dissemination of science of noninvasive ventilation leads to a more appropriate, scientific use of this equipment in the field of critical care.

Shirish Prayag MD FCCM
Shree Medical Foundation
Prayag Hospital
Pune, Maharashtra, India

Preface

Noninvasive ventilation (NIV), as a technique/intervention, is universally practiced by pulmonologists, intensivists, emergency physicians and anesthesiologists in different environments in varied conditions. Its use has expanded multifold over the years because of ease of application, cost effectiveness and flexibility. Indications have expanded, technology has improved leading to application of complex modes including dual modes, interface quality and choices have also improved thereby simplifying the application of technique. However, as a spin off, these added to the complexity, especially in view of choices of technology for delivery (ICU ventilators versus standalone NIV ventilators or by ventilators developed for home ventilation), how to optimize oxygenation and which mask (interface) to use to take care of patient's comfort with minimal leaks to maintain efficiency of ventilation. Noninvasive ventilations wider application lead to realization of limitation of the technique and potential harm. Practitioners frequently wonder how to nebulize, humidify the gas, correct patient ventilator asynchrony and use of sedation. Because of inherent reluctance for intubation, NIV is frequently used for prolonged periods in acute settings contributing to mortality and morbidity.

The ISCCM, the force and motivation behind the spread of critical care as a subspecialty in India, constituted a task force to relook at its previous guidelines on NIV in view of advances and new knowledge accumulated over the period under Dr Subhal Dixit and Dr Rajesh Chawla. During the formation of guidelines, it was realized that though there is an abundance of literature, but there is no Indian manual/monograph on noninvasive ventilation to guide the practitioners of this technique in the country, leading to concept and writing of this manual. There are 41 chapters in the manual under different section heads dealing with physiology, clinical applications, use in different types of respiratory failure, including end of life situations, and limitations, challenges as well as its use in pediatrics.

The editorial board is thankful to all the authors who have contributed in writing the chapters and sharing their knowledge and experiences. Dr Bharat Jagiasi, Dr Gunjan Chanchalani, Dr Khalid Ismail Khatib and Prof Banani Poddar deserve a special reference and thanks for their tireless work in helping shape the book in current format. We also extend our thanks to M/s Jaypee Brothers Medical Publishers, New Delhi, India, for ensuring the timely completion and publication of this manual.

Dhruva Chaudhry
on Behalf of Editorial Board
ISCCM Manual of Noninvasive Ventilation

Acknowledgments

As, President of Indian Society of Critical Care Medicine (ISCCM), it is my proud privilege to introduce the book *ISCCM Manual of Noninvasive Ventilation* to the critical care community.

With the ever-expanding field of critical care, an endeavor to strengthen the academics and ICU practices across the country, the ISCCM has come up with this book to serve as a bedside reference guide.

Noninvasive ventilation is the most popular way patients are ventilated in critical care units and its utility and indications have been well defined and accepted.

Experts from across the country have come together through the book to share their wide evidence based literature and knowledge in the field of noninvasive ventilation.

All the contributors are renowned critical care experts from leading institutions across India.

This book represents an invaluable resource for critical care professionals, and covers the full spectrum of noninvasive ventilation.

Intensivists, postgraduates across the country will find this book an invaluable reference text.

I would like to congratulate the Section Editors, Dr Khalid Ismail Khatib, Dr Bharat Jagiasi, Dr Gunjan Chanchalani and Dr Banani Poddar, on accomplishing the difficult task successfully.

I hope the book serves the purpose for critical care community in saving lives!

Best Wishes!!

Subhal Bhalchandra Dixit
MD IDCCM FICCM FCCM FICP
President ISCCM
2019-2020

Contents

Section 1: Introduction and Physiology

1. **Noninvasive Ventilation: Rationale and Definitions** 3
   Khalid Ismail Khatib, Subhal Bhalchandra Dixit
   Definitions *3*
   Advantages of Noninvasive Ventilation *4*
   Rationale for the Use of Noninvasive Ventilation *4*

2. **Heart–Lung Interactions during Noninvasive Ventilation** 5
   Jigeeshu Divatia, Jacob George Pulinilkunnathil
   Effects of Changes in Intrathoracic Pressure *5*
   Effects of Changes in Lung Volume *7*
   Ventricular Interdependence *8*
   Clinical Applications of Heart–Lung Interaction *9*

3. **Ventilators for Noninvasive Ventilation: Critical Care versus Noninvasive Home Ventilators** 13
   Deepak Govil, Ruchi Gupta Singla, Praveen Kumar G
   History and Development of NIV Ventilators *13*
   Current Domiciliary NIV Devices versus ICU Ventilators: What do We Know of the Machine We Use? *13*
   Understanding Noninvasive Ventilators *14*
   Alarms and Monitoring *16*
   Battery Backup *17*
   Noninvasive Ventilation in ICU Ventilators without NIV Mode *17*

4. **Modes of Ventilation for Noninvasive Ventilation Including Newer Modes** 19
   Gunjan Chanchalani, Minal Jariwala
   History *19*
   Classification *19*
   Modes *20*
   How to Choose the Right NIV Mode? *26*

5. **Noninvasive Ventilation Interfaces** 30
   Bharat Jagiasi, Leena Patil, Anand Srivastava
   Background *30*
   Interface *30*
   Practical Implications and Studies/Evidence *36*

6. **Noninvasive Ventilation: Adjuvant Therapies
   (Oxygenation, Humidification, Aerosol Therapies including Nebulization)** 40
   Akshaykumar Chhallani, Bharat Jagiasi
   Background *40*
   Oxygenation *40*
   Humidification *41*
   Aerosol Therapy *43*
   Bronchodilator Delivery by Metered-dose Inhaler *45*

7. **Noninvasive Ventilation: Indications, Contraindications, and Complications** 50
   Deven Juneja, Anish Gupta, Anjali Mishra
   Indications *50*
   Contraindications *56*
   Complications *57*

8. **Application of Noninvasive Ventilation: Algorithmic Approach
   (Initiation, Customization, and Troubleshooting)** 62
   Rajesh Chawla, Roseleen Kaur Bali, Aakanksha Chawla
   Application of Noninvasive Ventilation *62*
   Assess the Need of NIV *62*
   Initiation of NIV *64*
   Mode of Ventilation *64*
   Monitoring *67*

9. **Physiology of Type I and Type II Respiratory Failure** 72
   Khalid Ismail Khatib, Subhal Bhalchandra Dixit
   Pathophysiology *72*

Section 2: Noninvasive Ventilation: Disease Specific

10. **Practical Approach to Use of Noninvasive Ventilation in
    Acute Hypercapnic Respiratory Failure** 77
    Vivek Kumar, Abhu Muhushur, Ashish Shukla
    What is Acute Hypercapnic Respiratory Failure? *77*
    What are Common Causes of Acute Hypercapnic Respiratory Failure? *77*
    What is the Pathophysiology of Acute Respiratory Failure in COPD? *78*
    How does Noninvasive Ventilation Work in this Situation? *78*
    Complications of Noninvasive Ventilation Therapy *85*
    Evidence for NIV Use in Acute Exacerbation of Chronic Obstructive Pulmonary Disease *86*
    What do the Guidelines Say? *86*

11. **Noninvasive Ventilation in Acute Exacerbation of COPD:
    Rationale, Indications, and Factors for Failure** 89
    Sumit Ray, Shivangi Khanna
    Rationale of NIV in Acute Exacerbations of COPD *89*

Indications of NIV in COPD *90*
Failure of NIV *91*

12. Noninvasive Ventilation in Hypoxemic Respiratory Failure: Rationale, Indications, and Outcomes 96

Dhruva Chaudhry, Sateesh A

Rationale of Noninvasive Ventilation in Hypoxemic Respiratory Failure *96*
Noninvasive Ventilation Application in Hypoxemic Respiratory Failure with Different Clinical Settings *98*
Noninvasive Ventilation Setup in Hypoxemic Respiratory Failure *101*

13. Noninvasive Ventilation in Cardiogenic Pulmonary Edema 105

Rajesh Chandra Mishra, Sharmili Sinha, Gopal Raval, K Swarna Deepak

Pathophysiology of Cardiogenic Pulmonary Edema *105*
Heart-Lung Interaction during CPAP and How CPAP (NIV) Helps in Reversing these Physiological Changes *106*
How does Bilevel Positive Airway Pressure Work? *108*
CPAP Compared with BIPAP *108*
Practical Aspects of Noninvasive Ventilation in Cardiogenic Pulmonary Edema *109*

14. Noninvasive Ventilation in Acute Respiratory Distress Syndrome 113

Praveen Kumar G, Deepak Govil

Noninvasive Ventilation in Acute Respiratory Distress Syndrome *113*

15. Role of Noninvasive Ventilation in Postoperative Cases 119

Prasad Padwal, Rahul Pandit

Background *119*
Role of NIV in Abdominal Surgery *119*
Role of NIV in Bariatric Surgery *120*
Role of NIV in Spinal Surgery *120*
Role of NIV in Thoracic Surgery *120*
Role of NIV in Post-Lung Transplant *121*
Role of NIV in Atelectasis *121*

16. Noninvasive Ventilation in Obstructive Sleep Apnea 124

Kapil Zirpe, Kapil S Borawake

Obstructive Sleep Apnea *124*
Positive Airway Pressure Therapy *125*
Modes of Positive Airway Pressure *126*
Patient-Device Interface *130*
Accessory Features *131*
Assessing Adequacy of PAP Settings *132*

17. Noninvasive Ventilation in Neuromuscular Disease 134

Raymond Dominic Savio, Pratheema Ramachandran, Babu Abraham

Myopathies *134*
Diseases that Affect the Neuromuscular Junction *136*
Tetraplegia/Quadriplegia *138*

18. **Noninvasive Ventilation in Chest Wall Deformities and Chest Trauma** — 142
    Suneel Kumar Garg, Prashant Singh, Gunjan Chanchalani, Amit Goel
    Mechanism Underlying Respiratory Failure in Chest Wall Deformity *142*
    Place of NIV in Chest Wall Deformities *143*
    Noninvasive Ventilation in Trauma *145*

19. **Noninvasive Ventilation in Immunocompromised Patients and Patients on Palliative Care** — 149
    Supradip Ghosh, Ripenmeet Salhotra, Sonali Ghosh
    Noninvasive Ventilation in Immunocompromised Patients *149*
    Noninvasive Ventilation in Palliative Care *153*

20. **Noninvasive Ventilation in Pneumonia** — 156
    Vikas Marwah, Priyanka Singh, Amit Singh Vasan
    Evidence for Use of Noninvasive Ventilation in Pneumonia *156*
    Reasons for NIV Failure in ARF due to Pneumonia *157*

Section 3: Noninvasive Ventilation in Specific Situations

21. **Noninvasive Ventilation during Transport** — 163
    Suresh Ramasubban
    Interhospital Transfer *163*
    Intrahospital Transfer *164*

22. **Noninvasive Ventilation during Intensive Care Unit Procedures** — 169
    Sheila Nainan Myatra, Nishanth Baliga, Nirmalyo Lodh
    Preoxygenation *169*
    Bronchoscopy *171*
    Endoscopy and Transesophageal Echocardiography *172*
    Procedural Sedation *173*

23. **Ambulation on Noninvasive Ventilation in Critically Ill Patients** — 176
    Prashant Nasa, Aanchal Singh
    Effects of Bed Rest on Critically Ill Patients *176*
    Management of Intensive Care Unit-Acquired Weakness *177*
    Early Mobilization of Mechanically Ventilated Patients *177*
    Early Ambulation of Patient on Noninvasive Ventilation *177*
    Early Ambulation with Noninvasive Ventilation *178*
    Cost-Effectiveness of Early Mobilization *179*
    Future Directions *180*

24. **Sedation during Noninvasive Ventilation** — 183
    Subhal Bhalchandra Dixit, Khalid Ismail Khatib
    Indications for Sedation in Patients on Noninvasive Ventilation *183*

Drugs Used for Sedation during Noninvasive Ventilation *183*
Monitoring during Sedation for Patients on Noninvasive Ventilation *184*

25. Humidification and Aerosol Therapy in Noninvasive Ventilation — 186

Jayeshkumar Dobariya, Jigar Padalia, Milap Mashru

Humidification *186*
Points that Favor Humidification during Noninvasive Ventilation *186*
Some Points against the Use of Humidification in Noninvasive Ventilation *187*
Conclusion for Humidification In Noninvasive Ventilation *188*
Recommendations *188*
Aerosol Therapy in Noninvasive Ventilation *188*
Aerosol System *188*
Aerosol Deposition *188*
Factors Favoring Drug Delivery by Aerosol System *189*
Common Applications of Aerosol Therapy in Critical Care *190*
Factors Affecting Aerosol Therapy in Noninvasive Ventilation *190*
Recommendations (Good Practice Points) *193*

Section 4: Monitoring and Weaning

26. Monitoring of Patients on Noninvasive Ventilation — 197

Neetu Jain, Satya Ranjan Sahu, GC Khilnani

Requirements for Adequate Monitoring of Patient on NIV *198*

27. Capnography in Noninvasive Ventilation: Clinical Implications — 203

Jacob George Pulinilkunnathil, Nirmalyo Lodh, Swapna Chitra Vijayakumaran, Atul Prabhakar Kulkarni

Need for Capnography Monitoring during Noninvasive Ventilation *203*
Understanding the Capnography Waveform *204*
End-Tidal Capnography at the Bedside *205*
Transcutaneous CO_2 Monitoring *207*
Use of Continuous Capnography in Intensive Care Unit (ICU) *208*
Indications for Using Cutaneous Monitoring in Intensive Care Unit (ICU) *208*
Future Directions *208*

28. Weaning from Noninvasive Ventilation — 210

Palepu B Gopal, Lakshmi Sasidhar Puvvula

Indications for Noninvasive Ventilation *210*
Modes of Noninvasive Ventilation *210*

29. Noninvasive Ventilation in Failure to Wean from Invasive Ventilation, Postextubation Failure, and Tracheostomy — 214

Khusrav Beji Bajan

Noninvasive Ventilation as a Weaning Assist from Invasive Mechanical Ventilation *216*
Noninvasive Ventilation to Prevent Postextubation Respiratory Failure *216*
Noninvasive Ventilation and Tracheostomy *218*

Section 5: Problems with Noninvasive Ventilation

30. Skin Sore, Nutrition (RT Feeding), Gastric Insufflation, Physiotherapy: Lung Toileting, and Agitated Patients   223
Sachin Gupta, Deeksha Tomar

Skin Sores *223*
- Skin Lesions *223*
- Pathogenesis *224*
- Risk Factors *224*
- Stages of Pressure Ulcers *224*
- Measures to Prevent Pressure Sores *224*

Nutrition *227*
- Reasons for Underfeeding Patients on Noninvasive Ventilation *227*

Gastric Insufflation *228*

Physiotherapy *228*
- Techniques *228*

Agitated Patients *229*

Section 6: Home Ventilation

31. Home Ventilation: Essentials of Practice   233
Sandesh Kumar, Yash Javeri, Rohit yadav
- Equipment *233*
- Indications *234*
- Contraindications *235*
- Selection of Patient *236*
- Interface *236*
- Ventilator *236*
- Assessment of Patient Suitability of Domiciliary Use of Noninvasive Ventilation *237*
- Patient Education and Monitoring *237*

32. Discharge Criteria of Noninvasive Ventilation Dependent Patients   239
Bharat Jagtasi, Archana Suraj Thakur, Tushar Sontakke
- General Criteria *239*
- Device Criteria *240*
- Disease Specific Criteria *240*
- Social Criteria *241*
- Follow-up Criteria *242*
- Noninvasive Ventilation in Palliative Care *242*

33. Monitoring Accuracy of Home Ventilators and Telemonitoring of Patient on Home Bilevel Positive Airway Pressure   245
Ganshyam Jagathkar, Divija Sannapareddy, Rahul Agrawal
- Indications to Use Home Noninvasive Ventilation *245*
- What to Monitor? *245*

Telemonitoring *248*
Recommendation *249*

34. Home Ventilation in Long-term Noninvasive Ventilation Users — 251
Rajesh Pande, Maitree Pandey

Major Indications for Home Ventilation *251*
Congestive Heart Failure *254*

Section 7: High Flow Nasal Cannula

35. High Flow Nasal Cannula versus Noninvasive Ventilation — 259
Susruta Bandyopadhyay, Ansuman Mukhopadhyay

Hypoxemic Respiratory Failure *260*
Cardiogenic Pulmonary Edema *260*
In Postextubation Patients *260*
Preintubation Apneic Oxygenation *261*
In "Do Not Intubate" Patients *261*
Post-Cardiac Surgery Respiratory Failure *261*
Other Indications *262*

36. High Flow Oxygen Therapy: Disease Specific — 264
Sameer Jog, Jaikumar D Mulchandani, Carol D'silva

Equipment *264*
Physiological Effects and Mechanisms of Action *265*
Indications *266*
Contraindications *267*
Complications *268*
Essentials of Practice *268*
High Flow Nasal Cannula in Clinical Practice: Evidence *269*

37. Monitoring and Weaning in High Flow Nasal Cannula — 275
Simran Singh

Physiological Effects of High Flow Nasal Cannula *275*
Predictors of High Flow Nasal Cannula Treatment Failure in Patients with Acute Hypoxemic Respiratory Failure *276*
Predictors of High Flow Nasal Cannula Success *276*
Patient Monitoring *276*
Settings of High Flow Nasal Cannula *278*
Weaning from High Flow Nasal Cannula *279*

Section 8: Neonatology and Pediatrics

38. Noninvasive Ventilation in Neonates — 285
Kirti M Naranje, Anita Singh, Niranjan Thomas

Nasal Continuous Positive Airway Pressure *285*

Principle of Continuous Positive Airway Pressure *286*
Noninvasive Positive Pressure Ventilation *293*
Monitoring and Nursing Care *295*
Complications of Noninvasive Ventilation *297*
Bilevel Continuous Positive Airway Pressure *297*
Newer Methods *298*

39. Heated Humidified High Flow Nasal Cannula Therapy in Neonates and Children — 300

Rajeev Kumar Thapar, Safal Muhammed MK

Mechanisms of Action *301*
Limitations *301*
Indications of High Flow Nasal Cannula *302*
Administration of High Flow Nasal Cannula *303*

40. Home Respiratory Support in Children: What is Possible in India? — 306

Kana Ram Jat, Nitin Dhochak

History, Burden, and Indications of Home Respiratory Support *307*
Interface for Respiratory Support *308*
Equipment for Respiratory Support *309*
Ancillary Therapies *311*
Training of Care Providers and Titration of Therapy *312*
Weaning of Home Respiratory Support *313*
Follow-up and Outcome *313*

41. Noninvasive Ventilation in Acutely Ill Children — 316

Samriti Gupta, Jhuma Sankar

Background *316*
Physiologic Principles *317*
Indications and Contraindications of Noninvasive Ventilation *317*
Initiation and Management of Noninvasive Ventilation *318*
Measurement and Monitoring *320*
Noninvasive Ventilation Failure/Success *320*
Complications *321*
Use of NIV in Acute Care Setting in Pediatrics: Evidence and Outcomes *321*

Index — *327*

Section 1

Introduction and Physiology

1. Noninvasive Ventilation: Rationale and Definitions
2. Heart–Lung Interactions during Noninvasive Ventilation
3. Ventilators for Noninvasive Ventilation: Critical Care versus Noninvasive Home Ventilators
4. Modes of Ventilation for Noninvasive Ventilation Including Newer Modes
5. Noninvasive Ventilation Interfaces
6. Noninvasive Ventilation: Adjuvant Therapies (Oxygenation, Humidification, Aerosol Therapies including Nebulization)
7. Noninvasive Ventilation: Indications, Contraindications, and Complications
8. Application of Noninvasive Ventilation: Algorithmic Approach (Initiation, Customization, and Troubleshooting)
9. Physiology of Type I and Type II Respiratory Failure

Chapter 1

Noninvasive Ventilation: Rationale and Definitions

Khalid Ismail Khatib, Subhal Bhalchandra Dixit

INTRODUCTION

The use of noninvasive ventilation (NIV) has expanded to a number of diseases and situations with an aim to provide benefit to the patient and to prevent the complications associated with invasive mechanical ventilation (MV).[1] Positive pressure ventilation (whether provided invasively or noninvasively) has benefits like reducing work of breathing, increasing delivery of higher concentration of oxygen to the alveoli, and preventing closure of upper airways. Specific benefits of providing mechanical ventilation noninvasively are that it saves cost, allows patient to take breaks from treatment for eating and other daily activities, and is better tolerated and may be more convenient. The evidence for these benefits is overwhelming for a few diseases [cardiogenic pulmonary edema, hypercapnic respiratory failure due to acute exacerbation of chronic obstructive pulmonary diseases (COPD) and other causes, weaning from MV for COPD patients, etc.] while it is not so robust for some of the conditions in which NIV has been used [acute respiratory failure (ARF) due to severe bronchial asthma, viral pneumonias, de novo hypoxemic nonhypercapnic ARF, etc.].[1-4]

DEFINITIONS

Noninvasive ventilation: It is defined as mechanical ventilation provided without the use of invasive airway. It may be provided with positive or negative pressure. The most common and widely utilized method is providing NIV by positive pressure and for all practical purposes, when the term NIV is used, it denotes noninvasive positive pressure ventilation.[1]

Patient–ventilator interfaces: As NIV avoids the use of endotracheal intubation (ETI), it mandates the use of face masks, oronasal face masks, or helmets through which compressed gas is supplied to the patient by the ventilator. These devices are known as interfaces.

Inspiratory positive airway pressure (IPAP): It denotes peak inspiratory pressure during the phase of inspiration.

Expiratory positive airway pressure (EPAP): It denotes the pressure at the end of expiration. The EPAP is referred to as continuous positive airway pressure (CPAP) when IPAP = EPAP, and is denoted as PEEP when IPAP > EPAP.

Positive end-expiratory pressure (PEEP): It denotes the pressure maintained at the end of expiration.

Rise time: It is the time taken to reach the set pressure or the speed at which pressure rises to reach the set pressure. Flow of air depends on the rise time. Shorter the rise time more rapid is the flow.

ADVANTAGES OF NONINVASIVE VENTILATION

Noninvasive ventilation has the following advantages over invasive MV with respect to application for use, complications (infective or local), and advantages to the patient.
- Increased patient comfort due to reduced work of breathing
- Prevention of localized trauma to the upper airways
- Reduction of ventilator-associated pneumonia
- Reduction in sedation and its attendant complications
- Reduces length of ICU and hospital stay in some patients
- Preserves airway clearance of secretions

RATIONALE FOR THE USE OF NONINVASIVE VENTILATION[5]

Noninvasive ventilation results in the unloading of the respiratory muscles, improves the gas exchange at the alveolar level, and increases alveolar ventilation. The decreased load on the respiratory muscles decreases respiratory muscle fatigue. Increased alveolar ventilation decreases CO_2 levels and respiratory acidosis.

CONCLUSION

Noninvasive ventilation is used for beneficial effects in a variety of critically ill patients in various clinical scenarios. It has some advantages over invasive mechanical ventilation. It improves respiratory physiology and facilitates gas exchange.

REFERENCES

1. Nava S, Hill N. Non-invasive ventilation in acute respiratory failure. Lancet. 2009;374(9685):250-9.
2. Rochwerg B, Brochard L, Elliott MW, Hess D, Hill NS, Nava S, et al. Official ERS/ATS clinical practice guidelines: noninvasive ventilation for acute respiratory failure. Eur Respir J. 2017;50(2): pii: 1602426.
3. Pisani L, Corcione N, Nava S. Management of acute hypercapnic respiratory failure. Curr Opin Crit Care. 2016;22(1):45-52.
4. Brochard L, Lefebvre JC, Cordioli RL, Akoumianaki E, Richard JC. Noninvasive ventilation for patients with hypoxemic acute respiratory failure. Semin Respir Crit Care Med. 2014;35(4):492-500.
5. Tobin MJ. Advances in mechanical ventilation. N Engl J Med. 2001;344(26):1986-96.

Chapter

2

Heart–Lung Interactions during Noninvasive Ventilation

Jigeeshu Divatia, Jacob George Pulinilkunnathil

■ INTRODUCTION

Heart-lung interactions refer to the changes in cardiovascular physiology resulting from changes in lung volume and intrathoracic pressure (ITP) during respiration. The heart and lungs are enclosed in the thoracic cavity and are subjected to the surrounding intrathoracic pressure. Phasic changes in the intrathoracic pressure and lung volume during respiration affect the cardiac function. These interactions become more prominent with intermittent positive pressure ventilation (IPPV). This chapter describes physiological changes and the clinical applications of heart-lung interactions during noninvasive ventilation (NIV).

The major determinants of heart–lung interactions are:
- Changes in intrathoracic pressure
- Changes in lung volume
- Ventricular interdependence
- Changes in intra-abdominal pressure due to the movements of the diaphragm

■ EFFECTS OF CHANGES IN INTRATHORACIC PRESSURE

Venous Return

During spontaneous respiration, the intrathoracic pressure reduces with the onset of inspiration. The reduction in intrathoracic pressure is transmitted to the right atria. The gradient between mean systemic filling pressure (MSFP) and right atrial pressure (RAP) increases, resulting in increased venous return and an increase in RV preload **(Fig. 1)**. The increase in venous return is limited due to the collapse of the great veins at the root of the neck at extremes of ITP.

With positive pressure ventilation, the increase in ITP is transmitted to the right atrium and MSFP-RAP gradient reduces, resulting in a decreased venous return and reduced right ventricular (RV) output.[1] This effect is more significant in hypovolemic patients. Compensatory mechanisms include venoconstriction due to an increase in sympathetic tone secondary to lung inflation. This maintains the MSFP-RAP gradient and venous return. The descent of diaphragm during inspiration increases the intra-abdominal pressure, compresses the splanchnic circulation, and also aids in maintaining the venous return to thorax.[2]

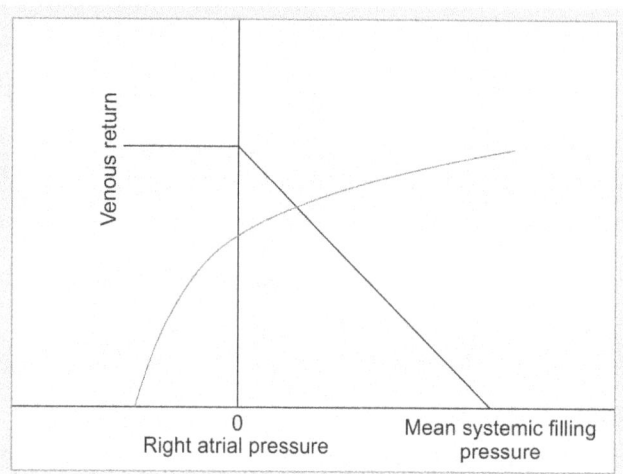

Fig. 1: Graph showing the relation between right atrial pressure, mean systemic filling pressure (MSFP), and venous return.

Ventricular Function

The ventricular output depends upon the preload, contractility, and afterload. The transmural pressure of the ventricle is the intraventricular pressure minus the intrathoracic pressure. During normal inspiration, the intrathoracic pressure is negative. During extreme tachypnea or removal of positive pressure support, the ITP becomes extremely negative, and the left ventricular (LV) and aortic transmural pressures increase, resulting in an increased afterload and impedance to left ventricular output. Simultaneously, a reduction in ITP increases venous return and intrathoracic blood volume.[3] Hence, during weaning from mechanical ventilation, as the spontaneous ventilation is being reduced, the venous return and the RV preload

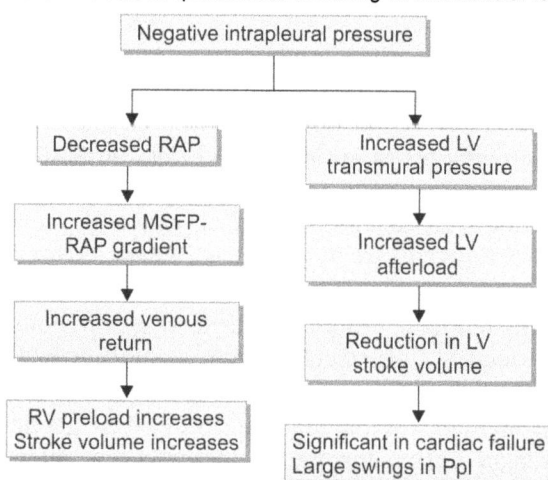

Flowchart 1: Effects of spontaneous breathing on biventricular function.

(RAP: right atrial pressure; LV: left ventricle; MSFP: mean systemic filling pressure; RV: right ventricle; Ppl: intrapleural pressure)

increase while the LV output is impeded by an increase in LV transmural pressure. This may result in weaning-induced pulmonary edema. The effects of intrathoracic pressure swings on biventricular function during spontaneous ventilation are summarized in **Flowchart 1**.

With IPPV, the venous return reduces and RV afterload increases, with a resultant reduction in right ventricular output and LV preload. The positive intrapleural pressure decreases the LV transmural pressure and afterload, thus improving ejection of the left ventricle.[3]

These physiological changes induced by IPPV are used to manage heart failure. The effects of IPPV on biventricular function are summarized in **Flowchart 2**.

Flowchart 2: Effects of intrathoracic pressure (ITP) during positive pressure ventilation on biventricular function.

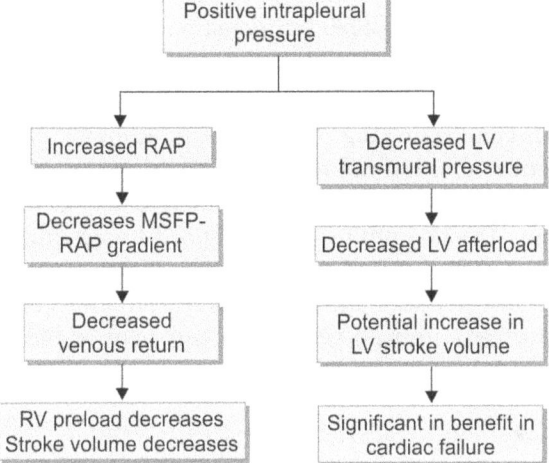

(RAP: right atrial pressure; LV: left ventricle; MSFP: mean systemic filling pressure; RV: right ventricle; Ppl: intrapleural pressure)

EFFECTS OF CHANGES IN LUNG VOLUME

Changes in Autonomic Tone

Inflation of the lungs with normal tidal volumes has a vagolytic effect resulting in tachycardia, whereas lung inflation with tidal volume >10 mL/kg can result in bradycardia with vasodilation. Positive pressure ventilation causes increased prostaglandin synthesis and reduced atrial natriuretic peptide (ANP) synthesis resulting in salt and water retention.[4]

Effects on the Cardiovascular System

During IPPV, as the lungs expand, the pulmonary vessels are squeezed, resulting in a transient increase in blood volume entering the left atrium. This effect is overtaken by the reduction in venous return, with a net reduction in preload to both ventricles. The inflated lungs compress the heart in the cardiac fossa and reduce the cardiac volume resulting in a reduction in diastolic compliance.[5]

During spontaneous breathing, the dilation of pulmonary vessels results in pooling of blood in the pulmonary circulation and reduced LV preload. Over the next few beats, increased venous return leads to increased right ventricular output with resultant increase in LV preload.

Effects on Pulmonary Vascular Resistance

At low lung volumes, extra-alveolar vessels get kinked with resultant increase in pulmonary vascular resistance (PVR). At high-lung volumes, PVR is increased as overdistended alveoli compress the alveolar capillaries. The net PVR is least at functional residual capacity (FRC) and increases above and below the FRC.[6] RV afterload is determined mainly by the PVR.

■ VENTRICULAR INTERDEPENDENCE

Both ventricles are enclosed together in the pericardium and separated by the interventricular septum. The phenomenon by which volume or pressure overloading of either ventricle affects the function of the other ventricle is called ventricular interdependence.

Series Effect

During IPPV, the phasic changes in lung volume and intrathoracic pressure result in changes in the RAP, venous return, and intrathoracic blood volume. During inspiration, there is a reduction in RV preload and RV stroke volume, which results in reduced LV preload after about three heart beats. The LV output is also reduced transiently provided it is preload-responsive. These phasic variations in LV stroke volume (stroke volume variation—SVV) or its surrogate arterial pulse pressure [systolic pressure variation (SPV) and pulse pressure variation (PPV), respectively] during ventilation can help to identify patients are fluid responsive (**Fig. 2**).

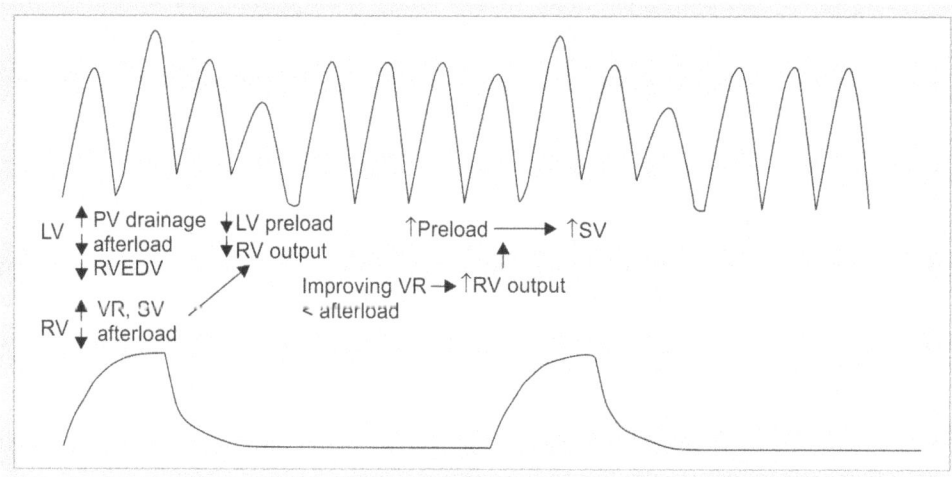

Fig. 2: Hemodynamic changes due to ventricular interdependence in series. (LV: left ventricle; RV: right ventricle; RVEDV: right-ventricular end-diastolic volume)

Parallel Effect

Normally, the LV pressure exceeds the RV pressure and the interventricular septum is usually central. During spontaneous breathing, in deep inspiration, the negative intrathoracic pressure results in increased venous return to the RA and preload of the RV.[7] If the RV is dilated, there is a shift of the septum into the LV cavity, reducing the left-ventricular end-diastolic volume (LVEDV) and stroke volume. If the there is a pericardial effusion that prevents expansion of the volume of the cardiac chambers, the LV diastolic compliance, LV filling, LVEDV, and LV output decrease, especially during inspiration, when the venous return and RV filling increase. This is manifested at bedside as an exaggerated drop in systolic pressure during inspiration in a spontaneously breathing patient, called pulsus paradoxus (**Fig. 3**).

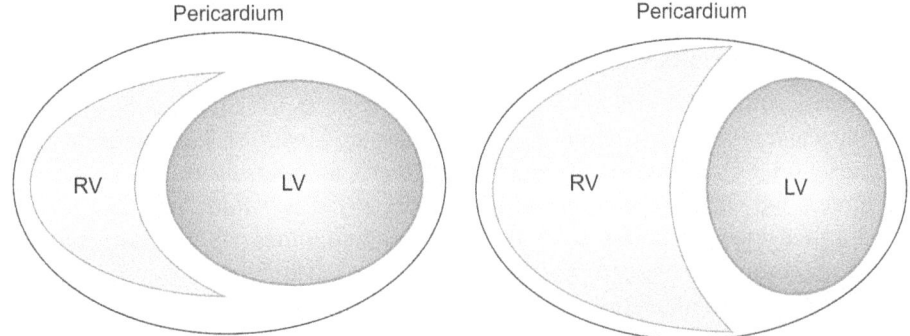

Fig. 3: Ventricular interdependence in parallel. (LV: left ventricle; RV: right ventricle)

CLINICAL APPLICATIONS OF HEART–LUNG INTERACTION

Pulsus Paradoxus

Pulsus paradoxus is an exaggerated physiological phenomenon based on ventricular interdependence. As ITP becomes negative during inspiration, the venous return increases and volume overload of the right ventricle results in a shift of the interventricular septum toward the left ventricle. This reduces the diastolic compliance of left ventricle, and reduces LVEDV and a fall in left ventricle stroke volume that manifests as a fall in systolic pressure. This systolic reduction in blood pressure during normal inspiration is further accentuated in patients with active breathing efforts with great negative swings of intrathoracic pressure and can be a marker of disease severity, e.g., status asthmaticus and pericardial diseases.[8]

Reverse Pulsus Paradoxus

A paradoxical increase in systolic pressure during inspiration followed by a decrease in systolic pressure during expiration is called reversed pulsus paradoxus. This is due to an augmentation in left ventricular function due to a significant reduction in left ventricular afterload in patients with relative hypervolemia such as LV systolic failure.

Kussmaul's Sign

During spontaneous breathing, inspiration results in reduced intrathoracic and right atrial pressure, increased MSFP-RAP gradient, and increased venous return. In conditions of poor RV compliance and increased RV afterload (pulmonary embolism), an increased venous return during inspiration will increase the right atrial pressure and central venous pressure (CVP). This paradoxical rise of CVP during inspiration is called Kussmaul's sign.[9]

Negative Pressure Pulmonary Edema

In cases where there is a markedly negative intrathoracic pressure—such as breathing against an obstructed glottis—there is a marked increase in the venous return. The left ventricular transmural pressure will increase significantly, and the left ventricular outflow is impeded. This combination of increased venous return associated with an increased impedance to left ventricular ejection results in increased intrathoracic blood volume, increased venous hydrostatic pressure, and pulmonary edema, called negative pressure pulmonary edema.[10]

Predicting Fluid Responsiveness

During respiration, there is a cyclic change in the intrathoracic pressure causing cyclic changes in right ventricular and left ventricular function. These are identified at the bedside as systolic pressure variation (SPV), stroke volume variation (SVV), and pulse pressure variation (PPV), and are increasingly used to determine fluid responsiveness.[11] Both PPV and SVV can be calculated at bedside by commercially available minimally invasive monitors using inbuilt mathematical algorithms.

However, during spontaneous breathing, as during noninvasive ventilation, these cyclical changes in intrathoracic pressure and lung volume are not of the same magnitude. PPV and SVV may remain falsely negative even in preload responders and cannot be used as predictors of fluid responsiveness. Similarly, the variation in vena cava diameter in accordance with respiration measured by bedside echocardiography, either at superior vena cava (SVC) or inferior vena cava (IVC) distal to the entry of portal vein, is unreliable in spontaneously breathing patients receiving noninvasive ventilation.

Management of Cardiogenic Pulmonary Edema

The pathophysiology of cardiogenic pulmonary edema (CPE) includes:
- Reduced left ventricular contractility, hypervolemia, and an increased afterload
- A low cardiac state resulting in tissue hypoxia that in turn increases myocardial stress and ischemia
- Wide swings of intrathoracic pressure with tachypnea that increases the venous return to the thorax. Positive pressure effectively acts on each step:
  - An increased intrathoracic positive pressure decreases the venous return and the preload of the heart
  - An increased intrathoracic positive pressure reduces the left ventricular transmural pressure, thereby reducing afterload and decreasing the impedance to the left ventricular ejection
  - As the respiratory muscles are also supported, the work of breathing reduces resulting in a reduction in the wide fluctuations of intrathoracic pressure. IPPV and PEEP maintain alveoli patent, augmenting oxygenation and reducing hypoxia-induced vasoconstriction and PVR.

In a large multicenter trial, 1,069 patients presenting to the emergency departments in the United Kingdom were randomized to receive standard oxygen therapy, continuous positive airway pressure (CPAP) (5–15 cm H_2O), or NIV (inspiratory pressure, 8–20 cm H_2O; PEEP, 4–10 cm H_2O). There was earlier improvement in symptoms of respiratory distress with CPAP and NIV compared to oxygen therapy; however, there was no difference in survival.[12]

Systematic reviews[13-17] have concluded that NIV decreases the need for intubation and hospital mortality, and although an early trial suggested greater risk of myocardial infarction with NIV than with CPAP,[18] there is no increase in the occurrence of acute myocardial infarction with NIV. The current European Respiratory Society/American Thoracic Society (ERS/ATS) clinical practice guidelines on noninvasive ventilation for acute respiratory failure[19] recommend either bi-level NIV or CPAP for patients with ARF due to cardiogenic pulmonary edema (strong recommendation, moderate certainty of evidence).

Pulmonary Edema of Weaning

When patients with borderline cardiac reserve are planned for weaning, as spontaneous breathing is resumed, the left ventricular afterload increases and the work of left ventricle increases. The reduction in intrathoracic pressure increases the venous return to the heart and the patient is at risk of pulmonary edema (*see* **Flowchart 1**). The net effect is an increased intrathoracic blood volume and decreased left ventricular function, both resulting in increased pulmonary hydrostatic pressure and pulmonary edema in patients with poor cardiac function. Development of pulmonary edema is associated with a drop in the lung volume and lung compliance, requiring greater respiratory effort for inspiration. These efforts in virtue of deep inspiratory efforts reduce the ITP and decrease the transmural pressure, thereby increasing the afterload. The increased afterload causes more pulmonary edema and the vicious cycle continues. In such patients, weaning or attempts to weaning cause an increased myocardial oxygen demand, increased respiratory muscle load, and increased oxygen demand due to pulmonary edema.[20] Such patients, if identified early, will benefit from reduction in preload and afterload or will require positive pressure support even after extubation, such as with NIV.

Cardiopulmonary Interactions that may Contribute to Lung Injury during NIV

The negative intrapleural pressure during a spontaneous breath results in higher alveolar transmural pressures with potential for volutrauma. Simultaneously, the transmural pressure across the pulmonary capillaries becomes more negative, resulting in increased pulmonary capillary blood flow and fluid shift from the capillaries into the pulmonary interstitium.[21]

In animal experiments, it has been shown that with a high-tidal volume, pulmonary blood flow and right ventricular cavity can be obliterated during inspiration and restored during expiration. This high flow–no flow–high flow cycle causes vascular shearing and endothelial injury. If, during NIV, high respiratory drive results in high tidal volumes then there is potential for lung injury by this mechanism. This may be mitigated, if NIV reduces work of breathing with a consequent reduction in tidal volume, by the maintenance of diaphragmatic tone that results in a counterbalancing PEEP.[22]

■ CONCLUSION

The heart–lung interactions occurring due to noninvasive ventilation can be beneficial or detrimental. These interactions can be successfully used for benefit in select cases such as cardiac failure. Early identification of patient's disease states and prediction of the possible heart–lung interactions are important for further hemodynamic monitoring and to optimize ventilatory management in critically ill patients.

REFERENCES

1. Henderson WR, Griesdale DEG, Walley KR, Sheel AW. Clinical review: Guyton—the role of mean circulatory filling pressure and right atrial pressure in controlling cardiac output. Crit Care. 2010;14(6):243.
2. Takata M, Wise RA RJ. Effects of abdominal pressure on venous return: abdominal vascular zone conditions. J Appl Physiol (1985). 1990;69(6):1961-72.
3. Grubler MR, Olivier W, David B, Stefan B. Basic concepts of heart-lung interactions during mechanical ventilation. Swiss Med Wkly. 2017;147(3738):1-14.
4. Pinsky MR. Heart-lung interactions. Curr Opin Crit Care. 2007;13(5):528-31.
5. Gomez H, Pinsky MR. Chapter 36: Effects of mechanical ventilation on heart-lung interactions. Effect of mechanical ventilation on heart-lung interactions. In: Tobin MJ (Ed). Principles and Practice of Mechanical Ventilation, 3rd edition. Columbus: McGraw-Hill Education; 2012.
6. Cherpanath TGV, Lagrand WK, Schultz MJ, Groeneveld ABJ. Cardiopulmonary interactions during mechanical ventilation in critically ill patients. Netherlands Hear J. 2013;21(4):166-72.
7. Jardin F, Vieillard-Baron A. Monitoring of right-sided heart function. Curr Opin Crit Care. 2005;11(3):271-9.
8. Hamzaoui O, Monnet X, Teboul JL. Pulsus paradoxus. Eur Respir J. 2013;42(6):1696-705.
9. Mansoor AM, Karlapudi SP. Kussmaul's Sign. N Engl J Med. 2015;372(2):e3.
10. Bhattacharya M, Kallet RH, Ware LB, Matthay MA. Negative-pressure pulmonary edema. Chest. 2016;150(4):927-33.
11. Michard F, Teboul JL. Using heart-lung interactions to assess fluid responsiveness during mechanical ventilation. Crit Care. 2000;4(5):282-9.
12. Gray A, Goodacre S, Newby DE, Masson M, Sampson F, Nicholl J, et al. Noninvasive ventilation in acute cardiogenic pulmonary edema. N Engl J Med. 2008;359(2):142-51.
13. Potts JM. Noninvasive positive pressure ventilation: effect on mortality in acute cardiogenic pulmonary edema: a pragmatic meta-analysis. Pol Arch Med Wewn. 2009;119(6):349-53.
14. Weng CL, Zhao YT, Liu QH, Fu CJ, Sun F, Ma YL, et al. Meta-analysis: noninvasive ventilation in acute cardiogenic pulmonary edema. Ann Intern Med. 2010;152(9):590-600.
15. Mariani J, Macchia A, Belziti C, Deabreu M, Gagliardi J, Doval H, et al. Noninvasive ventilation in acute cardiogenic pulmonary edema: a meta-analysis of randomized controlled trials. J Card Fail. 2011;17(10):850-9.
16. Vital FM, Ladeira MT, Atallah AN. Non-invasive positive pressure ventilation (CPAP or bilevel NPPV) for cardiogenic pulmonary oedema. Cochrane Database Syst Rev. 2013;5:CD005351.
17. Cabrini L, Landoni G, Oriani A, Plumari VP, Nobile L, Greco M, et al. Noninvasive ventilation and survival in acute care settings: a comprehensive systematic review and metaanalysis of randomized controlled trials. Crit Care Med. 2015;43(4):880-8.
18. Mehta S, Al-Hashim AH, Keenan SP. Noninvasive ventilation in patients with acute cardiogenic pulmonary edema. Respir Care. 2009;54(2):186-95.
19. Rochwerg B, Brochard L, Elliott MW, Hess D, Hill NS, Nava S, et al. Official ERS/ATS clinical practice guidelines: noninvasive ventilation for acute respiratory failure. Eur Respir J. 2017;50(2): pii: 1602426.
20. Teboul JL. Weaning-induced cardiac dysfunction: where are we today? Intensive Care Med. 2014;40(8):1069-79.
21. Yoshida T, Fujino Y, Amato MB, Kavanagh BP. Fifty Years of Research in ARDS. Spontaneous Breathing during Mechanical Ventilation. Risks, Mechanisms, and Management. Am J Respir Crit Care Med. 2017;195(8):985-92.
22. Katira BH. Ventilator-induced lung injury: Classic and Novel Concepts. Resp Care. 2019;64(6):629-37.

Chapter 3

Ventilators for Noninvasive Ventilation: Critical Care versus Noninvasive Home Ventilators

Deepak Govil, Ruchi Gupta Singla, Praveen Kumar G

INTRODUCTION

Noninvasive ventilation (NIV) is routinely used in various acute care settings for respiratory failure. With increase in number of domiciliary NIV prescriptions, critical care physicians are more likely to encounter patients either on home NIV admitted to the intensive care unit for various indications or discharge patients on domiciliary ventilation. This necessitates the treating physician to understand the principles of these tools and titrate the therapy to individual patient needs.

HISTORY AND DEVELOPMENT OF NIV VENTILATORS

Positive pressure ventilation began with NIV through mask and various other interfaces till the introduction of invasive ventilation. The first continuous positive airway pressure (CPAP) delivery system using nasal mask was developed in 1981 by Sullivan.[1,2]

The at-home/domiciliary NIV delivery devices were initially developed to provide volume-controlled ventilation. The first bi-level ventilator (Respironics BiPAP) was built in 1980s. It was a simple device providing expiratory positive airway pressure (EPAP) and inspiratory positive airway pressure (IPAP), functioning only in timed mode. The further development to basic design included sensitive trigger, addition of the S (spontaneous) mode, and the S/T mode. This was followed by rapid development of NIV machines with increased compactness and complexity. The automatic machines have a built-in sensor and a microprocessor to assess and analyze the patient's breathing pattern and deliver the breath according to it. Newer modes were added on, to improve patient comfort and to ensure definitive delivery of therapy.[1,2]

Intensive care unit (ICU) ventilators were primarily developed to provide invasive ventilation, but with greater demand and growing indications of NIV, most of the current ICU ventilators provide NIV modes.

CURRENT DOMICILIARY NIV DEVICES VERSUS ICU VENTILATORS: WHAT DO WE KNOW OF THE MACHINE WE USE?

The ICU ventilators are developed to comply with certain standardization and regulations. Portable NIV ventilators, though comply with broad standardization norms, are provided with greater degree of freedom for development and are patent protected. Hence, it has led to the current state where many models are available for domiciliary use with various modes of ventilation. The algorithm for many such modes for delivery and calibration remains undisclosed by the manufacturers, leading to confusion regarding there working principle. It becomes important to understand that despite the various names given, most of the modes work on the same basic principles of delivery. Clinicians need to familiarize themselves with the machines they commonly use in there settings.

UNDERSTANDING NONINVASIVE VENTILATORS

The intensivists are in general well versed with the ICU ventilators. These ventilators are driven by compressed gas and provide monitoring with graphical presentations and alarm mechanisms. Also, these are able to provide high and precise FiO_2 (fraction of inspired oxygen) delivery. The circuit has a separate inspiratory and expiratory limb to avoid rebreathing.

Mask interface may be used with conventional ICU ventilators to provide ventilation noninvasively. Usually, these are pressure-targeted mode of ventilation (either pressure support ventilation or pressure control ventilation) to allow for leak compensation through the mask. The mask used with ICU ventilators does not have an expiratory port or any other port for addition of oxygen. Inspiration and expiration are facilitated by dual limb circuit: one limb working as an inspiratory limb and one as the expiratory limb. The expiratory valve is placed near the ventilator. FiO_2 is set in the ventilator and hence can be titrated according to patient's requirement. Display interface is user friendly and airway pressure waveform recordings can be seen and adjusted real time.

On the contrary, the increasing number of portable home ventilators and modes has posed a challenge to the physician to understand the basic working principles of these machines. Simply put, NIV, like ICU ventilators provide a positive pressure at the patient's airway with a turbine or a pump, which are regulated by real-time pressure sensors in the control unit to deliver the prescribed therapy.

The volume delivered to the patient depends upon the pressure generated across the system, which is the sum of the positive pressure generated by NIV and the pressure generated by the inspiratory muscles of the patient.

The NIV central unit is provided with feedback sensors. Across the large spectrum of NIV ventilators available, all have pressure sensors to sense the pressure delivered at the patient's airway. This data then is integrated with the flow pattern during the breath and is run through the algorithms, which are specific to the mode and machine taking into account the leak in system, dead space in the circuit, compliance of the circuit, etc. The result of the final run through the algorithm is used by the ventilator to tune the pump, in order to deliver adequate pressure and flows. The exact algorithm and their implication on actual delivery of therapy remain a gray area.

It becomes important to note that the feedback algorithm takes into account the circuit characteristics, hence the circuit, mask, and expiratory port used should be the one recommended by the manufacturer for that machine.[3]

The NIV ventilators need to be assessed based on the following features:[4]
- *Gas supply*: Conventional ICU ventilators are run by compressed gas; whereas, at-home NIV machines use either an electronic turbine or a compressor to pressurize the gas.

- *Circuit*: All the conventional ICU ventilators use dual limb circuits, one forms the inspiratory limb and other forms the expiratory limb. On the contrary, most of the home ventilators function on single limb circuit. To prevent rebreathing on a single limb, an expiratory port is always incorporated in the circuit, thereby causing intentional leak. The expiratory port can be either provided in the interface or in the limb of the circuit. Continuous baseline flow during expiratory phase allows the expiratory gases to be expelled through the port and thus avoids rebreathing. It has been shown that an EPAP of at least 4 cmH$_2$O is needed to prevent rebreathing. The amount of rebreathing is least when the expiratory port is on the interface rather than on the circuit.[5]
- *Inspiratory trigger and flow*: Inspiratory triggers need to be sensitive enough to allow early recognition of inspiratory efforts to start pressurization of circuit. Refer to Table 1 for various types of triggers present in ICU and at-home ventilators. Significant leak in the circuit can cause autotriggering, especially, if the ventilator is set on flow trigger.

    Miyushi et al. found, in an experimental study, that in the presence of increasing degrees of air leak, the trigger function of two bi-level ventilators that had unchangeable trigger sensitivity (Respironics BiPAP Vision and BiPAP S/T-D) outperformed that of two conventional ICU ventilators with adjustable trigger sensitivity (Nellcor Puritan Bennett 7200ae and Puritan Bennett 840).[6] Other studies have also shown repeatedly that BiPAP machines for wide range of variability at least perform similar to conventional ICU ventilators.[7-11]
- *Air leak compensation*: Newer ventilators allow flow adjustments to compensate for some amount of the leaks in the system.

    Also, pressure-targeted ventilation to an extent compensates for the leaks and delivers adequate tidal volumes. Volume-targeted ventilation, however, is unable to do so and delivered tidal volume will be lower than the set tidal volumes.[12]

    Intensive care ventilators used for NIV measure the leak in the circuit as the difference between volumes delivered and expired, and provide leak compensation accordingly. Also, flow triggers and cancellation criteria are continuously adapted according to leak in most ventilators.
- *Deleterious effects of major leaks*:
    - Inability to achieve effective pressure and volumes to be delivered
    - Sleep disturbances
    - *Auto triggering*: In case of massive leaks, the flow drop due to it may be recognized as an inspiratory effort thereby triggering an untimely respiratory cycle and causing asynchrony.
- *Cycling to expiration*: In the ICU ventilators, noninvasive mode of ventilation is flow cycled. The threshold flow at which inspiration is cycled to expiration can be set by the user, depending on patient needs. Flow cycling is default method of cycling in home ventilators, where breath is cycled to expiration when the flow reaches default thresholds. In certain ventilators (Respironics BiPAP Vision), expiratory cycling is on auto mode or autofunction and is analyzed with every breath and autoadjusted.
- *Oxygen supply*: Most at-home NIV machines do not have oxygen–air blender to deliver fixed FiO$_2$. Oxygen may be entrained in the circuit. The delivered FiO$_2$ hence will depend on:
    - Where O$_2$ is entrained, it is the most important factor determining the FiO$_2$ delivered for given flow

- Gas and oxygen flows
- Leak in the circuit
- *Ventilatory settings*: Lower the EPAP and IPAP setting, higher is the FiO_2 delivered
- Breathing patterns
- Position of exhalation valve

In an experimental setting, Waugh and De Kler found that, with a bi-level ventilator and the leak port inside the mask, the FiO_2 was higher with lower IPAP and EPAP settings, and when O_2 was added at the ventilator outlet instead of the mask inlet.[13]

In an in vitro analysis done by Schwartz et al., the highest oxygen concentration was achieved with oxygen added to the mask, with the leak port in the circuit, and with the lowest settings of inspiratory and expiratory positive airway pressure.[14]

- *Backup respiratory rate*: Backup rate is provided in all ICU ventilators and is an important safety feature when patient is in pressure support ventilation. The latest NIV machines are now provided with backup rate to avoid apnea.
- *Modes*: NIV modes in detail are beyond the scope of this chapter and are discussed elsewhere.

A note to be made of EPAP and IPAP on domiciliary BiPAP versus the pressure support and positive end-expiratory pressure (PEEP) in ICU ventilators. This can be explained graphically as given in **Figure 1**.

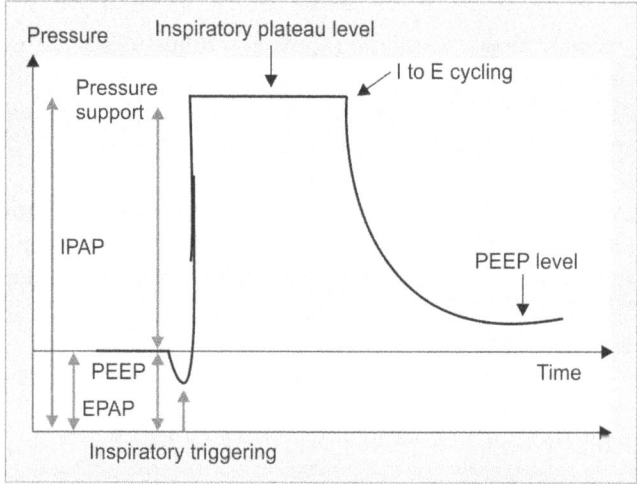

Fig. 1: Inspiratory positive airway pressure (IPAP) and expiratory positive airway pressure (EPAP) on at-home ventilators versus pressure support and positive end-expiratory pressure (PEEP) on intensive care unit (ICU) ventilators.

ALARMS AND MONITORING

With leak being an integral part of NIV ventilation, the most important variable to be measured is the expired tidal volume. This can be accurately measured in ICU ventilators and with the dual limb circuit.

With the domiciliary NIV machines, inspiratory tidal volume indicated includes the air leak through the circuit and hence is not a reflection of delivered tidal volume. The single limb circuit with an expiratory port cannot accurately measure the expired tidal volume. The algorithm used by the manufacturers to give this value is not still validated.

BATTERY BACKUP

Battery backup of any NIV system should be noted, especially if the patient is acutely dependent on NIV or patient requires transportation.

The various differences between NIV mode on ICU ventilators and at-home ventilators are summarized in **Table 1**.

Table 1: Difference between noninvasive ventilation (NIV) mode on intensive care unit (ICU) ventilator and at-home ventilators.

Characteristics	ICU ventilators	At-home NIV machine
Gas supply and pressurization	Use highly pressurized gas supply	➤ Have a compressor or electronic turbine to pressurize the room air. ➤ Stable pressures are not assured, especially when high ventilatory performance is required. ➤ No guarantee of stable pressurization, especially at higher pressures
Circuit tubings	*Dual limb*: One inspiratory other expiratory limb	➤ Typically single limb circuit ➤ Few newer machines with dual limb circuit
Circuit expiratory port	Expiratory valve in the ventilator	➤ Intentional leak in the mask or near it ➤ One way expiratory valve
Trigger	➤ Flow-based trigger, ➤ Time trigger in control mode ➤ Advanced ventilators like (NAVA) may include neural signal as trigger.	➤ Flow-based trigger ➤ Pressure-based trigger (no longer used) ➤ Time trigger (T/timed mode)
Cycling	➤ *Support mode*: Flow cycling ➤ *Control mode*: Time cycling	➤ Flow cycling
Oxygen supply	➤ Pressurized oxygen into the air oxygen blender	➤ Mostly without blender ➤ Newer model with blenders available
FiO_2 delivery	➤ Higher FiO_2 and fixed FiO_2 may be delivered	➤ Variable FiO_2 performance
Alarms and monitoring	Advance monitoring and graphical representation with highly sensitive alarms	➤ Provided with basic alarms and monitoring, which greatly vary
Alarms utility	Provide better monitoring and care in acute settings	Very sensitive alarms to leaks may not be useful as some amount leak acceptable

FiO_2: Fraction of inspired oxygen

NONINVASIVE VENTILATION IN ICU VENTILATORS WITHOUT NIV MODE

The ICU ventilators are commonly used to provide NIV. However, when a mask interface is used, the leaks generated may cause variable triggering, cycling, and therapy delivery. In an ICU ventilator when NIV mode is activated, the flow increase to compensate increase in leak is noted.

In a bench study, Vignus et al. evaluated eight ICU ventilators for delivery of NIV with and without leak and with and without NIV mode activation. On most ventilators, it was noted that without activating the NIV mode, leaks lead to increase in trigger delay and workload, a decrease in pressurization, and delayed cycling. In most of the ventilators, most of the issues were ameliorated by activation of NIV mode; however, the performance was greatly variable. Hence, when NIV is applied using ICU ventilator without NIV mode, these aspects need to be taken into consideration.[15]

CONCLUSION

Wide variation exists between ICU ventilators and domiciliary ventilators. With ever increasing modes and complexity, it becomes even more important for the treating physician to understand the working principles of the machine at hand to tailor-make ventilation according to patient needs.

REFERENCES

1. David J Pierson. History and epidemiology of noninvasive ventilation in the acute-care setting. Respiratory Care. 2009;54 (1):40-50.
2. Kacmarek RM. The Mechanical Ventilator: Past, Present, and Future. Respiratory Care. 2011; 56(8):1170-80.
3. Farré R, Navajas D, Montserrat JM. Technology for noninvasive mechanical ventilation: looking into the black box. ERJ Open Res. 2016;2: 00004-2016.
4. Scala R, Naldi M. Ventilators for noninvasive ventilation to treat acute respiratory failure. Respiratory Care. 2008;53(8):1054-80.
5. Schettino GP, Chatmongkolchart S, Hess DR, Kacmarek RM. Position of exhalation port and mask design affect CO_2 rebreathing during noninvasive positive pressure ventilation. Crit Care Med. 2003;31(8):2178-21.
6. Miyoshi E, Fujino Y, Uchiyama A, Mashimo T, Nishimura M. Effects of gas leak on triggering function, humidification, and inspiratory oxygen fraction during noninvasive positive airway pressure ventilation. Chest. 2005;128(5):3691-98.
7. Lofaso F, Brochard L, Thierry H, Hubert L, Haref A, Isabey D. Home versus intensive care pressure support devices. Experimental and clinical comparison. Am J Respir Crit Care Med. 1996;153(5): 1591-99.
8. Bunburaphong T, Imaka H, Nishimura M, Hess D, Kacmarek RM. Performance characteristics of bilevel pressure ventilators. A lung model study. Chest. 1997;111(4):1050-60.
9. Tassaux D, Strasser F, Fonseca S, Dalmas E, Jolliet P. Comparative bench study of triggering, pressurization and cycling between the home ventilator VPAP II and three ICU ventilators. Intensive Care Med. 2002;28(9):1254-61.
10. Richard JC, Carlucci A, Breton L, Langlais N, Jaber S, Maggiore S, et al. Bench testing of pressure support ventilation with three different generations of ventilators. Intensive Care Med. 2002;28(8): 1049-57.
11. Lofaso F, Brochard L, Touchard D, Hang T, Harf A, Isabey D. Evaluation of carbon dioxide rebreathing during pressure support ventilation with airway management system (BiPAP) devices. Chest. 1995;108(3):772-78.
12. Claudio Rabec. Ventilator modes and settings during non-invasive ventilation: effects on respiratory events and implications for their identification. Thorax. 2011;66:170-8.
13. Waugh JB, De Kler RM. Inspiratory time, pressure setting, and site of supplemental oxygen insertion affect delivered oxygen fraction with the Quantum PSV noninvasive positive pressure ventilation. Respir Care. 1999;44(5):520-23.
14. Schwartz AR, Kacmarek RM, Hess DR. Factors affecting oxygen delivery with bi-level positive airway pressure. Respir Care. 2004; 49(3):270-75
15. Vignaux L, Taussaux D, Jolliet P. Performance of noninvasive ventilation modes on ICU ventilators during pressure support: A bench model study. Intensive Care Med. 2007;33(8):1444-51.

Chapter 4

Modes of Ventilation for Noninvasive Ventilation Including Newer Modes

Gunjan Chanchalani, Minal Jariwala

INTRODUCTION

When noninvasive ventilator (NIV) was introduced in the 1980s, number of modalities were few, with very limited settings. Currently there are over 30 brands of ventilators, offering multiple settings and modes, with a vast varying terminology.

HISTORY

The use of NIV dates back to the early 1930s, during the latter years of polio epidemic, when rocking beds[1] and pneumobelts[2] were developed. Later, negative pressure ventilation was used noninvasively with the development of Tank ventilators, Jacket ventilator, and Cuirass. In the 1980s, positive pressure noninvasive ventilators were introduced, which were initially volume limited. Pressure targeted ventilators appeared in early 1990s, and with a predominant shift to the use of same.

CLASSIFICATION

A ventilator mode is described by the method of interaction of the ventilator with the patient and the method by which the inspiratory support is delivered to the patient. Each mode can be described by three components:
1. The way the ventilator initiates the breath (trigger sensitivity)
2. The control variable within the inspiratory cycle
3. The variable which ends the inspiration (cycling variable).

Trigger: The triggering function of the ventilator is how the ventilator recognizes the inspiratory effort of the patient.

Trigger can be of following types:
- *Pressure-based trigger:* The ventilator detects the drop in the pressure in the proximal airways. This trigger is present in most of the old ventilators.
- *Flow-based trigger:* Most recent ventilators have this type of trigger. There is a continuous bias flow in the ventilator circuit during the expiratory phase of the respiratory cycle and the ventilator detects an inspiratory flow change. Flow trigger is present in most recent ventilators, as it reduces the trigger delay duration between the patient's inspiratory effort and the initiation of the breath by the ventilator.[3]

Air leaks cause either ineffective triggering or auto-triggering by mimicking inspiratory flow or by dropping the pressure below the trigger threshold.

Control variable: The inspiration is mainly pressure-limited in most NIV, few old ones do have volume-limited ventilators as well. Currently hybrid modalities have been introduced to achieve the desired ventilation.

Cycling: Cycling from inspiration to expiration can be either flow-cycled or time-cycled.
- *Flow-cycled*: When the inspiratory flow drops to the pre-set percentage of the peak inspiratory flow, the ventilator switches to expiration. Air leaks may delay cycling, as higher flows are delivered to maintain the desired pressure limit. Increasing the percentage of peak inspiratory flow prevents the delay in cycling in chronic obstructive pulmonary disease (COPD) patients and thus asynchrony.[4]
- *Time-cycled*: The operator either sets the inspiratory time, I:E ratio, and RR. The ventilator cycles when a preset time criterion is reached.

The modes of noninvasive ventilation can be classified as under **Flowchart 1.**

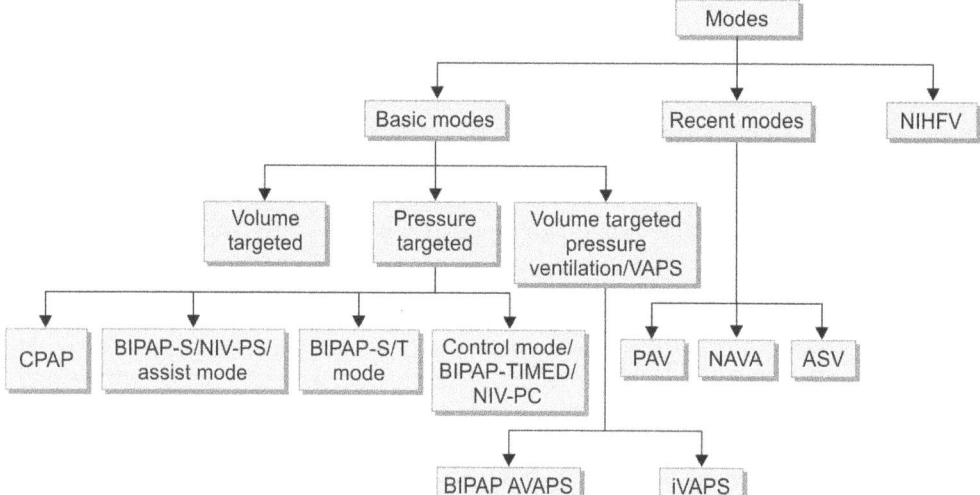

Flowchart 1: Basic classification of modes of NIV

(ASV: adaptive servo ventilation; AVAPS: average volume assured pressure support; BIPAP-S: bilevel positive airway pressure spontaneous mode; iVAPS: intelligent volume assured pressure support; NIV: noninvasive ventilator; NIHFV: noninvasive high-frequency ventilator; NAVA: neurally-adjusted ventilatory assist; PAV: proportional assisted ventilation; VAPS: volume assured pressure support)

MODES

A. Basic Modes

1. Volume-targeted Ventilation Mode/Volume Assist-Control Mode

This mode is used quite less as compared to the pressure-limited modes. The ventilator delivers a set tidal volume (TV), inspiratory flow over a set time. The pressure to achieve the TV varies, depending on the airway resistance, lung compliance, and patient effort.[5]

It is a flow-triggered, volume-limited, flow-cycled/time-cycled mode.

Setting: TV of 6–8 mL/kg ideal body weight (IBW). May be used as assisted mode, where patient triggers his own breath, or as a controlled mode at a preset rate, if no trigger is recognized.

Indication: It can be used in patients with unstable respiratory mechanics, wherein pressure targeted modes fail to achieve the desired volume.

Limitations: Cannot compensate adequately for air leaks causing failure to deliver the set TV, and also auto-triggering of premature breaths.[6]

- Higher peak pressures may be generated to achieve the target volume causing patient discomfort, more leaks and gastric insufflation.
- Does not adjust to the varying patient demand, as the volume and resultant flow is preset. This may not satisfy a dyspneic patient, thereby increasing the work of breathing (WOB) and causing patient discomfort.

2. *Pressure-targeted Ventilation*

   In this mode, the ventilator generates a pre-set positive pressure gradient in the airways for a given time, which creates airflow across the airway. In the initial part of inspiration, this gradient is large, creating a higher flow rate. As the gradient narrows toward the end of inspiration, the flow decelerates, until no gradient exists.

   Thus, the TV generated in the pressure-targeted modes is determined by the difference between the inspiratory and expiratory pressure [inspiratory positive airway pressure (IPAP) and expiratory positive airway pressure (EPAP)], inspiratory time, patient's pulmonary mechanics (airway resistance and lung compliance) and effort.[5]

   Pressure-targeted ventilation is usually better tolerated due to higher peak inspiratory flow rates, which meets the patient's demand and maintains patient comfort.[7] Newer advances in this mode offer better compensation for unintentional leaks and adjustable sensitivities for trigger and cycling, which further enhance the patient–ventilator synchrony.

   Limitation: TV delivered varies from breath to breath and is reduced with increased airway resistance and poor lung compliance.

   a. *Continuous positive airway pressure:* CPAP maintains a constant set pressure throughout the respiratory cycle (both inspiration and expiration), without assisting the inspiration. Hence, the patient needs to have an intact respiratory drive, and ability to maintain adequate minute ventilation. Both the respiratory rate and the depth of respiration are controlled by the patient. The patient's effort is recognized by pressure and flow sensors, which adjust the inspiratory and expiratory flow to maintain the preset pressure throughout the cycle.

      This positive pressure stents opens the airways, opens the under-ventilated alveoli, and increases the functional residual capacity. This helps to improve oxygenation by reducing the right-to-left intrapulmonary shunt, and also improves lung mechanics.[8] In COPD patients, this pressure counterbalances the auto-positive end-expiratory pressure (PEEP), thus reducing the inspiratory threshold load on the patient, his WOB, and dyspnea.[9] In congestive heart failure (CHF) patients, it decreases the LV afterload, LV transmural pressure, and improves cardiac output.[10]

      Setting: Pressures of 5–12 cm H_2O are used commonly. Patient should have a good respiratory drive.

Indications:[11]
- In obstructive sleep apnea (OSA), maintains a patent upper airway
- In CHF, augments the cardiac output
- Post-extubation, in obese patients
- In infants, used for tracheomalacia and infections like acute bronchiolitis, pneumonia.

Advantage: Low cost, no asynchrony

Limitations:
- It provides no inspiratory assistance, hence not as effective in reducing the respiratory muscle WOB.
- Contraindicated in COPD and asthma with severe air trapping, and in patients with poor respiratory effort.[11]

b. **BIPAP-S mode (spontaneous) /NIV-PS/ Assist mode**: The terms BIPAP and NIV are often used interchangeably. This mode is most frequently used in clinical practice.[12] It is a flow/pressure-triggered, pressure-limited, and flow-cycled mode.

In this mode, a greater pressure is provided during inspiration, compared to expiration, thus assisting inspiration. This helps to lower the inspiratory effort, unload the respiratory muscles, improve gas exchange, and reduce dyspnea. A flow or pressure trigger sensitivity recognizes the patient's effort and increases the pressure to the set IPAP during inspiration. When the inspiratory flow drops to a pre-determined percentage level, the ventilator cycles to the set EPAP level to permit exhalation.

The patient initiates each breath and there is no preset rate. The TV varies with each breath and is multifactorial depending on the level of IPAP, patient's inspiratory effort, and the lung elastance and airway resistance. Higher EPAP is needed to improve oxygenation and higher PS helps to deliver higher TV.[13]

The terminology used varies as per the ventilator. In the portable home ventilator, this mode is referred as BIPAP-S mode; EPAP and IPAP are used for expiratory and inspiratory cycle pressures, respectively. In the ICU ventilators, this mode is labeled as NIV-PS mode, terminology PEEP is used for EPAP, and PS plus PEEP is equal to IPAP.

Setting: Inspiratory trigger sensitivity, a target inspiratory pressure, and cycling trigger (percentage of the peak inspiratory flow). Initially low pressures should be used to allow patient tolerance (EPAP/PEEP of 3–5 cm H_2O with an inspiratory pressure of 8–10 cm H_2O). These pressures should be gradually increased to achieve a tidal volume of 6–8 mL/kg of IBW, improve dyspnea, and decrease patient distress.

The main limitations of this mode are patient–ventilator asynchrony, setting the ideal trigger setting, poor tidal volume delivery, and tachypnea.

The major reasons for asynchrony during the use of this mode are the pressure support level and the degree of air leak.[14] The air leak prevents the required reduction in the inspiratory flow to cycle the ventilator to expiratory phase. Use of proper size and fitting of the interface, and reducing the pressure settings to as much as possible, helps minimize the air leak. Some noninvasive ventilators allow adjustment of the expiratory flow trigger and raising the expiratory trigger threshold may help improve patient–ventilator synchrony by avoiding prolonged inspiration. Also switching to pressure-limited, time-cycled mode helps improve synchrony. Newer ventilators compensate for leaks with an inbuilt algorithm and thus minimize the asynchrony.

c. *BIPAP-Spontaneous/timed (ST) mode (earlier known as Assist/Control or A/C mode)*: Older ventilators termed this mode as Assist/Control or A/C-mode. In this mode, the ventilator assists the spontaneously breathing patient. But if there is no trigger detected over a preset interval, then it initiates a machine triggered breath by increasing the pressure to the IPAP level. It then cycles to expiration after a pre-determined percentage of inspiratory time.

It is a flow/machine-triggered, pressure-limited, and flow/time-cycled mode.

Settings: IPAP, EPAP, respiratory rate, inspiratory time (IPAP%).

Advantages:
- More patient comfort than a controlled mode.
- Ensures adequate ventilation in patients with an unreliable respiratory effort, by having a preset back-up RR.

d. *Control mode/BiPAP-Timed mode /NIV-PC*: This mode is flow/pressure triggered in spontaneous breathing patient and time-triggered for controlled breaths, pressure-limited and either flow- or time-cycled. The ventilator maintains the set RR of the patient, irrespective of the patient effort.

Setting: Inspiratory and expiratory pressures are set similar to the PS mode. The respiratory rate is set and the inspiratory time is set as either absolute time or as I:E ratio.

This mode helps to improve patient–ventilator asynchrony that occurs due to air leak or failure to cycle in COPD patients with a delayed drop in inspiratory flows, as it is also time-cycled.[15,16]

This mode is preferred in patients with central respiratory depression, and in patients in whom adequate CO_2 washout cannot be achieved despite high inspiratory pressures and TV. This mode provides complete rest to the respiratory muscles.

Limitations: Risk of overventilation is high. Some patients find it difficult to tolerate, due to asynchrony.

3. *Volume-targeted Pressure Ventilation/Volume-assured Pressure Support*

This modality was developed to assure the delivery of required target TV with the features of pressure-limited ventilation mode. The ventilator delivers a pressure-limited breath, and detects the TV delivered. If this TV is below the pre-determined target level, it changes to a flow-cycled breath, and subsequently adjusts its pressure level to achieve the set TV.[5]

a. *BIPAP-AVAPS (Average volume assured pressure support)*: AVAPS securely delivers the target volume by automatically changing the PS level.

Main indication: COPD and hypoventilation syndrome.

Setting: Target TV, range of pressures during inspiration, expiratory pressure (EPAP) and a back-up respiratory rate, inspiratory time. The ventilator chooses the lowest inspiratory pressure within the set range to achieve the targeted TV.

Advantage: Since it delivers an assured TV and thus minute ventilation, it helps in faster and more reliable correction of hypercarbia.[17]

However, a recent multicenter RCT[18] failed to demonstrate any significant difference in CO_2 levels, intubation or in-hospital mortality with the use of AVAPS as compared to PS mode.

Limitation:
- If higher TV is generated above the desired range, the support is reduced causing fatigue.
- In patients with low lung compliance, increased inspiratory pressure is needed.
- Air leaks may prevent achieving the desired PS level and hence the desired TV.[19]

b. *Intelligent volume assured pressure support ventilation (iVAPS)*: iVAPS targets achieving the predetermined VA (alveolar ventilation in L/min), irrespective of the changing patient effort, and lung mechanics. VA is calculated by subtracting the estimated dead space from the target MV. The dead space is estimated by using height.[20]

The ventilator constantly monitors the patient's airflow and RR, and the estimated VA is derived. Along with the PS level, it also automatically adjusts the backup respiratory rate within a range, to achieve the target alveolar ventilation and to optimize patient comfort. Similarly, if the achieved VA is higher, PS is decreased. This adjustment is done based on an in-built intelligent algorithm. iVAPS uses two-thirds of the set backup RR during spontaneous respiration, and the set RR during apnea.[20]

Setting: Maximum and minimum PS level, target alveolar ventilation, backup RR, trigger, cycle, inspiratory time maximum and minimum.

Advantages:
- Can help predict COPD exacerbations, by monitoring ventilation trends.
- Titration is easier despite disease progression, as the patient's ventilator demand is met.

Limitations:
- In patients with large physiological dead space (emphysema), the estimated VA is much higher than the actual VA. Thus, in emphysema, a higher target VA needs to be set to achieve adequate actual VA.[20]
- In COPD patients and in patients with unintentional leak, hyperinflation is common.
- Disruption of sleep occurs due to excess over-titration of PS.

B. Recent Ventilator Modes

Newer modes of NIV are developed to match the physiological pattern of breathing of the patient, and help to improve patient–ventilator synchrony. These modes have closed-loop control systems for intra- and inter-breath control of breath assistance to optimize patient's WOB.

1. *Proportional-assisted Ventilation*

   This mode is similar to the PS mode, but it offers the advantage of better synchrony than the PS mode and prevents over/under assistance.[21] It is a patient-triggered, pressure-limited, and flow-cycled mode.

Chapter 4: Modes of Ventilation for Noninvasive Ventilation Including Newer Modes

Setting: The operator has to set the percentage of assistance (that has to be provided for the flow and volume, based on the pulmonary resistance and elastance), PEEP, and FiO_2.

The ventilator tracks the patient's inspiratory flow and volume based on the equation of motion, and delivers proportional flow and volume to meet the demand.[22] The ventilator thus follows the breathing pattern of the spontaneously breathing patient and provides the set fixed proportional assistance. So, if the patient's inspiratory flow increases, proportionally the assistance is increased. This helps to meet the patient's demand and thus prevents the increase in the respiratory rate.[23]

Studies have failed to prove any benefit in reducing intubation rates, hospital stay or mortality, however they do report better patient comfort and patient–ventilator synchrony with the use of PAV with NIV.[24,25]

It is better tolerated by COPD patients, as it closely follows their respiratory pattern, and has decreased risk of disproportionate support level and auto-PEEP.[23]

Limitations:
- Difficulty in measuring pulmonary resistance and elastance in NIV.
- Fails to provide support in patients with auto-PEEP.
- Cannot be used in patients with poor respiratory drive and neuromuscular weakness.

2. *Neurally-adjusted Ventilatory Assist*

Neurally-adjusted ventilatory assist (NAVA) helps to improve both trigger as well as cycle asynchrony. An EMG electrode is inserted in the lower esophagus and placed close to the diaphragmatic aperture. This electrode detects the electrical activity at the initiation of contraction of the diaphragmatic muscles as an index of initiation of respiratory effort and signals the ventilator to initiate the flow without delay. The whole of the breathing process from the initiation to the end of the inspiratory cycle is controlled by the patient's respiratory center.[23] The ventilator is triggered, limited as well as cycled by the diaphragmatic electrical activity signal detected by the multi-array electrode.

This mode provides the maximum degree of coordination with the triggering of the ventilator and the highest degree of compatibility with the patient's inspiratory cycle, as it tracks the electrical activity of the diaphragm and not the inspiratory flow.

In COPD patients with auto-PEEP, NAVA helps achieve better synchrony.[26] Studies have however failed to show any significant improvement in NIV success rate, or hospital stay and mortality.[27]

Setting: NAVA gain (the support is determined as a multiplication of the signal activity by the electrical activity). Cycling- is usually set at 80% of the maximum inspiratory electrical activity.

Advantages: The assistance provided is not affected by the pulmonary mechanics like airway resistance, elastance, intrinsic PEEP or air leak.[28]

Limitations:
- Data on use of NAVA with noninvasive ventilation is limited, and hence its clinical impact cannot be assessed.
- The need for placement of an esophageal catheter device.[23]

3. *Adaptive Servo Ventilation*

Adaptive servo ventilation (ASV) mode was initially designed for CSA patients. It can also be used for chronic heart failure patients with Cheyne stokes breathing (CSB), OSA, and CSA[23]. This mode is different from the adaptive support ventilation of invasive ventilators.

In patients with normal respiration, ASV provides continuous pressure throughout the respiratory cycle like a CPAP. But when it detects apnea, it increases the inspiratory pressure to the maximum set pressure to deliver a breath. In patients with CSB, it provides lower support during the hyperventilation and increasing PS and RR when the respiratory effort is waning.

The device detects the patient's airflow continuously, and adjusts its respiratory parameters based on in-built algorithms, to maintain a stable breathing.[29]

Setting: Maximum PS, back-up RR, EPAP

When compared CPAP, ASV has shown to decrease the number of apnea-hypopnea index <10 in 89.7% patients, as compared to 64.5% reduction with CPAP.[30] SERVE-HF trial reported a higher risk of cardiovascular death in patients with use of ASV mode, in patients with CHF and EF <45%.[31]

Limitations:
- Should be avoided in patients with CHF who have coexisting sleep disorders and low EF <45%.[23]
- Cannot be used in patients with decreased respiratory drive (e.g. congenital central alveolar hypoventilation).

C. Noninvasive High-frequency Ventilation

Noninvasive high-frequency ventilation (NIHFV) is a commonly used in infants for noninvasive ventilation. A high respiratory rate (80–1,600/min) with low flows (less than the anatomical dead space—2 mL/kg) is delivered to maintained a high MAP.[32]

It is a flow-regulated, time-cycled mode that provides subphysiologic tidal volumes at a very high frequency, controlled-pressure delivery of low-frequency breathing cycles with a controlled pressure delivery of low-frequency breathing cycles. The TV and gas exchange is affected by the pressure amplitude and inspiratory time, and the interface.

It is used in neonates and infants as a rescue method to avoid intubation, when other modes of NIV fail.

HOW TO CHOOSE THE RIGHT NIV MODE?

In order to achieve the maximum clinical and physiological benefit, choosing the right NIV mode and appropriate settings is crucial. Choice of mode is mainly decided by factors like operator familiarity and experience, etiology, and severity of the disease process and the breathing effort by the patient.

The following suggestions may help guiding the choice of mode as per the disease state:
- Patients with good spontaneous respiratory drive usually benefit well from CPAP mode to improve oxygenation.

- Pressure-targeted modes are preferred over volume-targeted to deliver ventilation in presence of air leaks, as they help to maintain TV better.[33]
- In patients who need high pressures for chest inflation (restrictive disease, severe chest deformity, obese), volume-controlled ventilation mode is more effective.[34]
- PSV mode/assist mode is usually most commonly used and well tolerated by most patients. Flow triggering is preferred over pressure triggering in assisted modes, as it reduced WOB more and provides better patient-ventilator synchrony[35]. It is found to be highly beneficial in COPD exacerbations treatment, and in preventing re-intubation.[36,37]
- In patients with cardiogenic pulmonary edema, both CPAP and NIV-PS have been found to be effective.[38]
- In post thoracic and upper abdominal surgical patients, CPAP has shown to reduce respiratory complications.[39,40]
- In post-traumatic patients with acute respiratory failure, a meta-analysis of 10 studies showed that NIV-PS mode significantly improved oxygenation, reduced intubation rate and infectious complications, as compared to CPAP mode. However, no difference in mortality was found.[41]

A special mention needs to be made here about high flow nasal oxygen as it is now increasingly being used in critically ill patients not cooperating for NIV, in hypoxemic acute respiratory failure.[34] It is not really a mode of NIV, but a special oxygen therapy. It does not provide any respiratory support, but creates a low level of PEEP/CPAP and helps reduce airway resistance by using high flows of oxygen.

SUMMARY

Now-a-days there are vast and varying options of noninvasive ventilators and modes, with each company having different terminology for the same mode. This creates lot of confusion amongst the clinicians in daily practice. However, to navigate successfully, one must have a clear understanding of the modes and goals of ventilation to be achieved.

REFERENCES

1. Eve FC. Actuation of the inert diaphragm. Lancet. 1932;2:995-7.
2. Adamson JP, Lewis L, Stein JD. Application of abdominal pressure for artificial respiration. JAMA. 1959;169:1613-7.
3. Aslanian P, El Atrous S, Isabey D, Valente E, Corsi D, Harf A, et al. Effects of flow triggering on breathing effort during partial ventilatory support. Am J Respir Crit Care Med. 1998;157(1):135-43.
4. Tassaux D, Gainnier M, Battisti A, Jolliet P. Impact of expiratory trigger setting on delayed cycling and inspiratory muscle workload. Am J Respir Crit Care Med. 2005;172(10):1283-9.
5. Rabec C, Rodenstein D, Leger P, Rouault S, Perrin C, Gonzalez-Bermejo J, et al. Ventilator modes and settings during non-invasive ventilation: effects on respiratory events and implications for their identification. Thorax. 2011;66(2):170-8.
6. Vignaux L, Tassaux D, Carteaux G, Roeseler J, Piquilloud L, Brochard L, et al. Performance of noninvasive ventilation algorithms on ICU ventilators during pressure support: a clinical study. Intensive Care Med. 2010;36(12):2053-9.
7. Windisch W, Storre JH, Sorichter S, Virchow JC Jr. Comparison of volume- and pressure-limited NPPV at night: a prospective randomized cross-over trial. Respir Med. 2005;99(1):52-9.

8. Katz JA, Marks JD. Inspiratory work with and without continuous positive airway pressure in patients with acute respiratory failure. Anesthesiology. 1985;63(6):598-607.
9. Petrof BJ, Legaré M, Goldberg P, Milic-Emili J, Gottfried SB. Continuous positive airway pressure reduces work of breathing and dyspnea during weaning from mechanical ventilation in severe chronic obstructive pulmonary disease. Am Rev Respir Dis. 1990;141:281-9.
10. Naughton MT, Rahman MA, Hara K, Floras JS, Bradley TD. Effect of continuous positive airway pressure on intrathoracic and left ventricular transmural pressures in patients with congestive heart failure. Circulation. 1995;91(6):1725-31.
11. Venessa P, Sharma, S. (2018). Continuous Positive Airway Pressure (CPAP).
12. Ozsancak Ugurlu A, Sidhom SS, Khodabandeh A, Ieong M, Mohr C, Lin DY, et al. Use and outcomes of noninvasive positive pressure ventilation in acute care hospitals in Massachusetts. Chest. 2014;145(5):964-71.
13. L'Her E, Deye N, Lellouche F, Taille S, Demoule A, Fraticelli A, et al. Physiologic effects of noninvasive ventilation during acute lung injury. Am J Respir Crit Care Med. 2005;172(9):1112-8.
14. Vignaux L, Vargas F, Roeseler J, Tassaux D, Thille AW, Kossowsky MP, et al. Patient-ventilator asynchrony during non- invasive ventilation for acute respiratory failure: a multicenter study. Intensive Care Med. 2009;35(5):840-6.
15. Vignaux L, Vargas F, Roeseler J, Tassaux D, Thille AW, Kossowsky MP, et al. Patient-ventilator asynchrony during noninvasive ventilation: the role of expiratory trigger. Intensive Care Med. 1999;25(7):662-7.
16. Hess DR. Patient-ventilator interaction during noninvasive ventilation. Respir Care. 2011;56(2): 153-65.
17. Briones Claudett KH, Briones Claudett M, Chung Sang Wong M, Nuques Martinez A, Soto Espinoza R, Montalvo M, et al. Noninvasive mechanical ventilation with average volume assured pressure support (AVAPS) in patients with chronic obstructive pulmonary disease and hypercapnic encephalopathy. BMC Pulm Med. 2013;13:12.
18. Cao Z, Luo Z, Hou A, Nie Q, Xie B, An X, et al. Volume-targeted versus pressure-limited noninvasive ventilation in subjects with acute hypercapnic respiratory failure: a multicenter randomized controlled trial. Respir Care. 2016;61(11):1440-50.
19. Luján M, Sogo A, Pomares X, Monsó E, Sales B, Blanch L. Effect of leak and breathing pattern on the accuracy of tidal volume estimation by commercial home ventilators: a bench study. Respir Care. 2013;58(5):770-7.
20. Johnson K, Johnson D. Treatment of sleep-disordered breathing with positive airway pressure devices: technology update. Medical Devices: Evidence and Research. 2015;8:425-37.
21. Masip J, Peacock WF, Price S, Cullen L, Martin-Sanchez FJ, Seferovic P, et al. Indications and practical approach to non-invasive ventilation in acute heart failure. Eur Heart J. 2018;39(1):17-25.
22. Younes M, Puddy A, Roberts D, Light RB, Quesada A, Taylor K, et al. Proportional assist ventilation. Results of an initial clinical trial. Am Rev Respir Dis. 1992;145(1):121-9.
23. Seyfi S, Amri P, Mouodi S. New modalities for noninvasive positive pressure ventilation: A review article. Caspain J Intern Med. 2019;10(1):1-6.
24. Gay PC, Hess DR, Hill NS. Noninvasive proportional assist ventilation for acute respiratory insufficiency. Comparison with pressure support ventilation. Am J Respir Crit Care Med. 2001;164(9): 1606-11.
25. Elganady AA, Beshey BN, Abdelaziz AAH. Proportional assist ventilation versus pressure support ventilation in the weaning of patients with acute exacerbation of chronic obstructive pulmonary disease. Egypt J Chest Dis Tuberc. 2014;63(3):653-60.
26. Liu L, Xia F, Yang Y, Longhini F, Navalesi P, Beck J, et al. Neural versus pneumatic control of pressure support in patients with chronic obstructive pulmonary diseases at different levels of positive end expiratory pressure: a physiological study. Crit Care. 2015;19:244.

27. Piquilloud L, Tassaux D, Bialais E, Lambermont B, Sottiaux T, Roeseler J et al. Neurally adjusted ventilatory assist (NAVA) improves patient-ventilator interaction during noninvasive ventilation delivered by face mask. Intensive Care Med. 2012;38(10):1624-31.
28. Sinderby C, Beck J. Proportional assist ventilation and neurally adjusted ventilatory assist—better approaches to patient ventilator synchrony? Clin Chest Med. 2008;29(2):329-42.
29. Javaheri S, Brown LK, Randerath WJ. Positive airway pressure therapy with adaptive servoventilation: part 1: operational algorithms. Chest. 2014;146(2):514-23.
30. Morgenthaler TI, Kuzniar TJ, Wolfe LF, Willes L, McLain WC 3rd, Goldberg R. The complex sleep apnea resolution study: a prospective randomized controlled trial of continuous positive airway pressure versus adaptive servo-ventilation therapy. Sleep. 2014;37(5):927-34.
31. Cowie MR, Woehrle H, Wegscheider K, Angermann C, d'Ortho MP, Erdmann E, et al. Adaptive servo-ventilation for central sleep apnea in systolic heart failure. N Engl J Med. 2015;373(12):1095-105.
32. Fischer HS, Rimensberger PC. Early noninvasive high-frequency oscillatory ventilation in the primary treatment of respiratory distress syndrome. Pediatr Pulmonol. 2018;53(2):126-7.
33. Mehta S, McCool FD, Hill NS. Leak compensation in positive pressure ventilators: a lung model study. Eur Respir J. 2001;17(2):259-67.
34. Bello G, Ionescu Maddalena A, Giammatteo V, Antonelli M. Noninvasive options. Crit Care Clin. 2018;34(3):395-412.
35. Nava S, Ambrosino N, Bruschi C, Confalonieri M, Rampulla C. Physiological effects of flow and pressure triggering during noninvasive mechanical ventilation in patients with chronic obstructive pulmonary disease. Thorax. 1997;52(3):249-54.
36. Chandra D, Stamm JA, Taylor B, Ramos RM, Satterwhite L, Krishnan JA, et al. Outcomes of noninvasive ventilation for acute exacerbations of chronic obstructive pulmonary disease in the United States, 1998-2008. Am J Respir Crit Care Med. 2012;185(2):152-9.
37. Appendini L, Purro A, Patessio A, Zanaboni S, Carone M, Spada E, et al. Partitioning of inspiratory muscle work-load and pressure assistance in ventilator-dependent COPD patients. Am J Respir Crit Care Med. 1996;154(5):1301-9.
38. Rochwerg B, Brochard L, Elliott MW, Hess D, Hill NS, Nava S, et al. Official ERS/ATS clinical practice guidelines: noninvasive ventilation for acute respiratory failure. Eur Respir J. 2017;50(2):1602426.
39. Chiumello D, Chevallard G, Gregoretti C. Non-invasive ventilation in postoperative patients: a systematic review. Intensive Care Med. 2011;37(6):918-29.
40. Jaber S, Lescot T, Futier E, Paugam-Burtz C, Seguin P, Ferrandiere M, et al. Effect of noninvasive ventilation on tracheal reintubation among patients with hypoxemic respiratory failure following abdominal surgery: a randomized clinical trial. JAMA. 2016;315(13):1345-53.
41. Chiumello D, Coppola S, Froio S, Gregoretti C, Consonni D. Noninvasive ventilation in chest trauma: systematic review and meta-analysis. Intensive Care Med. 2013;39(7):1171-80.

Chapter 5

Noninvasive Ventilation Interfaces

Bharat Jagiasi, Leena Patil, Anand Srivastava

■ BACKGROUND

Noninvasive ventilation (NIV) has an important role in modern day ventilation whether it is for acute condition or chronic. However, the success of NIV depends largely on the interface.[1] Good interface can improve the tolerance to NIV and the efficacy of NIV.[2-7] Kramer et al. reported that NIV fails in 18% of patients because of mask discomfort.

Non-invasive ventilation refers to the administration of ventilatory support without using an invasive artificial airway (endotracheal tube or tracheostomy tube).

■ INTERFACE

A point, where two systems, subjects, or organizations meet and interact, is known as interface. The success of the interaction depends on the interface. In this Chapter, the word interface means any oral, nasal, oronasal, and full face device used to deliver ventilation.

In this context, there are two systems—the man and the machine (i.e., the ventilator) and we are going to focus on the point through which they interact, i.e., interface.

During acute respiratory failure, treatment efficacy takes precedence over patient comfort whereas for long-term treatment, patient comfort does matter. Hence various types of interfaces are devised and used in practice.

Choice of interface is important factor for NIV success or failure.

Characteristics of Ideal Interface

No interface is ideal. The discussion about ideal interface is to define what is ideal interface.

Ideal interface is defined as standard or principle, which fulfills set criteria. The aim of defining the ideal is for comparing various interfaces, choosing from the available options and also developing better ones' **(Box 1)**.

> **Box 1:** Characteristics of ideal interface.
> ➢ Leak free
> ➢ Nontraumatic
> ➢ Minimal dead space
> ➢ Low resistance to airflow
> ➢ Good stability

Contd...

Contd...

> **Box 1:** Characteristics of ideal interface.
> - Nondeformable
> - Light weight
> - Long lasting
> - Nonallergic
> - Low cost
> - Easy to manufacture
> - Available in various sizes
> - Ideal securing system

Physiological Aspects

Noninvasive ventilation is type of positive pressure ventilation (pressure support or pressure control), wherein tidal volume is provided to the patient, once trigger is sensed by the machine. The tidal volume delivered to the patient is affected by leaks, dead space, and patient machine synchrony apart from the ventilator settings.

- *Leaks:* It is the most common problem faced by patient as well as caregivers which leads to discomfort, inadequate ventilation, and asynchrony. Leaks can be of two types:
  1. Intentional—these are present in single limb circuits e.g. home bilevel positive airway pressure (BiPAP)], where the machine does not have an expiratory limb or valve. These are created to prevent rebreathing.
  2. Nonintentional—leaks between skin and mask. These happen mostly due to ill-fitting or improperly secured masks. There is a common tendency of fixing these leaks by overtightening the straps. This leads to patient discomfort and skin ulceration.

  Newer methods to reduce leaks include mask support ring, hydrogel or foam seals, lip seal, and chin strap.

  Here I would like to share two bench mark studies:
  1. Mehta et al.[8]—they compared and evaluated positive pressure ventilators used to administer NIV, including pressure-targeted and volume-targeted devices. They demonstrated that leak compensation depends on ventilator mode, leak size, inspiratory air flow capabilities, and inspiratory time. Also pressure-targeted modes are able to sustain delivered tidal volume regardless of leaks better than volume targeted one.
  2. Louis et al.[9]—the results of the study showed that leaks lead to asynchrony with the machine.

- *Dead space:* Volume of air not involved in gaseous exchange either because it remains in conducting airways or it reaches alveoli that are not adequately perfused. Therefore it can be divided into physiological and anatomical dead space.[10,11-13]

  The third kind of dead space of our concern is apparatus dead space. It is the part of gasses, in the breathing circuit, that is rebreathed by the patient. Typically, it lies beyond the point of separation of inspiratory and expiratory part of tubings. The effect of dead space on ventilation depends on fresh gas flow rates and type of ventilation (i.e., spontaneous or controlled).

  It has been seen that increasing the fresh gas flow rate or providing pressure support decreases the dead space effect on ventilation.

Section 1: Introduction and Physiology

- *Asynchrony:* Asynchrony is more common with NIV than with invasive ventilation.[14] Of all the interfaces, asynchrony is most common with helmets.[15,16]
- *Patient comfort:* Problems faced by patients include—air leaks, ocular irritation and lacrimation, headache, skin breakdown or ulceration, and claustrophobia.[17,18] Most common site for skin ulceration—bridge of the nose which can be avoided by preventing excessive fit while accepting small amount of air leaks[19] in comparison to oronasal mask, there is decreased skin ulceration with the use of helmets.
    - *Efficacy:* Selection of right interface has a measure impact on the efficacy of NIV. Generally, Oronasal masks are preferred in acute respiratory failure,[20] while nasal masks are more comfortable for long-term and domiciliary NIV.[21]

Types of Interfaces

The development of various types of interfaces is largely driven by the need for ventilation in patients with obstructive sleep apnea (OSA) or chronic obstructive pulmonary disease (COPD). Most of the masks used are readymade (modular once are also available) and finding the right one for the patient determines the success of the therapy.

Various types of interfaces are:
- Oral interfaces (mouthpiece and bite plates) **(Fig. 1)**
- Nasal interfaces (nasal mask, nasal pillows, and nasal sling) **(Fig. 2)**
- Oronasal **(Fig. 3)**
- Full face **(Fig. 4)**
- Helmet **(Fig. 5)**

Most common used interface is oronasal mask.

Oral Interfaces

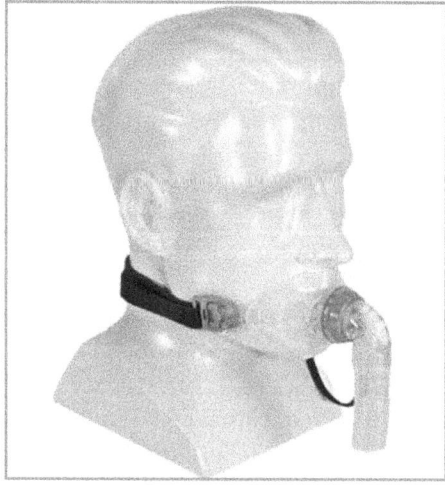

Fig. 1: Oral interfaces.

- Mouthpiece and bite plates are two types of oral interfaces.
- It can be used easily during the daytime but cumbersome to use during the night time.

- These devices are usually used in patients requiring long-term ventilation such neuromuscular diseases (NMDs) and cystic fibrosis.[22-24]
- One study suggests that mouthpiece is as effective as full face mask in reducing the inspiratory effort in patients receiving NIV for acute respiratory failure.[25]
- *Side effects:*
  - Difficult to maintain position
  - Salivation
  - Chances of gagging or vomiting
  - Gastric distension
  - Orthodontic deformation

Nasal Interfaces

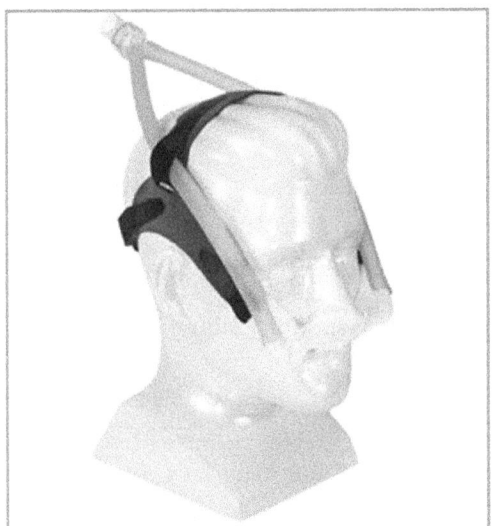

Fig. 2: Nasal interfaces.

Preferable for patients with OSA or COPD (long-term ventilation)
- Advantages:
  - Less claustrophobia
  - Mouth remains uncovered (easy speech and allows cough)
  - Less gastric distension
  - Less vomiting
  - Less chances of asphyxia (free mouth)
  - Free eyes (less lacrimation, can wear specs)
- Contraindications:
  - Edentulous
  - Respiration through mouth
  - Oral surgery especially soft palate

- *Disadvantage:*
  - Vt monitoring unreliable
  - Limited efficacy in case of increased nasal resistance[26]

Oronasal Mask

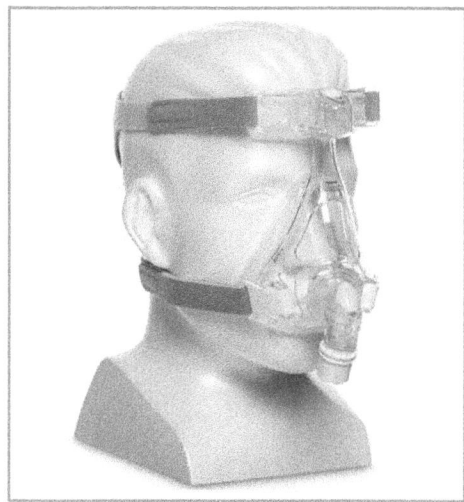

Fig. 3: Oronasal mask.

- Most commonly used in acute respiratory failure because these patients tend to breathe through mouth.
- Masks are transparent, easy to adjust, and available in various sizes.
- Masks usually are made from two parts:
  1. *Cushion:* Forms the seal with the patients face
     a. Is soft nontraumatic and prevents air leak.
     b. Made from polyvinyl chloride, polypropylene, silicon, silicon elastomer, or hydrogel.
  2. *Frame:* Stiff material, makes it nondeformable and stable.
     a. Made from polyvinyl chloride, polycarbonate, and thermoplastic.
     b. The mask frame has several attachment points for the head gear.
- *Advantages:*
  - Fewer air leaks than nasal
  - Less patient cooperation is required.
- *Contraindications:*
  - Face injury or deformity or surgery
  - Claustrophobia
  - Vomiting
- *Disadvantages:*
  - Skin damage

Full Face Mask

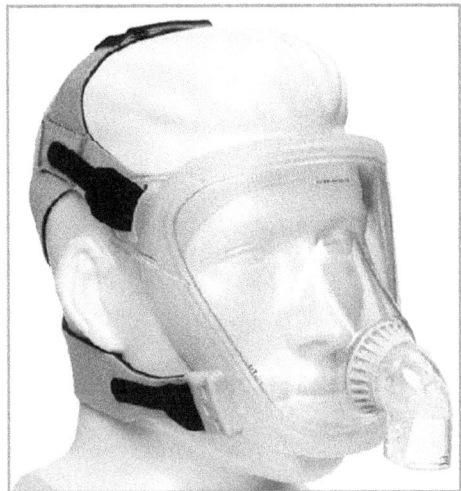

Fig. 4: Full face mask.

These are similar to oronasal mask. Only difference being that the cuff seals around the perimeter of the face, therefore there is no pressure on areas that are prone for pressure injury with oronasal mask. These masks also have antiasphyxia valve.

Helmet

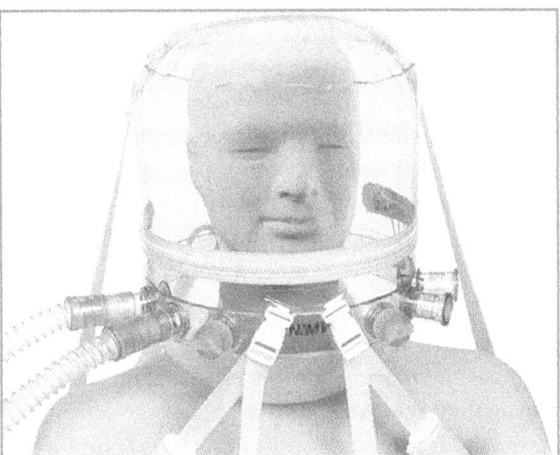

Fig. 5: Helmet.

Helmet has two parts:
1. Hood
2. Collar—neck/shoulder

There are two ports. One is for entry and the other is for exit of oxygen

It is commonly used for hyperbaric oxygen therapy.

Advantages:
- Less dependent on facial contours
- Needs no/less patient cooperation
- Better comfort
- Lower risk of skin damage

Contraindications:
- Claustrophobia
- Tetraplegia
- Tidal volume monitoring
- Restriction of head and neck movements

PRACTICAL IMPLICATIONS AND STUDIES/EVIDENCE

The success of NIV depends on:
- Indication of application
- Ventilatory technique/mode used
- NIV interface adopted

Noninvasive interfaces most widely used are oronasal and nasal mask.

Except for the acute care setting (where oronasal mask was used), nasal mask was previously often used only for chronic ventilation but with the advent of a portable, bilevel, pressure support ventilators for obstructive sleep apnea, nasal masks could be used even in acute setting.

Independent of the course of evolution, various centers started using their ICU ventilators to provide NIV. The difficulties caused by leaks in these earlier ventilators called for the use of oronasal masks, which had to be tightly fitted, resulting in a significant risk of skin breakdown and ulceration.

As NIV became better established, both interfaces and ventilators evolved, allowing it to be more patient centered and comfortable. Currently, the clinician is presented with a variety of potential interfaces, including mouthpieces, nasal masks, nasal pillows, orofacial masks, full face masks (sometimes referred to as total face masks) and helmets.

Studies

Holanda et al.[27] designed their trial to determine the relative incidence, type, and intensity of short-term adverse effects related to three interfaces (nasal mask, oronasal mask, and full face mask), as well as evaluating their relative comfort.

They found no differences among the masks in terms of comfort scores or of their effects on respiratory rate, heart rate, and oxygen saturation. End-tidal CO_2 levels were lowest for the full face mask and highest for the nasal mask. No differences in adverse effects were observed. Full face mask did not cause any pain or air leaks but lead to claustrophobia and oronasal dryness thus suggesting that humidification be considered when the full face mask is used. Overall, it supports the use of the full face mask as a reasonable alternative to the nasal or oronasal mask, especially if there are problems related to pain about the bridge of the nose or air leaks into the eyes.

The question every clinician ideally would like to have answered is this: "which interface is the best to use for my patient in acute respiratory failure to ensure optimal compliance with NIV and thus avoid intubation and ventilation?"

Here we would like to address this question by taking reference of the studies done by Anton A et al.[28] and Kwok H et al.[29] while Anton A et al. found no difference between the interfaces, although only 14 patients were used, it was Kwok H et al. who demonstrated that in acute respiratory failure mask intolerance was greater with nasal mask, primarily due to persistent air leakage through the mouth.

■ SUMMARY

Although the potential of the interface to influence patient tolerance of NIV, as well as to alter its benefits, is generally accepted, evidence in the literature supporting one interface over another is limited.

Most studies provide only indirect information, since they involve healthy individuals or clinically stable patients, neither of which represents the population of interest to the clinician. The findings of one study support the common belief that, in the dyspnoeic patient, nasal masks are less well tolerated than are oronasal masks.

How to reduce the risk of skin damage during noninvasive ventilation (Fig. 6)?

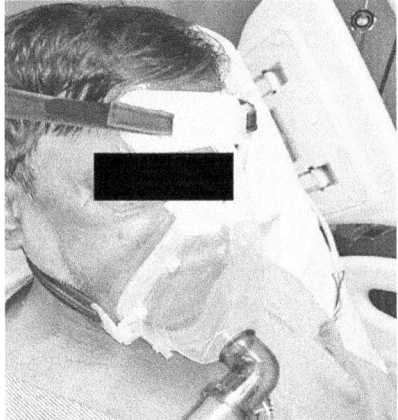

Fig. 6: Skin damage during noninvasive ventilation.

- Use various types of interfaces altering intermittently.
- Use proper harness and tightening bands.
- Skin and mask hygiene are to be strictly followed.
- Use nasal-forehead spacer (to reduce the pressure on the bridge of the nose).
- Use forehead pads (to obtain the most comfortable position on the forehead).
- Cushioning system between mask prong and forehead is to be tried.
- Remove patients' dentures when making impression for molded mask
- In home care, replace the mask according to the patients' daily use
- Skin pad (Restore, Hollister, Libertyville, Illinois; or Duoderm, Bristol-Myers Squibb, Princeton, New Jersey)

REFERENCES

1. Navalesi P, Fanfulla F, Frigerio P, et al. Physiologic evaluation of noninvasive mechanical ventilation delivered with three types of masks in patients with chronic hypercapnic respiratory failure. Crit Care Med. 2000;28:1785-90.
2. Bott J, Carrol MP, Conway JH, et al. Randomised controlled trial of nasal ventilation in acute ventilator failure due to chronic obstructive airways disease. Lancet. 1993;341:1555-7.
3. Kramer N, Meyer TJ, Meharg J, et al. Randomized, prospective trial of noninvasive positive pressure ventilation in acute respiratory failure. Am J Respir Crit Care Med. 1995;151:1799-806.
4. Brochard L, Mancebo J, Wysochi M, et al. Noninvasive ventilation for acute exacerbation of chronic obstructive pulmonary disease. N Engl J Med. 1995;333:817-22.
5. Plant PK, Owen JL, Elliot MW. A multicentre randomised controlled trial of the early use of noninvasive ventilation in acute exacerbation of chronic obstructive pulmonary disease on general respiratory wards. Lancet. 2000;335:1931-5.
6. Antonelli M, Conti G, Rocco M, et al. A comparison of noninvasive positive-pressure ventilation and conventional mechanical ventilation in patients with acute respiratory failure. N Engl J Med. 1998;339:429-35.
7. Nava S, Ambrosino N, Clini E, et al. Noninvasive mechanical ventilation in the weaning of patients with acute respiratory failure due to chronic obstructive pulmonary disease: a randomized controlled trial. Ann Intern Med. 1998;128:721-8.
8. Mehta S, McCool FD, Hill NS. Leak compensation in positive pressure ventilators: a lung model study. Eur Respir J. 2001;17:259-67.
9. Louis B, Leroux K, Isabey d, et al. Effect of manufacturer-inserted mask leaks on ventilator performance. Eur Respir J. 2010;35:627-36.
10. Saatci E, Miller DM, Stell IM, et al. Dynamic dead space in face masks used with noninvasive ventilators: a lung model study. Eur Respir J. 2004;23:129-35.
11. Fraticelli AT, Lellouche F, L'Her E, et al. Physiological effects of different interfaces during noninvasive ventilation for acute respiratory failure. Crit Care Med. 2009;37:939-45.
12. Cuvelier A, Pujol W, Pramil S, et al. Cephalic versus oronasal mask for noninvasive ventilation in acute hypercapnic respiratory failure. Intensive Care Med. 2009;35:519-26.
13. Fodil R, Lellouche F, Mancebo J, et al. Comparison of patient-ventilator interfaces based on their computerized effective dead space. Intensive Care Med. 2011;37:257-62.
14. Vignaux L, Vargas F, Roeseler J, et al. Patient-ventilator asynchrony during non-invasive ventilation for acute respiratory failure: multicenter study. Intensive Care Med. 2009;35:840-6.
15. Moerer O, Fischer S, Hartelt M, et al. Influence of two different interfaces for noninvasive ventilation compared to invasive ventilation on the mechanical properties and performance of a respiratory system: a lung model study. Chest. 2006;129:1424-31.
16. Vargas F, Thille A, Lyazidi A, et al. Helmet with specific settings versus facemask for noninvasive ventilation. Crit Care Med. 2009;37:1921-8.
17. Schonhofer B, Sortor-Leger S. Equipment needs for noninvasive mechanical ventilation. Eur Respir J. 2002;20:1029-36.
18. Gregoretti C, Confalonieri M, Navalesi P, et al. Evaluation of patient skin breakdown and comfort with a new face mask for non-invasive ventilation: a multi-center study. Intensive Care Med. 2002;28:278-84.
19. Calderini E, Confalonieri M, Puccio PG, et al. Patient-ventilator asynchrony during noninvasive ventilation: the role of expiratory trigger. Intensive Care Med. 1999;25:662-7.
20. Soo Hoo GH, Santiago S, Williams AJ. Nasal mechanical ventilation for hypercapnic respiratory failure in chronic obstructive pulmonary disease: determinants of success and failure. Crit Care Med. 1994;22:1253-61.
21. Mojoli F, Iotti GA, Gerletti M, et al. Carbon dioxide rebreathing during non-invasive ventilation delivered by helmet: a bench study. Intensive Care Med. 2008;34:1454-60.

22. Bach JR, Alba AS, Bohatiuk G, et al. Mouth intermittent positive pressure ventilation in the management of post-polio respiratory insufficiency. Chest. 1987;91(6):859-64.
23. Bach JR, Alba AS, Saporito L. Intermittent positive ventilation via mouth as an alternative to tracheostomy for 257 ventilator users. Chest. 1993;103(1):174-82.
24. Madden BP, Kariyawasam H, Siddiqi AJ, et al. Noninvasive ventilation in cystic fibrosis patients with acute or chronic respiratory failure. Eur Respir J. 2002;19(2):310-3.
25. Lellouche F, Fraticelli A, Taille´ S, et al. Physiological evaluation of five interfaces during noninvasive ventilation in healthy subjects (abstract). Intensive Care Med. 2002;28:A180.
26. Ohi M, Chin K, Tsuboi T, et al. Effect of nasal resistance on the increase in ventilation during noninvasive ventilation (abstract). Am J Respir Crit Care Med. 1994;149:A643.
27. Holanda MA, Reis RC, Winkeler GF, et al. Influence of total face, facial and nasal masks on short-term adverse effects during noninvasive ventilation. J Bras Pneumol. 2009;35(2):164-73.
28. Antón A, Tárrega J, Giner J, et al. Acute physiologic effects of nasal and full-face masks during noninvasive positive-pressure ventilation in patients with acute exacerbations of chronic obstructive pulmonary disease. Respir Care. 2003;48(10):922-5.
29. Kwok H, McComack J, Cece R, et al. Controlled trial of oronasal versus nasal mask ventilation in the treatment of acute respiratory failure. Crit Care Med. 2003;31(2):468-73.

Chapter 6

Noninvasive Ventilation: Adjuvant Therapies (Oxygenation, Humidification, Aerosol Therapies including Nebulization)

Akshaykumar Chhallani, Bharat Jagiasi

BACKGROUND

Noninvasive ventilation (NIV) is administration of ventilator support without using an invasive artificial airway. NIV is subdivided into negative pressure ventilation and noninvasive positive pressure ventilation (NIPPV).

Bilevel positive airway pressure (BIPAP) and continuous positive airway pressure (CPAP) are two most commonly used modes during NIV.

Bilevel positive airway pressure machines deliver air flow to the airway at a prescribed pressure in a similar way as a C-PAP machine; the difference is that there are two pressure levels in BIPAP.

Two most common adjunct therapies also known as add-on care that is given in addition to the primary or initial therapy to maximize its effectiveness.

Adjunct therapies are often required during NIV to address special needs such as preventing hypoxemia, stabilizing gas exchange, adequate humidification, and delivery of inhaled medications to relieve bronchospasm.

This overview describes the rationale and examines the evidence supporting adjunctive therapies during NIV.

OXYGENATION

Oxygen is an essential element for human survival. It has become a mainstay of treatment for critically ill patients. The main emphasis is to prevent hypoxemia. It is the treatment for hypoxemia and not breathlessness as it seems to be a knee jerk reaction to mere presence of a serious illness.

Supplemental oxygen is frequently added to bilevel NIV circuit for adequate oxygenation. In critically ill, ideally it is recommended to keep an arterial hemoglobin oxygen saturation between 88 and 95% and arterial oxygen partial pressure (PaO_2) between 55 and 80 mm Hg with least inspiratory oxygen fraction (FiO_2).[1]

NIV ventilators entrain room air and most of machines have the facility to provide oxygen directly into mask **(Fig. 1)**.

It can be added between mask and exhalation port or just distal to exhalation port or at ventilator outlet.[2]

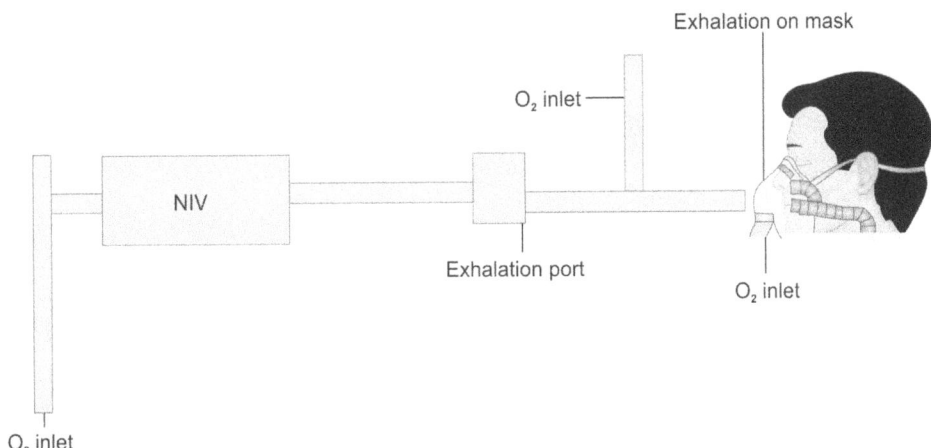

Fig. 1: Facility to provide oxygen.

Flow adjusted nasal cannula can also be used for oxygenation.[3]

The target FiO_2 (what patient is receiving) depends upon flow rate of air from the ventilator, the extent of leak, and the respiratory rate and breathing pattern of the patient in addition to external oxygen. The highest value of FiO_2 is reached with an active valve circuit with oxygen injected close to mask, a nose mask instead of nose mouth mask and with minimum expiratory positive airway pressure (EPAP).[4]

HUMIDIFICATION

The human airway has an important role in heating and humidifying inspired gas, and recovering heat and moisture from expired gas. Absolute humidity (AH) is the measure of water vapor (moisture) in the air regardless of temperature. Relative humidity (RH) also measures water vapor but relative to temperature of air.

In order to optimize gas exchange and protect lung, the human airway must provide gas at core temperature and 100% RH at the alveolar surface.

NIV delivers inspired air at very significant high-flow rates, which may overwhelm the natural humidification mechanism. The appropriate application of humidification during NIV is poorly understood. The need for humidification of gas in NIV is controversial.[5]

In a prospective clinical investigations of 24 patients with acute respiratory failure (ARF), arterial pressure of carbon dioxide ($PaCO_2$) was significantly higher with HME (heat and moisture exchanger) than HH (heated humidifier).

This study showed the effect of HME, dead space may decrease efficiency of NIV in patients with ARF.[6]

Randomized crossover study in nine patients receiving NIV for moderate to severe ARF concluded that the use of HME lessens the efficacy of NIV in reducing effort compared to HH.[7]

Respiratory humidification is a way of artificial warming and humidification of respiratory gas. The term respiratory gas conditioning stands for warming, humidification, and purification of respiratory gas. Inadequate gas conditioning may have a negative impact on patients' compliance to NIV treatment especially in chronic users as it can cause anatomical and functional deterioration of nasal mucosa.

Effects of Inefficient Gas Conditioning during NIV
- Metaplastic changes and keratinization of nasal mucosa
- Increase work of breathing
- Increase nasal airway resistance (NAWR)
- Decrease comfort and compliance to NIV[6]

Air Leak
In contrast to invasive ventilation, NIV uses an open circuit which is inherently leaky. Air leak during NIV may be between mask and skin, mouth leaks with nasal ventilation or nose leaks with mouth piece ventilation. This causes unidirectional nasal flow, so heat and moisture recovered from expired air is less. This will cause drop in AH.

During NIV, a large mouth leak from a nasal mask can cause an increase in NAWR.

Following factors pay vital role to maintain airway humidity during NIV:
- Inspiratory flow
- Inspired oxygen fraction
- % of leak
- Type of ventilators
- Interface
- Pressure and temperature of inhaled gas
- Type of humidification used

Types of Humidification Devices
Presently available options for humidification are either HH and or HME filter.[7] Technically, both produce AH levels which is adequate for the physiological functioning of upper airway.

During NIV, significant advantages are seen with HH as compared with HME **(Table 1)**.

Table 1: Difference between heated humidifier (HH) and heat and moisture exchanger (HME).

Parameter	HH (heated humidifier)	HME (heat and moisture exchange)
Dead space	Limited or no effect	Increase dead space
Work of breathing	Less	More as compared to HH
Heavy secretions	Preferred	Better to avoid
Electricity requirement	Yes	No
Convenience to use	Yes	Cumbersome

It seems that HH is superior to HME during acute NIV but this is probably not true in chronic users.

Heated Humidifier

Either these are Passover or bubble humidifiers. Bubble diffusion humidifier provides humidified oxygen or any other gas by allowing the gas to bubble through reservoir of water.

Passover humidifiers are named such as because the air literally passes over the water in the humidifier. It will passively add moisture.[8] Passover HH should be used to treat or prevent nasal congestion and improve patient compliance.

Bubble humidifier and HMEs found to cause increase work of breathing and airway resistance

Still there is insufficient data to make a recommendation for need and type of humidification in a patient on NIV.[9]

The choice of humidifier should be made according to the clinical context, user friendly status, potential possible complications, and cost factor.[10]

AEROSOL THERAPY

It is crucial and very common to use aerosol therapy during NIV.

An aerosol is a suspension of fine solid particles or liquid droplets in the air or another gas. Medical aerosol is any suspension of liquid or solid drug particles in a carrier gas.

Evidence does not support aerosol delivery without discontinuation of NIV.-

Mode of Ventilator

The effect of mode of ventilator on aerosol delivery is not very clear.

Continuous positive airway pressure and Bi-PAP are the two modes, which are commonly used during NIV.

Parkes and Bersten determined the efficacy of bronchodilator therapy during CPAP delivered by face mask.[11]

In a limited study of nine patients, they studied the response to incremental dose of inhaled bronchodilators with jet nebulizer alone (control) and the jet nebulizer with CPAP and a tight fitting face mask.

CPAP significantly reduced total aerosol delivery to the face mask from 6.85 (1.52) to 1.3 (0.37)%.

Despite a reduction in aerosol presented to the proximal airway when CPAP was delivered by face mask, the bronchodilator response to inhaled beta 2-agonist in stable asthmatic subjects was not affected

In a randomized clinical trial, Pollack CV compared the effect of beta-adrenergic agonist.

Aerosol in treating acute bronchospasm either with nasal BiPAP or small volume nebulizer (SVN).[12]

This study concluded the response to initial ED (emergency department) management of bronchospasm, as measured by PEFR (Peak expiratory flow rate) was better with aerosol delivered by BiPAP than with those delivered by SVN.

Maccari JG showed equivalent deposition of inhaled substance in healthy lungs when spontaneous breathing (SB), CPAP, and bi level were compared.[13]

Aerosol Deposition and Particle Size

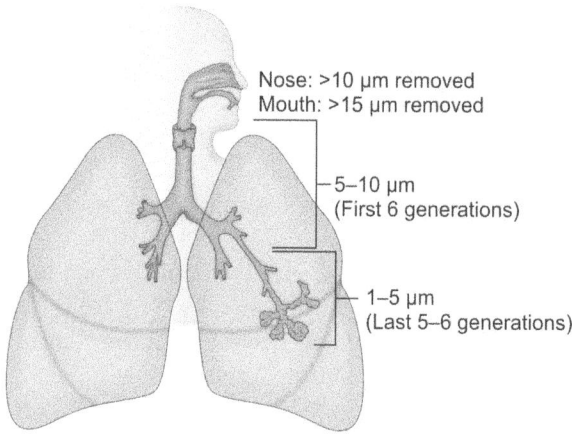

Fig. 2: Aerosol deposition and particle size.

Particle size plays an important role in lung deposition along with particle distribution and velocity. Particle size 1–5 μm easily reaches lung peripheries, 5–10-μm size particle deposits in the large bronchi while 10-100 μm deposit in nasopharynx **(Fig. 2)**.

Aerosol Equipment for NIV

Nasal mask can be used comfortably during NIV for aerosol therapy. The helmet and total face mask may expose patient's eyes to flow from NIV; hence, it is advisable not to use these devices for aerosol delivery during NIV.

Position of Aerosol Generator During NIV

Unlike invasive ventilation, placing the nebulizer near the ventilator reduces aerosol delivery during NIV. The best position of aerosol generator is in between leak port and mask **(Fig. 3)**.

The leak port allows gas washout during expiration and its position impacts the efficiency of aerosol device during NIV.

More aerosols are delivered when the leak port is in the circuit instead of mask.

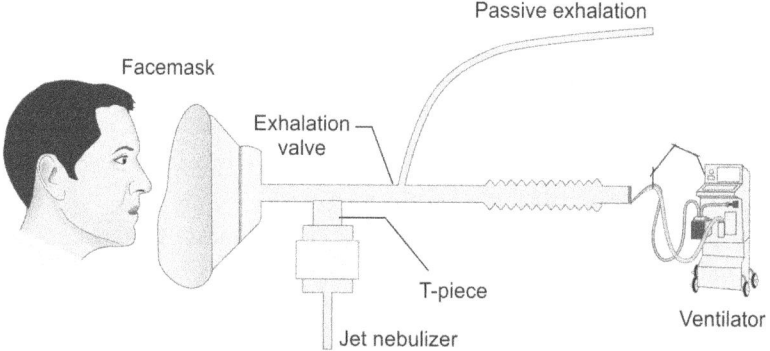

Fig. 3: Nebulization during spontaneous breathing, CPAP and bi-level positive pressure.

Newer generation critical care ventilators had special mode for NIV. These have inspiratory and expiratory valves and separate hoses for inspiratory and expiratory gases. The same method is followed for aerosol delivery in newer generations critical care ventilators as of invasive ventilation.

Ventilator Pressures

When using a nebulizer, more aerosol is delivered with a higher level of pressure support and less aerosol is delivered with higher level of expiratory pressure.

There is no definite evidence to recommend either single limb or double limb circuit for effective aerosol delivery.

Types of Aerosol Generator

- Pressurized metered-dose inhaler (pMDI)
- Small volume nebulizer
- Drug dose inhaler

*Pressurized metered-dose inhaler (**Fig. 4**)*: It is a portable light and compact drug device that dispenses multiple doses by a metered valve. It requires hand breath coordination. Several types of commercially available adapters can be used to connect pMDI canister to the ventilator circuit.

BRONCHODILATOR DELIVERY BY METERED-DOSE INHALER

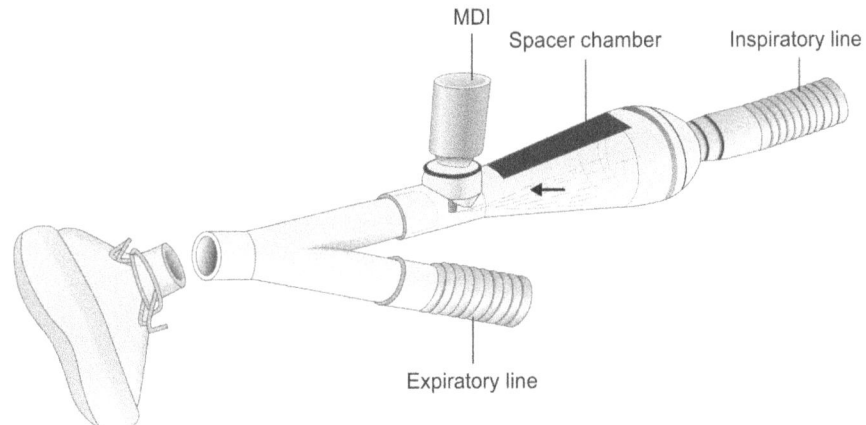

Fig. 4: Schematic representation of metered-dose inhaler (MDI) adapted to the spacer device in the inspiratory limb of ventilator circuit.

Small Volume Nebulizer (Table 2)

SVN can be categorized into two types
1. Jet/pneumatic nebulizer
2. Ultrasonic nebulizer

Table 2: Small volume nebulizer.

Advantages	Disadvantages
Minimal patient coordination required	Needs electricity or compressed gas
Drug, dose, and concentration can be modified	Poor portability
Can deliver combination	Risk of drug exposure to eyes
Can be used in all age groups	Cleaning and assembly

Jet Nebulizer (Fig. 5)

This is portable instrument, which requires an electrical battery power source to convert liquid drug solution or suspension in the aerosol.

Jet nebulizers are based on venturi principle. It works on changes in pressure. The liquid formulation containing drug particles along with the compressed air within inhaler chamber passes through a very narrow tube and enters a wide area, the increase in the volume compressed air leads to reduction of its pressure and anastomoses the liquid into microsize droplets.

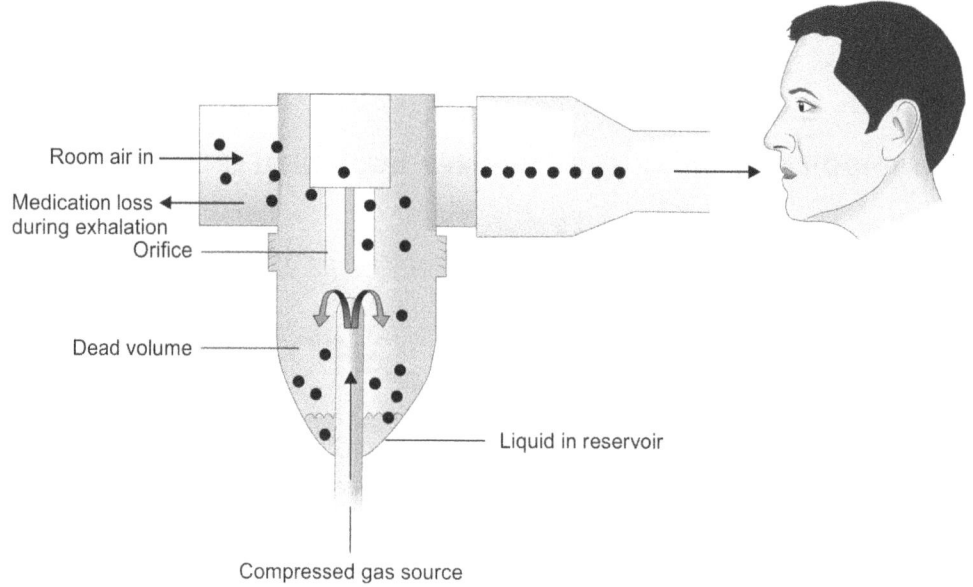

Fig. 5: Aerosol delivery device.

Theoretically nebulizer driven by air can worsen hypoxemia, if it improves the ventilation to nonperfused lung parenchyma. Patient should simultaneously receive supplement oxygen if compressor is used. Ideally oxygen mains should drive nebulizer.[14]

Types of Pneumatic/Jet Nebulizer (SVN)[15]

- Pneumatic jet nebulizer with reservoir tube
- Jet reservoir with collection bag
- Breath enhanced jet nebulizer

Aerosol delivery with the jet nebulizer is lower than pMDI and the mesh nebulizer. Aerosol deposition obtained with the mesh nebulizer is greater than the pMDI because of the higher nominal dose used with the nebulizer. Despi, Nava, et al. showed a significant bronchodilator effect in stable patients with COPD receiving bronchodilators through pMDI with spacer during NIV.[16] Therefore, pMDIs can be effectively used in patients receiving NIV.

Aerosol drug delivery with vibrating mesh nebulizers was three-to fivefold greater than that with jet nebulizers because of a smaller dead volume of mesh nebulizers.[17]

Dead volume, known as residual volume, is the amount of drug remaining in the nebulizer cup at the end of therapy.

Common Drugs Used for Nebulization (Table 3)[18]

- Adrenergic bronchodilators, e.g., Adrenaline
- Catecholamine derivatives, e.g., Beta-agonist like Salbutamol
- Anticholinergic bronchodilators, e.g., Tiotropium and Tipratropium bromide, Glycopyrrolate
- Inhaled steroids, e.g., Budesonide

Table 3: Common drugs used for nebulization.

Drug	Route	Dosage	Frequency
Adrenaline	Neb 1%	0.25–0.5 mL	QID
Salbutamol	Neb, MDI 0.5	100 µg	TID/QID
Levosalbutamol	Neb	0.63–1.25 mg	TID/QID
Terbutaline	MDI	2 puffs	QID
Ipratropium bromide	MDI Neb	250 µg	QID
Budesonide	Neb	0.5 mg	BID

Dry Powder Inhaler

- It delivers medication to the lung in the form of dry powder.
- Its effectiveness depends upon the inhalation force of patient hence it is rarely used in critically ill patients.

Ultrasonic Nebulizer

- It produces ultrasound waves.
- This electronic device produces current which is used to produce high-frequency vibration that breaks up water into an aerosol mist.

Steps and Techniques for Correct Use of Jet Nebulizer

Jet nebulizer is connected by a T piece directly to the mask. Avoid common mistake to connect the HME filter proximal to nebulizer so that nebulized particles are not stuck up in HME.

While using pMDI, a spacer is placed between the mask and circuit and pMDI is actuated into spacer and synchronized with initiation of inhalation.

Ideally nebulizer should be kept vertical during treatment

Patient needs to breath normally with occasional deep breaths.
Occasionally, tapping the side of nebulizer helps the solution drop to where it can be misted.[19]
When to stop nebulizer?
Newer nebulizer has microprocessor which will automatically turn off it once drug dose is complete.

Evidence suggests that once sputter starts, very low additional drug is inhaled. Hence some clinicians recommend to stop nebulization 1 minute after sputtering starts. Nebulizer should be changed every 24 hours. If it is labeled as single patient use, then it should be discarded accordingly.

Infection Control[20]

Cleaning instructions for the jet nebulizer:
- Wash your hand before and after handling equipment thoroughly.
- Dissemble nebulizer parts after every treatment.
- Rinse the mask, nebulizer cup with either sterile or distilled water for at least half a minute or 1 minute.
- Do not wash nebulizer tubing or compressor.
- Shake of excessive water.
- Air dry on an absorbent towel.

Cleaning Once or Twice a Week

- Remove plastic tubing from compressor
- Wash all parts except tubing
- Follow manufactures' instructions:
  - 3% hydrogen peroxide for 30 minutes or
  - 70% isopropyl alcohol for 5 minutes

▎KEY POINTS

- Supplemental oxygen is required to treat hypoxemia.
- Because of deleterious effect of dry air, humidification is essential during NIV.
- Correct application of humidification may help to prevent NIV-induced dryness.
- There is insufficient data to recommend timing of humidification in acute and chronic conditions and also type of humidifier in different clinical scenario.
- Aerosol therapy is commonly used during NIV.
- Beta-agonist, anticholinergic, and inhaled steroids are widely used in ICU for nebulization purpose.
- The effectiveness of aerosol therapy is technique and instrument dependent.

▎REFERENCES

1. Ferguson ND. Oxygen in the ICU Too much of good thing? JAMA. 2016;316(15):1553-4.
2. Kaul S, Stell S, Chinn S, et al. The effect of entrainment site and inspiratory pressure on the delivery of oxygen therapy during noninvasive mechanical ventilation in acute COPD patients. Euro Res Rev. 2006;15:190-1.

3. Hoofs M, Hagmeijer R, Duiverman ML. Inspired oxygen fraction during non invasive ventilation: The influence of flow rates, masks, exhalation ports & ventilator setting. Euro Resp J. 2018;52:PA2377.
4. Esquinas A, Nava S, Scala R, et al. Humidification & difficult endotracheal intubation in failure of non invasive mechanical ventilation (NIV). Preliminary results. Am J Respir Crit Care Med. 2008;177:a644.
5. Richard GN, Cistulli PA, Ungar RG, et al. Mouth leak with nasal continuous positive airway pressure increases nasal airway resistance. Am J Respir Air 1996;154:182-6.
6. Jaber S, Chanques G, Matecki S, et al. Comparison of the effects of heat and moisture exchangers and heated humidifiers on ventilation and gas exchange during non-invasive ventilation. Intensive Care Med. 2002;28:1590-4.
7. Lellouche F, Maggiore SM, Deye N, et al. Effect of the humidification device on the work of breathing during noninvasive ventilation. Intensive Care Med. 2002;28:1582-9.
8. Hill N. Complication of non invasive positive pressure ventilation. Respir care. 1997;42:432.
9. Esquinas Rodriguez AM, Scala R, Soroksky A, et al. Humidifiers during non-invasive ventilation: Key topics and practical implications. Crit Care. 2012;16(1):203.
10. Branson RD, Gentile MA. Is Humidification always necessary during noninvasive ventilation in the hospital. Respir Care. 2010;55(2):209-16.
11. Parkes SN, Bersten AD. Aerosol kinetics and bronchodilator efficacy during continuous positive airway pressure delivered by face mask. Thorax.1997;52:171-5.
12. Pollack CV Jr, Fleisch KB, Dowsey K. Treatment of acute bronchospasm with beta-adrenergic agonist aerosols delivered by a nasal bilevel positive airway pressure circuit. Ann Emerg Med. 1995;26:552-7.
13. Maccari JG, Teixeira C, Savi A, et al. Nebulization during spontaneous breathing, CPAP, and bi-level positive-pressure ventilation: A randomized analysis of pulmonary radioaerosol deposition. Respir Care. 2014;59:479-84.
14. Udwadia F, Udwadia ZF, Kohli AF, et al. Asthma management. Principles of Respiratory Medicine. New Delhi: Jaypee Brothers Medical Publishers; 2010.
15. American Association for Respiratory care. (2017). A Guide to Aerosol Delivery Devices for Respiratory Therapist, 4th Edition. [online] Available from http://www.aarc.org/education/online-courses/aerosol-devices/ [Last accessed December, 2019].
16. Nava S, Karakurt S, Rampulla C, et al. Salbutamol delivery during non-invasive mechanical ventilation in patients with chronic obstructive pulmonary disease: A randomized, controlled study. Intensive Care Med. 2001;27:1627-35.
17. Ari A. How to optimize aerosol drug delivery during noninvasive ventilation: What to use, how to use it, and why? Eurasian J Pulmonol. 2019;21:1-8.
18. Chang DW. Pharmacotherapy for mechanical ventilation. Clinical Application of Mechanical Ventilation. United States: Cengage Learning; 2013. pp. 455-89.
19. Ari A. Aerosol therapy in pulmonary critical care. Respir Care. 2015;60(6):858-79.
20. American Association for Respiratory Care. AARC Clinical Practice Guideline: selection of an aerosol delivery device. Respir Care. 1992;37(8):891-7.

Chapter 7

Noninvasive Ventilation: Indications, Contraindications, and Complications

Deven Juneja, Anish Gupta, Anjali Mishra

■ INTRODUCTION

The use of noninvasive ventilation (NIV) has increased dramatically in the past few years and it has become an integral tool for the management of respiratory failure in the intensive care units (ICUs). Increased availability, improving ventilator technology and better understanding, has made it an accepted alternative to invasive mechanical ventilation (IMV) in certain cases. Even the evidence base for use in different clinical scenarios has increased considerably in recent years. NIV is not suited for all respiratory conditions and the key to successful application of NIV is in understanding its limitations with timely escalation to IMV in cases of failure. In conditions which respond quickly to therapy, NIV may serve as an important adjunct to standard medical therapy.

■ INDICATIONS

The indications of NIV vary depending upon the underlying cause, severity of disease and associated complications. There are certain potential factors which are associated with successful application of NIV (**Box 1**).[1]

Box 1: Potential predictors of success in noninvasive positive pressure ventilation.

- Young adults
- Low APACHE scores
- Conscious, oriented, GCS > 8
- Intact dentition
- Moderate hypercarbia ($PaCO_2$ > 45 mm Hg, < 92 mm Hg)
- Moderate acidemia (pH between 7.10–7.35)
- Improvements in gas exchange and hemodynamic parameters within first 2 hours of NIV application

(APACHE: acute physiology and chronic health evaluation; GCS: Glasgow coma scale; NIV: noninvasive ventilation)

A trial of NIV should be given in all patients with a disease known to respond to NIV in the absence of contraindications. The maximum numbers of randomized controlled trials (RCTs) have been done in patients with chronic obstructive pulmonary disorder (COPD). However, there are a multitude of studies describing the use of NIV in various other medical disorders (**Box 2**).

Chapter 7: Noninvasive Ventilation: Indications, Contraindications, and Complications

Box 2: Potential medical disorders which may benefit with use of noninvasive ventilation.

Indications for NIV for respiratory failure in the following conditions
- Acute exacerbation of COPD
- Cardiogenic pulmonary edema
- Acute asthma
- Immunocompromised patients
- De novo ARF
- Perioperative/Postoperative cases
- Trauma
- Palliative care
- Viral illness
- Neuromuscular diseases or chest wall deformity
- Postextubation
- Weaning in progress

(ARF: acute respiratory failure; COPD: chronic obstructive pulmonary disease; NIV: noninvasive ventilation)

Acute Exacerbation of Chronic Obstructive Pulmonary Disease

Acute exacerbation of COPD (AECOPD) with hypercapnic respiratory failure is a common cause for hospital admission. Respiratory acidosis develops when the capacity of the respiratory muscle pump is exceeded with failure to achieve adequate alveolar ventilation. As a result, there is increase in arterial carbon dioxide ($PaCO_2$) and consequent respiratory acidosis. NIV is the preferred initial mode of ventilation in patients of AECOPD with hypercapnic respiratory failure. The success rate of NIV has been shown in RCTs to be around 80–85%. NIV helps to improve oxygenation, acute respiratory acidosis, and reduces the work of breathing. It also helps to reduce the incidence of ventilator associated pneumonia (VAP) and the length of ICU and hospital stay. The classic indications of NIV in patients with AECOPD is:[2]

- Acute or acute-on-chronic respiratory acidosis with respiratory distress—to prevent endotracheal intubation and IMV. In patients who present with tachypnea and a pH of 7.25–7.35 (without metabolic acidosis), the use of NIV is associated with a favorable outcome. An improvement in pH and/or respiratory rate are predictors of successful outcome with improvement usually evident in 1–4 hours.[3]
- Prevention of acute respiratory acidosis, i.e., $PaCO_2$ is normal or elevated but pH is normal. It is mainly used to reduce the work of breathing.
- In "do not intubate (DNI)" status patients for symptomatic relief.

Noninvasive Ventilation for Acute Hypercapnic Respiratory Failure due to Acute Exacerbation of Chronic Obstructive Pulmonary Disease

Bilevel NIV [bilevel positive airway pressure (BiPAP)] has been shown to prevent intubation in a subgroup of AECOPD patients with pure respiratory acidosis (pH 7.25–7.35).[4] NIV has also shown to reduce the rates for intubation, ICU and hospital length of stay and improvement in survival with reduced rate of infections.

Bilevel Noninvasive Ventilation as an Alternative to First-line Endotracheal Intubation

Studies which have compared NIV to endotracheal intubation and IMV have shown that use of NIV is associated with fewer re-admission rates, reduced VAP rates and shorter duration of mechanical ventilation and ICU stay.[5] Based on the studies, recommendation is to use NIV for patients with hypercapnic respiratory failure secondary to AECOPD.[6] A trial of NIV should be given to all patients unless clinical condition does not permit.[6]

Noninvasive Ventilation for ARF due to AECOPD Exacerbation to Prevent the Development of Respiratory Acidosis

Randomized controlled trials have failed to show any benefit with NIV to prevent respiratory acidosis. In some studies, it has shown to reduce the rates of intubation but with no effect on mortality. Hence, it is suggested to not use NIV in patients with AECOPD with ARF without respiratory acidosis.[6]

Cardiogenic Pulmonary Edema

Respiratory failure in patients with cardiogenic pulmonary edema (CPE) occurs due to high capillary pressures and consequent alveolar flooding with/without left ventricular (LV) dysfunction. Alveolar flooding reduces respiratory system compliance. In this context NIV helps to improve respiratory mechanics by decreasing the negative pressure swings generated by the respiratory muscles. Thus, NIV helps to reduce LV afterload and LV work.[7]

A number of systematic reviews and meta-analysis have been published, wherein it was concluded that NIV decreased the rate of intubation and reduced in hospital mortality and NIV was not associated with increase in rates of myocardial infarction.[8,9] It is important to note that none of the trials included patients with acute coronary syndrome and/or cardiogenic shock and hence, these recommendations do not apply to these subgroup of patients.

Single-center RCTs have been conducted to evaluate the use of CPAP or NIV to treat CPE in the prehospital setting. Pooled analysis of the trials demonstrated a decrease in hospital mortality and need for intubation. An improvement in dyspnea and oxygenation was also noted. However, these trials were heterogeneous with respect to their design and patient selection and hence, application of the results to the population at whole is difficult.[10]

Acute Asthma

The pathophysiological feature of asthma is airway hyperresponsiveness leading to reversible bronchoconstriction. This leads to increase in the resistive workload with increase in respiratory muscle work. In addition, hyperinflation reduces the efficiency of respiratory muscles with eventual fatigue leading to hypercapnia.[11] NIV helps to reduce the work of breathing, improves ventilation and oxygenation, and decreases the feeling of dyspnea.

There is limited data with respect to use of NIV in acute asthmatics with respiratory failure as the number of patients requiring ICU admission is small. It has been shown that use of CPAP in patients with induced asthma improved energy utilization by decreasing the pressure-time product, thus, translating to improvement in respiratory mechanics and breathing pattern. A number of uncontrolled studies have shown improvement of physiological parameters when comparing NIV with routine care in exacerbations of asthma.[12] However, RCTs and meta-analysis have not shown any difference in clinical outcomes.[12] A large retrospective study conducted by Stefan MS et al. showed reduced in-hospital mortality and shorter length of hospital stay in patients who received NIV as compared to IMV.[13] Even though NIV has shown to improve forced expiratory volume in 1 second (FEV1) and peak expiratory flow rate, pooled analyses have failed to show a reduction in mortality, intubation rate or ICU length of stay.

Since, data is limited no recommendation has been made with respect to use of NIV in acute asthma.[6] However, there is a subgroup of patients who have asthma-COPD overlap syndrome (ACOS) and BiPAP may be considered in these patients.

Immunocompromised Patients

The most common indication for ICU admission in immunocompromised patients is ARF. NIV is the first-line approach for patients with mild-to-moderate ARF. Gristina GR et al. in their multicenter study investigated the impact of NIV use in hematological patients and concluded that use of NIV was an independent predictor of survival.[14] A meta-analysis by Huang HB et al. has shown NIV to improve short-term outcomes, reduce the need for intubation, and ICU length of stay.[15]

Acute Respiratory Failure in the Postoperative Setting

Abdominal surgery, anesthesia, and postoperative pain can lead to diaphragm dysfunction leading to atelectasis, reduced lung volume, hypoxemia and respiratory failure. Diaphragm dysfunction can last up to 7 days. NIV has shown a favorable role in ARF after abdominal, thoracic, and cardiac surgeries. It has been shown to improve ventilation and aeration with reduction in atelectasis during the postoperative period, especially after major abdominal surgeries. Studies on management of respiratory failure with NIV after abdominal surgery have shown a reduction in rate of reintubation and healthcare associated infections.[16] In supradiaphragmatic surgery NIV has shown to reduce the need for reintubation and reduced in-hospital mortality.[17] A Cochrane review concluded that use of NIV in patients after upper abdominal surgery may reduce rate of intubation and ICU length of stay. However, they could not elicit any mortality benefit.[18] However, in postoperative patients presenting with respiratory failure, surgical complications such as anastomotic leaks, sepsis (intra-abdominal) should be addressed first and then NIV should be initiated.

Chest Trauma

Trauma patients are a diverse patient population with varying respiratory needs. The severity of respiratory dysfunction and impairment of gas exchange along with associated injuries determine the type of respiratory support needed in these patients. The mechanisms of ARF following trauma are divided into direct and indirect causes. Direct injury refers to damage to the rib cage, airways, lung parenchyma, diaphragm or pulmonary vasculature (rib fractures, flail chest, pulmonary contusions, pneumothorax, hemothorax, etc.) while indirect injury refers to capillary leakage and altered surfactant composition with leakage of edema fluid and infiltration with inflammatory cells into the alveoli. Indirect injury is secondary to nonthoracic trauma and is mainly associated with shock, sepsis, acute pancreatitis, massive blood transfusions, and coagulation abnormalities. Both the mechanisms may ultimately result in acute respiratory distress syndrome (ARDS). The role of NIV in chest trauma patients may be broadly divided into NIV in flail chest trauma and non-flail chest trauma.

Noninvasive Ventilation in Flail Chest Trauma

Respiratory failure in these cases is secondary to intrapulmonary shunt, ventilation-perfusion mismatch (V/Q), pneumothorax, hemothorax, and atelectasis. Till date only two RCTs have compared NIV with IMV in patients with flail chest. An RCT conducted by Bolliger et al. compared CPAP with IMV in 69 patients and concluded that CPAP was associated with shorter duration of treatment and ICU length of stay and lower rate of infections.[19] Another RCT conducted by Gunduz et al. showed higher PaO_2 levels in the NIV group in the first 2 days.[20] Another RCT comparing NIV with high flow nasal oxygen showed higher rate of intubation in the latter group in chest trauma related hypoxemia.[21]

Noninvasive Ventilation in Non-flail Chest Trauma

The role of NIV in blunt chest trauma has been evaluated in various studies. A prospective observational study by Xirouchaki et al. showed improvement in gas exchange and respiratory rates with NIV and avoided IMV in a majority (18 of 22) of the cases.[22] Similarly, Vidhani et al. conducted a retrospective study and concluded that patients with pulmonary contusions and PaO_2/FiO_2 < 300 were safely managed with NIV.[23] A large meta-analysis of patients with blunt chest trauma concluded that the early use of NIV in selected patients may prevent intubation and decrease complications and ICU length of stay.[24]

Pandemic Viral Illness

The role of NIV in viral disease leading to ARF is controversial. At present there is no RCT which has evaluated the efficacy of NIV in pandemic viral disease. However, a number of observational studies have reported a high failure rate with NIV. A prospective multicenter study reported a failure rate of 60% with NIV for respiratory failure in influenza A (H1N1) patients.[25] Among those who responded well were those with low Acute Physiology and Chronic Health Evaluation (APACHE) II, low sequential organ failure assessment (SOFA), absence of acute kidney injury/renal failure, no vasopressor requirement and involvement of two or less quadrants on chest X-ray. NIV responsive patients had a shorter ICU and hospital stay, and shorter ventilation time. However, mortality rates were comparable in both the groups.

De Novo Acute Respiratory Failure

De novo respiratory failure refers to respiratory failure occurring in the absence of any preexisting respiratory disease. This subset of patients is categorized by hypoxemia ($PaO_2/FiO_2 \leq 300$), tachypnea (RR > 30–35 breaths/min) and new onset of respiratory disease (pneumonia, ARDS). The objective of NIV in these cases is to improve oxygenation, ventilation, reduce work of breathing and prevent intubation. However, the efficacy of NIV in reducing the work of breathing in hypoxemic patients is not well documented. NIV has shown to reduce the inspiratory effort in ARDS patients.[26] Theoretically, delivery of higher inspiratory pressures will translate into delivery of higher tidal volumes. This leads to high transpulmonary pressures and high tidal volumes which can further exacerbate lung injury. Also, application of lung protective ventilation via NIV is difficult and unpredictable. Higher pressures lead to increased air leaks and gastric distension. Studies on role on NIV in de novo ARF have shown it to reduce the rate of intubation. The potential problem with NIV use in these patients is a delay in intubation.[27] Also, of note is that NIV failure is associated with higher rate of postintubation complications and is an independent predictor mortality. Hence, it is imperative to carefully select patients for NIV use and manage them under close monitoring.

Neuromuscular Diseases or Chest Wall Deformity

Neuromuscular diseases (NMDs) or chest wall deformity (CWD) are classified as restrictive chest disorders which may lead to chronic respiratory failure. However, these patients may frequently require hospitalizations due to acute decompensation and may even present with hypercapnic respiratory failure. NIV use may improve quality of life and outcome of these patients especially if they have none to moderate bulbar weakness.[28]

Several measures have been advocated to assess the underlying diaphragmatic weakness and hence the need for initiating NIV. These include measurement of transdiaphragmatic or esophageal pressure, supine and upright FVC, maximum inspiratory pressure (PImax), overnight oximetry, and $PaCO_2$. However, no single test has been shown to be ideal in diagnosing or defining diaphragmatic weakness and hypoventilation. The current European guidelines suggest use of FVC < 80%, for initiating NIV support.[29] It is further recommended that NIV should be initiated early, before development of acidosis.[30]

Postextubation from Invasive Mechanical Ventilation

Postextubation respiratory failure is a common clinical problem with reported incidence rates to the tune of 23.5%. Reintubation is reported to be associated with poor prognosis and increased mortality.[31] NIV may help to prevent respiratory failure in postextubation cases or prevent reintubation in cases of postextubation respiratory failure. Studies have failed to show a significant difference with respect to rates of reintubation when NIV was compared to standard oxygen therapy. However, in the high-risk group (advanced age, preexisting comorbidities), studies have shown that NIV use is associated with reduced rates of reintubation and ICU mortality. Hence, the ERS/ATS recommendations have made a conditional recommendation to use NIV to prevent postextubation respiratory failure only in the high-risk group.[6] NIV for treatment of respiratory failure postextubation has been evaluated in multiple studies. Esteban et al. in their multicenter RCT showed no benefit with NIV on rates of reintubation, ICU mortality, hospital mortality and length of stay in ICU and hospital.[32] However, a higher ICU mortality was reported in the same study in the NIV group, possibly due to delay in intubation. A meta-analysis confirmed no benefit with NIV to prevent re-intubation or reduce mortality.[33] Hence, as per the current evidence, NIV should not be used for patients with postextubation respiratory failure.

Noninvasive Ventilation in Palliative Care

With death approaching, relief of pain and comfort of the patient become an important aspect of care. Worsening of breathlessness is commonly seen and families expect symptomatic relief for this symptom. The task force appointed by society of critical care medicine has classified patients into three types, type 1, 2, and 3. Type 2 and 3 patients categorize palliative care.[34] Type 2 patients do not want intubation but want salvage therapy in the form of noninvasive maneuvers to continue with a goal for surviving hospital stay. Type 3 patients seek only symptomatic relief and have no survival goal. NIV is an effective modality of therapy in these cases. RCTs have evaluated a role of NIV in palliative care and found improvement in dyspnea and better cognition secondary to reduced need for morphine.[35] The acceptance rate for NIV was similar to that of oxygen therapy signifying that NIV did not lead to troubling complications. Hence, it is suggested to use NIV for palliation in the patients with terminal cancer or other terminal conditions.

Weaning Patients from Invasive Mechanical Ventilation

In a Cochrane review, NIV was associated with a decrease in mortality, reduced rates of VAP, reduced ICU and hospital length of stay and duration of IMV.[36] A reduction in the proportion of weaning failure was also noted. However, this analysis included mostly patients with hypercapnic respiratory failure especially COPD. Similarly, a meta-analysis revealed a reduced length of ICU stay, reduced rates of reintubation and pneumonia in postsurgical patients.[37] No effect on ICU mortality was reported. A recent meta-analysis showed a reduced hospital mortality in the NIV weaning group in COPD patients but the effect was less certain in mixed ICU population.[38] A reduced ICU length of stay, duration of mechanical ventilation, and reduced rates of VAP were also noted. Hence, NIV may facilitate weaning from IMV in hypercapnic respiratory failure but no recommendation can be made about its use in hypoxemic patients.

CONTRAINDICATIONS

The contraindications to NIV can be divided into absolute and relative (**Table 1**).[39]

Table 1: Contraindications to noninvasive ventilation.	
Absolute	**Relative**
➢ Cardiac or respiratory arrest ➢ Facial trauma, deformity ➢ Facial burns ➢ Upper airway obstruction ➢ Life-threatening organ failure (nonrespiratory) ➢ Recent esophageal anastomosis ➢ Coma ➢ Arrhythmia with hemodynamic instability	➢ Uncooperative patient (confused, agitated) ➢ Inability to protect the airway or clear secretions ➢ Impaired consciousness (GCS < 8) ➢ Hemodynamic instability ➢ Acute pneumothorax ➢ Vomiting

(GCS: Glasgow Coma Scale)

Noninvasive ventilation is supposed to supplement spontaneous breathing. Hence, cardiac or respiratory arrest are absolute contraindications to the use of NIV. However, in cases of respiratory arrest a trial of NIV may be given but only under supervision. Any form of facial trauma, burn or deformity may make application of NIV interface difficult and hence, NIV is contraindicated in these cases. Hemodynamically unstable arrhythmias need cardioversion and IMV may be preferred.

A number of contraindications have not necessarily resulted in a poor outcome with NIV but have actually been a part of exclusion criteria in clinical trials. For example, coma is associated with loss of airway reflexes and is considered an absolute contraindication to NIV. However, a study on patients with GCS < 8 reported similar outcomes with NIV when

Chapter 7: Noninvasive Ventilation: Indications, Contraindications, and Complications

compared to more alert patients.[40] Similarly, patients who are confused, agitated, and have cognitive impairment do make application of NIV difficult but do not exclude its use.

Tension pneumothorax is an absolute contraindication but a trial of NIV can be given in patients with acute pneumothorax. One prerequisite is to drain the pneumothorax prior to administering NIV and close monitoring is warranted. Vomiting is considered a contraindication as patients with poor airway reflexes are prone to aspiration. The risk of vomiting should be assessed in each individual and NIV use should be individualized. Nasogastric tube insertion with gastric emptying may help to alleviate the risk.

It is important to emphasize that the presence of contraindications (relative) necessitate close monitoring and supervision in an ICU. A trial of NIV may be given and any indication of NIV failure should prompt insertion of an advanced airway and invasive mechanical ventilation.

■ COMPLICATIONS

Every effective therapy has its own set of risks and potential complications. With the increasing application of NIV, a number of studies and trials are now assessing its complications. Broadly the complications can be classified into major and minor (**Table 2**).[30,41]

Table 2: Complications of noninvasive ventilation.

Minor complications		Major complications	
Problems	Incidence	Problems	Incidence
Discomfort related to mask	30–50%	Aspiration pneumonia	~5%
Carbon dioxide rebreathing	50–100%	Hemodynamic instability (hypotension)	Rare
Skin rash and erythema	20–34%		
Nasal bridge ulceration/pressure sore	5–10%	Barotrauma	Rare
Airway dryness	10–20%	Mucus plugging	Infrequent
Nasal congestion	20–50%		
Gastric insufflation	5–40%		
Patient–ventilator dyssynchrony	13–100%		
Claustrophobia	5–20%		

Minor Complications

Mask Intolerance

Mask related discomfort is the most common problem encountered while using nasal or oronasal masks. An optimal mask fit with the right size mask and minimal air leak has to be ensured. Skin rashes and erythema is fairly common with the oronasal and nasal mask occurring in 30–50% of patients within a few hours, but a more serious complication with a long-term use is nasal bridge ulceration (5–10%).[30,41] Painful ulcerations may be severe enough leading to NIV failure. An improper overtight application is usually a failed attempt at avoiding air leak at the expense of causing skin trauma. Measures to reduce these complications include intermittent breaks with alternative modes of oxygen delivery (interfaces) and balancing the strap tension to restrict air leak under acceptable limits. Use of protective barriers such as nasal pillows, gel masks or masks with soft silicone seals are advocated. Topical steroids or antibiotics may be applied in cases of infected wounds.[30]

Complications Related to Pressure and Flow

Pressure related problems and complications include patient discomfort, air leak, ear or sinus pain and gastric insufflation. Large air leaks decrease the effective FiO_2 delivered, increases ventilator auto triggering, and rebreathing of CO_2. Air leaks may be less with pressure-controlled mode as compared to volume-controlled ventilation. Reducing inspiratory pressure and tidal volume may also aid in reducing air leaks. Gastric insufflations may occur in 5–40% of patients on NIV, who may complain of excessive flatulence having used NIV overnight. There is a serious risk of vomiting and pulmonary aspiration of gastric contents which may be avoided by keeping the pressures to <25 cm H_2O and placement of a nasogastric tube.[30,41]

Flow related concerns include nasal mucosal dryness and congestion with incidence of 10–20% and 20–50%, respectively.[41] Topical corticosteroids, nasal decongestants, topical saline and water based nasal gels can be used to alleviate these symptoms. Usually nasal and oral dryness is a result of air leak through the mouth resulting in loss of the nasal mucosa's capacity to heat and humidify inspired air. However, the controversy regarding the routine use of supplemental humidification in all patients subjected to NIV largely remains unanswered. Currently the British Thoracic Society (BTS) guidelines recommend humidification only in cases of upper airway dryness or when secretions are difficult to expectorate.[30] Eye irritation may also be caused by the air leak on the side of nose.

Patient Ventilator Dyssynchrony

This involves trouble with the synchronization of patients' inspiratory efforts with the triggering and cycling of the ventilator. Up to 12–23% of ARF patients on NIV, face problems related to auto and double triggering, premature or late cycling and ineffective breaths.[42] Reassuring the patient and curbing anxiety may help. Making ventilatory adjustments to pressure support and positive end-expiratory pressure (PEEP), ensuring adequate inspiratory time and readjusting rise time and inspiratory trigger sensitivity may ameliorate asynchrony to a large extent. Keeping a check on air leak also limits patient ventilator dyssynchrony (PVD). PVD has been estimated to be present in 24–43% of ARF patients as measured by the global asynchrony index.

Major Complications

Delay in Intubation and Risk of Aspiration Pneumonia

Patient selection and monitoring play a crucial role in avoiding NIV failure. Cautious implementation is recommended in cases with excessive gastric distension, nausea/vomiting, ileus and gastroesophageal reflux, where risk of aspiration is higher. Although largely underreported in RCTs, aspiration pneumonia has been documented in 5% of patients on NIV. However, the reported percentage of nosocomial pneumonia still remains lower than IMV.[41] Keeping the patient nil per orally until stabilized and placing them in sitting or semi-sitting positions may help.

Barotrauma

Barotrauma is a known complication of positive pressure ventilation. But the incidence is much less as compared to endotracheal intubation since the inflation pressures rarely exceed 25 cm H_2O. An acute pneumothorax may be life-threatening and needs to be promptly detected. The group of patients susceptible to barotrauma include patients with COPD, bullous lung disease, interstitial lung diseases, injury secondary to pneumonia, cystic fibrosis, and neuromuscular disorders. Minimum effective inspiratory pressures should be kept in these patients. The risk can further be reduced by using pressure-controlled ventilation, targeting the peak inspiratory pressure to less than 30 cm H_2O, optimizing the inspiratory and expiratory times to avoid breath stacking and applying a PEEP not exceeding the auto PEEP.[41]

Hemodynamic Effects

Mechanical ventilation increases the intrathoracic pressure that affects the venous return (reduces preload) and ventricular filling. CPAP reduces cardiac output and stroke volume, without changing heart rate or blood pressure and increases systemic vascular resistance. The hemodynamic effects are exaggerated in patients with severe disease who are already hypotensive or fluid depleted, and in patients with underlying cardiac disease or poor left ventricular functions.[41] NIV should also be avoided in uncontrolled ischemia or arrhythmias until the patient is stabilized.

Sedation-related Issues

Using appropriate sedation reduces agitation and improves patient compliance. Inadequate sedation may contribute to anxiety and poor patient-ventilator synchrony, resulting in increased work of breathing. However, sedation may increase the risk of hypoventilation, aspiration, and even hypotension. The BTS guidelines recommend the use of sedation with close monitoring in an HDU/ICU setting only. No significant studies till date have been published to establish the superior efficacy of either of the drugs used for sedation like opiates, benzodiazepines or dexmedetomidine.

CONCLUSION

Noninvasive ventilation is an important tool in the management of patients with respiratory failure. Conventionally its use was limited to patients with acute hypercapnic respiratory failure. However, with better understanding the application of this important tool has become more common with trials being conducted in patients with hypoxemic respiratory failure also. The judicious use of NIV has made it an effective alternative to IMV in certain patient populations. However, proper knowledge of its indications, contraindications, and complications is imperative for its appropriate utilization and improving patient outcomes.

REFERENCES

1. International Consensus Conferences in Intensive Care Medicine: noninvasive positive pressure ventilation in acute respiratory failure. Organized jointly by the American Thoracic Society, the European Respiratory Society, the European Society of Intensive Care Medicine, and the Société de Réanimation de Langue Française, and approved by ATS Board of Directors, December 2000. Am J Respir Crit Care Med. 2001;163(1):283-91.

2. Nava S, Navalesi P, Conti G. Time of noninvasive ventilation. Intensive Care Med. 2006;32:361-70.
3. Carrera M, Marin JM, Antón A, Chiner E, Alonso ML, Masa JF, et al. A controlled trial of noninvasive ventilation for chronic obstructive pulmonary disease exacerbations. J Crit Care. 2009;24: 473, e7-14.
4. Keenan SP, Powers CE, McCormack DG. Noninvasive positive-pressure ventilation in patients with milder chronic obstructive pulmonary disease exacerbations: a randomized controlled trial. Respir Care. 2005;50:610-6.
5. Conti G, Antonelli M, Navalesi P, Rocco M, Bufi M, Spadetta G, et al. Noninvasive vs. conventional mechanical ventilation in patients with chronic obstructive pulmonary disease after failure of medical treatment in the ward: a randomized trial. Intensive Care Med. 2002;28:1701-7.
6. Rochwerg B, Brochard L, Elliott MW, Hess D, Hill NS, Nava S, et al. Official ERS/ATS clinical practice guidelines: noninvasive ventilation for acute respiratory failure. Eur Respir J. 2017;50(2): p. ii. 1602426.
7. Lenique F, Habis M, Lofaso F, Dubois-Randé JL, Harf A, Brochard L. Ventilatory and hemodynamic effects of continuous positive airway pressure in left heart failure. Am J Respir Crit Care Med. 1997;155:500-5.
8. Vital FM, Ladeira MT, Atallah AN. Noninvasive positive pressure ventilation (CPAP or bilevel NPPV) for cardiogenic pulmonary oedema. Cochrane Database Syst Rev. 2013;5:CD005351.
9. Cabrini L, Landoni G, Oriani A, Plumari VP, Nobile L, Greco M, et al. Noninvasive ventilation and survival in acute care settings: a comprehensive systematic review and meta-analysis of randomized controlled trials. Crit Care Med. 2015;43:880-8.
10. Roessler MS, Schmid DS, Michels P, Schmid O, Jung K, Stöber J, et al. Early out-of-hospital noninvasive ventilation is superior to standard medical treatment in patients with acute respiratory failure: a pilot study. Emerg Med J. 2012;29:409-14.
11. Leatherman J. Mechanical ventilation for severe asthma. Chest. 2015;147:1671-80.
12. Lim WJ, Mohammed Akram R, Carson KV, Mysore S, Labiszewski NA, Wedzicha JA, et al. Noninvasive positive pressure ventilation for treatment of respiratory failure due to severe acute exacerbations of asthma. Cochrane Database Syst Rev. 2012;12:CD004360.
13. Stefan MS, Nathanson BH, Lagu T, Priya A, Pekow PS, Steingrub JS, et al. Outcomes of noninvasive and invasive ventilation in patients hospitalized with asthma exacerbation. Ann Am Thorac Soc. 2016;13:1096-104.
14. Gristina GR, Antonelli M, Conti G, Ciarlone A, Rogante S, Rossi C, et al. Noninvasive versus invasive ventilation for acute respiratory failure in patients with hematologic malignancies: a 5-year multicenter observational survey. Crit Care Med. 2011;39:2232-9.
15. Huang HB, Xu B, Liu GY, Lin JD, Du B. Use of noninvasive ventilation in immunocompromised patients with acute respiratory failure: a systematic review and meta-analysis. Crit Care. 2017;21(1):4.
16. Jaber S, Lescot T, Futier E, Paugam-Burtz C, Seguin P, Ferrandiere M, et al. Effect of noninvasive ventilation on tracheal reintubation among patients with hypoxemic respiratory failure following abdominal surgery: a randomized clinical trial. JAMA. 2016;315:1345-53.
17. Auriant I, Jallot A, Herve P, Cerrina J, Le Roy Ladurie F, et al. Noninvasive ventilation reduces mortality in acute respiratory failure following lung resection. Am J Respir Crit Care Med. 2001;164:1231-5.
18. Faria DAS, da Silva EMK, Atallah ÁN, Vital FMR. Noninvasive positive pressure ventilation for acute respiratory failure following upper abdominal surgery. Cochrane Database Syst Rev. 2015;10:CD009134.
19. Bolliger CT, Van Eeden SF. Treatment of multiple rib fractures. Randomized controlled trial comparing ventilatory with nonventilatory management. Chest. 1990;97:943-8.
20. Gunduz M. A comparative study of continuous positive airway pressure (CPAP) and intermittent positive pressure ventilation (IPPV) in patients with flail chest. Emerg Med J. 2005;22:325-9.
21. Hernandez G, Fernandez R, Lopez-Reina P, Cuena R, Pedrosa A, Ortiz R, et al. Noninvasive ventilation reduces intubation in chest trauma-related hypoxemia: a randomized clinical trial. Chest. 2010;137:74-80.

22. Xirouchaki N, Kondoudaki E, Anastasaki M, Alexopoulou C, Koumiotaki S, Georgopoulos D. Noninvasive bilevel positive pressure ventilation in patients with blunt thoracic trauma. Respiration. 2005;72:517-22.
23. Vidhani K, Kause J, Parr M. Should we follow ATLS guidelines for the management of traumatic pulmonary contusion: the role of noninvasive ventilatory support. Resuscitation. 2002;52:265-8.
24. Duggal A, Perez P, Golan E, Tremblay L, Sinuff T. Safety and efficacy of noninvasive ventilation in patients with blunt chest trauma: a systematic review. Crit Care. 2013;17(4):R142.
25. Masclans JR, Perez M, Almirall J, Lorente L, Marqués A, Socias L, et al. Early noninvasive ventilation treatment for severe influenza pneumonia. Clin Microbiol Infect. 2013;19:249-56.
26. L'Her E, Deye N, Lellouche F, Taille S, Demoule A, Fraticelli A, et al. Physiologic effects of noninvasive ventilation during acute lung injury. Am J Respir Crit Care Med. 2005;172:1112-8.
27. Brochard L, Lefebvre JC, Cordioli RL, Akoumianaki E, Richard JC. Noninvasive ventilation for patients with hypoxemic acute respiratory failure. Semin Respir Crit Care Med. 2014;35:492-500.
28. Vrijsen B, Testelmans D, Belge C, Robberecht W, Van Damme P, Buyse B. Noninvasive ventilation in amyotrophic lateral sclerosis. Amyotroph Lateral Scler Frontotemporal Degener. 2013;14(2):85-95.
29. Andersen PM, Abrahams S, Borasio GD, de Carvalho M, et al. EFNS guidelines on the clinical management of amyotrophic lateral sclerosis (MALS)—revised report of an EFNS task force. Eur J. Neurol. 2012;19(3):360-75.
30. Davidson AC, Banham S, Elliott M, Kennedy D, Gelder C, Glossop A, et al. BTS/ICS guideline for the ventilatory management of acute hypercapnic respiratory failure in adults. Thorax. 2016;71:ii, 1.
31. Thille AW, Harrois A, Schortgen F, Brun-Buisson C, Brochard L. Outcomes of extubation failure in medical intensive care unit patients. Crit Care Med. 2011;39:2612-8.
32. Esteban A, Frutos-Vivar F, Ferguson ND, Arabi Y, Apezteguía C, González M, et al. Noninvasive positive-pressure ventilation for respiratory failure after extubation. N Engl J Med. 2004;350:2452-60.
33. Lin C, Yu H, Fan H, Li Z. The efficacy of noninvasive ventilation in managing postextubation respiratory failure: a meta-analysis. Heart Lung. 2014;43:99-104.
34. Curtis JR, Cook DJ, Sinuff T, White DB, Hill N, Keenan SP, et al. Noninvasive positive pressure ventilation in critical and palliative care settings: understanding the goals of therapy. Crit Care Med. 2007;35:932-9.
35. Nava S, Ferrer M, Esquinas A, Scala R, Groff P, Cosentini R, et al. Palliative use of noninvasive ventilation in end-of-life patients with solid tumours: a randomised feasibility trial. Lancet Oncol. 2013;14:219-27.
36. Burns KE, Meade MO, Premji A, Adhikari NK. Noninvasive ventilation as a weaning strategy for mechanical ventilation in adults with respiratory failure: a Cochrane systematic review. CMAJ. 2014;186:E112-E122.
37. Glossop AJ, Shephard N, Bryden DC, Mills GH. Noninvasive ventilation for weaning, avoiding reintubation after extubation and in the postoperative period: a meta-analysis. Br J Anaesth. 2012;109(3):305-14.
38. Yeung J, Couper K, Ryan EG, Gates S, Hart N, Perkins GD. Noninvasive ventilation as a strategy for weaning from invasive mechanical ventilation: a systematic review and Bayesian meta-analysis. Intensive Care Med. 2018;44(12):2192-204.
39. NICE clinical guidance [CG12]. (2004). Chronic obstructive pulmonary disease—Management of chronic obstructive pulmonary disease in adults in primary and secondary care. [online] Available from http://www.nice.org.uk/guidance/cg12. [Last accessed Jan., 2020].
40. Diaz GG, Alcaraz AC, Talavera JCP, Pérez PJ, Rodriguez AE, Cordoba FG, et al. Noninvasive positive-pressure ventilation to treat hypercapnic coma secondary to respiratory failure. Chest. 2005;127:952-60.
41. Carron, M, Freo, U, BaHammam, AS, Dellweg D, Guarracino F, Cosentini R, et al. Complications of noninvasive ventilation techniques: a comprehensive qualitative review of randomized trials. Br J. Anaesth. 2013;110(6):896-914.
42. Vignaux L, Vargas F, Roeseler J, Tassaux D, Thille AW, Kossowsky MP, et al. Patient–ventilator asynchrony during noninvasive ventilation for acute respiratory failure: a multicenter study. Intensive Care Med. 2009;35:840-6.

Chapter 8

Application of Noninvasive Ventilation: Algorithmic Approach (Initiation, Customization, and Troubleshooting)

Rajesh Chawla, Roseleen Kaur Bali, Aakanksha Chawla

▮ INTRODUCTION

Noninvasive positive-pressure ventilation (NIPPV) increases spontaneous ventilation using the tight-fitting nasal or oronasal mask without using a conduit, i.e., an endotracheal intubation or tracheostomy tube. This can be used in a large number of conditions. The application of noninvasive ventilation (NIV) should never be continued when endotracheal intubation is clearly indicated.

▮ APPLICATION OF NONINVASIVE VENTILATION

Whenever you want to apply NIV, initial step would be to quickly examine the patient in detail. Look for vital parameters, hemodynamic instability, level of sensorium, and oxygenation. If SpO_2 is low, oxygen should be started. Oxygen should be titrated to keep SpO_2 at 88–92% in respiratory failure. Check arterial blood gas (ABG) and get other investigations like hemogram, kidney functions tests, serum electrolytes, blood and sputum culture, and chest skiagram. Start disease-specific management like antibiotics, bronchodilators (salbutamol and ipratropium nebulization), and corticosteroids.

▮ ASSESS THE NEED OF NIV

Before application of NIV, it is important to assess the requirement of NIV in that patient. In addition to the ongoing medical treatment, NIV should be applied to a patient in acute respiratory failure (ARF), depending on the clinical criteria (**Box 1**), provided there are no contraindications. NIV should only be considered, if there is sufficient evidence of its effectiveness in that particular disease condition (**Box 2**).

Box 1: Clinical criteria.

- Moderate-to-severe respiratory distress
- Increased respiratory rate > 25 breaths/min
- Use of accessory muscle or abdominal paradox
- Blood gas derangement pH < 7.35, $PaCO_2$ > 45 mm Hg
- PaO_2/FiO_2 < 300 or SpO_2 < 92% with FiO_2 0.5

Chapter 8: Application of Noninvasive Ventilation: Algorithmic Approach...

Box 2: Effectiveness for noninvasive ventilation (NIV) in acute respiratory failure (ARF) from different causes.

Causes of ARF	Level of evidence
➢ Acute exacerbation of chronic obstructive pulmonary disease (AECOPD)	A
➢ Weaning (AECOPD)	A
➢ Cardiogenic pulmonary edema (CPE)	A
➢ Immunocompromised patient	B
➢ Obesity hypoventilation syndrome and acute hypercapnic respiratory failure (AHRF)	B
➢ Neuromuscular disease/chest wall disease with AHRF (acute hypoxemic respiratory failure)	B
➢ Mild acute respiratory distress syndrome (ARDS)	B
➢ Postoperative respiratory failure	B
➢ Trauma	B
➢ Preintubation oxygenation	B
➢ Endoscopy	B
➢ Asthma exacerbations	C
➢ Postextubation respiratory failure in COPD	C
➢ Do-not-intubate status	C
➢ Pneumonia	C

(A: strong; B: intermediate; C: weak)

Contraindications of NIV are described in **Box 3**.

Box 3: Contraindications.

- ➢ Inability to protect the airways—comatose patients, patients with bulbar involvement, confused and agitated patients, and upper airway obstruction
- ➢ Hemodynamic instability—life-threatening arrhythmia, patients on very high doses of vasopressors, and recent myocardial infarction
- ➢ Facial abnormalities, facial burns, facial trauma, and facial anomaly
- ➢ Severe gastrointestinal symptoms—vomiting, obstructed bowel; recent gastrointestinal surgery, upper gastrointestinal bleeding
- ➢ Life-threatening hypoxemia and massive hemoptysis
- ➢ Copious secretions
- ➢ Conditions in which NIV has not been found to be effective
- ➢ NIV should only be applied in ARF if there is evidence for its efficacy in that disease state

(ARF: acute respiratory failure; NIV: noninvasive ventilation)

Noninvasive ventilation is initiated mostly in the emergency department, intensive care unit (ICU), and high-dependency unit (HDU). NIV has been found to be most effective in chronic obstructive pulmonary disease (COPD). NIV should be initiated in COPD when pH < 7.35 and pCO_2 > 45 mm Hg persist or develop despite optimal medical therapy. Severe acidosis is not a contraindication to NIV so long as the expertise to perform safe endotracheal intubation is readily available. The lower the pH the more chances of failure. One should not delay intubation when it is indicated.

Current guidelines recommend CPAP or bilevel NIV for patients with ARF due to cardiogenic pulmonary edema. There is uncertainty of evidence to recommend the use of NIV for ARF due to asthma. NIV can be used for patients with postoperative ARF. NIV is recommended for dyspneic patients for palliation in the setting of terminal congestive heart failure (CHF), terminal COPD, advanced cancer, and other terminal diseases. NIV has been applied for chest trauma patients with ARF with success. NIV is recommended to prevent postextubation respiratory failure only in high-risk patients. NIV should not be used in the treatment of all patients with established postextubation respiratory failure.

INITIATION OF NIV

Protocol for application of NIV: For successful NIV, it is important to coordinate the patient, interface, and ventilator. NIV can be delivered via the standard ICU ventilator found in most ICUs or a portable pressure ventilator.
- Patient interface—many interfaces like nasal, oronasal mask, full face mask, nasal prongs (pillows), and helmet can be used for the application of NIV. Oronasal mask is preferred in ARF. In one study of 26 patients with a COPD exacerbation complicated by hypercapnia compared three interfaces. Patients were randomly assigned to receive NIV via face mask, nasal mask, or nasal prongs (pillows). The face mask resulted in the greatest physiologic improvement, but the nasal mask was best tolerated. Recent studies have shown that application of NIV through helmet is associated with increased survival in patients of hypoxemic respiratory failure.
- The helmet allows patients to talk, read, and drink through a straw, and it minimizes complications such as nasal bridge skin necrosis, and gastric distension helmet and requires high flow and short inspiratory time to pressurize rapidly.

MODE OF VENTILATION

Noninvasive ventilation can be applied using portable pressure ventilators or conventional ICU ventilators. NIV can be applied using the same modes that are used for invasive mechanical ventilation; however, certain modes are used more frequently.
- In portable pressure ventilators bilevel positive airway pressure (BPAP) can be given in spontaneous or spontaneous/timed mode for application of NIV. Pressure support (PS)/pressure control/volume control modes are used more commonly when conventional ventilators are used for NIV application. Conventionally for the application of NIV in ARF, pressure targeted modes are the modes of choice. Both PS and pressure control modes are effective. Pressure modes are preferred because there are many advantages of pressure-targeted modes like pressure delivered is constant and pressure-targeted ventilation compensates for air leak.
- During application of NIV through portable pressure ventilator in spontaneous mode, when patient initiates a breath, he gets pressure from the machine which is called inspiratory positive airway pressure (IPAP) which is applied all through inspiration. When the flow falls to a predetermined value set on the ventilator, patient gets a pressure which is applied all through expiration which is called expiratory positive airway pressure (EPAP). IPAP improves ventilation and increases tidal volume and helps in carbon dioxide (CO_2) removal. EPAP improves oxygenation, opens up the upper airway and neutralize auto positive end-expiratory pressure (PEEP). PS applied is the difference between IPAP and EPAP (PS = IPAP – EPAP).

Application of NIV Using Portable Pressure Ventilators

Explain the therapy and its benefit to the patient in detail. Also, discuss the possibility of intubation.

- Choose the correct size of interface. There are many types of interfaces like nasal mask, oronasal mask, total face mask, and helmet. The oronasal mask is preferred in ARF. It is important to select proper size mask. Use the smallest possible mask.
- Set the NIV portable pressure ventilator in spontaneous or spontaneous/timed mode.
- Try to set machine parameters which are comfortable for the patient.
- Always set the backup respiratory rate 2-3 less than patient respiratory rate.
- Set I:E ratio 1:2 in COPD and 1:1 in obesity hypoventilation syndrome (OHS), neuromuscular disease (NMD), and chest wall disease (CWD).
- Rise time is the time taken from EPAP to IPAP. In obstructive patients, set rise time 100-400 ms (1-4) and in restrictive disease patient, set rise time 300-600 ms (from 3 to 6)
- Set max inspiratory time 0.8-1.2 sec (COPD) and 1.2-1.4 sec in OHS, NMD, and CWD
- Now start titration with very low settings, low IPAP of 8 cm H_2O with 4 cm H_2O of EPAP. The difference between IPAP and EPAP should be at least 4 cm H_2O at all times.
- To start with administer oxygen at 2 L/min.
- Hold the mask with the hand over the face. Do not fix it.
- Increase EPAP by 1-2 cm increments until the patients' inspiratory efforts are able to trigger the ventilator.
- If the patient is making inspiratory effort and the ventilator does not respond, it indicates that the patient has not generated enough respiratory effort to counter auto-PEEP and trigger the ventilator (in COPD patients). Increase EPAP further until this happens. Most of the patients require EPAP of about 4-6 cm H_2O. Patients who are obese or have obstructive sleep apnea require higher EPAP to trigger the ventilator.
- When the patients' effort is triggering the ventilator, leave EPAP at that level.
- Now, start increasing IPAP in increments of 1-2 cm up to a maximum pressure, which the patient can tolerate without discomfort and there is no major mouth or air leak.
- Now, secure interface with head straps. Avoid excessive tightness. If the patient has a nasogastric tube, put a seal connector in the dome of the mask to minimize air leakage.
- After titrating the pressure, increase oxygen to bring oxygen saturation to around 88-92% in hypercapnic respiratory failure. Oxygen should be entrained as close to the patient as possible. Adjust regularly oxygen flow required to maintain SpO_2 between 88-92%.
- As the settings may be different in wakefulness and sleep, readjust them accordingly.
- Close monitoring and the capability to initiate endotracheal intubation and other resuscitation measures should be available in the same center where NIV is being initiated. Start NIV preferably in the ICU or in the emergency room in ARF.
- Humidification is not routinely required. Heated humidification can be used in cases of mucosal dryness or if respiratory secretions are thick and tenacious.
- If the patient is dependent on NIV, bronchodilator drugs can be given via a nebulizer inserted into the ventilator tubing.

Application of NIV Using a Critical Care Ventilator

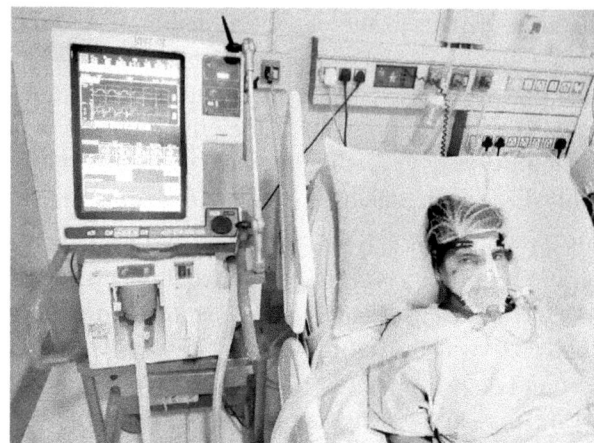

Fig. 1: Application of noninvasive ventilation through standard ICU ventilator.

There are several advantages of using NIV through standard ICU ventilator like one can give precise and high concentration of oxygen. Separate inspiratory and expiratory tubing decrease the rebreathing of CO_2. Large mask leaks and/or patient disconnections are appreciated quickly and it has better alarms and monitoring features **(Fig. 1)**.

- The first step is to select a ventilator, which is capable of fulfilling the needs of the patient.
- Explain the therapy to the patient.
- Choose the NIV mode. PS or pressure control modes are preferred. In selected patients, such as those suffering from NMDs, volume assists or volume control mode may be used.
- Choose an appropriate interface.
- Silent ventilator alarms
- Keep FiO_2 at 0.5.

Using Pressure Support Approach

- Start with low settings such as inspiratory PS at 5-6 cm H_2O and PEEP at 4 cm H_2O.
- Initiate NIV while holding the mask in place and confirm optimum fit. If it is big or small or loose, change it.
- Hold the mask. Do not fix the headgear.
- Now, increase PEEP until inspiratory efforts are able to trigger the ventilator.
- If the patient is making inspiratory effort and the ventilator does not respond, it indicates that the patient has not generated enough respiratory effort to counter auto-PEEP and trigger the ventilator (in COPD patients). Increase PEEP further until this happens.
- Once the patients' inspiratory efforts trigger the ventilator, start increasing PS further, keeping the patients' comfort in mind (reduced respiratory rate, reduced use of respiratory accessory muscle, etc.). Ensure that there are no major leaks.
- When there is significant mouth leak, there may be asynchrony. In that case, pressure control will be the preferred mode of NIV and the T_i can be set to avoid asynchrony.
- Increase fraction of oxygen concentration to maintain oxygen saturation between 88 and 92% at all times.

Chapter 8: Application of Noninvasive Ventilation: Algorithmic Approach...

- Secure interface with the headgear. It should be tight, but not overtight. Small leaks are acceptable.
- A pressure support/control of more than 25 cm is rarely required in COPD, but higher pressures can be used when using NIV for other indications. PEEP is usually titrated between 5 and 10 cm H_2O to improve triggering and oxygenation.

■ MONITORING

The patient must be monitored very closely clinically **(Box 4)**. All this must be documented every 15 minutes for the first hour in the clinical notes.

Box 4: Monitoring of NIV in ARF.

- Mask comfort
- Tolerance of ventilator settings
- Respiratory distress
- Respiratory rate
- Sensorium
- Accessory muscle use
- Abdominal paradox
- Ventilator parameters
- Air leaking
- Adequacy of pressure support
- Adequacy of PEEP
- Tidal volume (5–7 mL/kg)
- Patient–ventilator synchrony
- Continuous oximetry (until stable)
- ABG, baseline and 1–2 h, then as indicated

(ABG: arterial blood gas; ARF: acute respiratory failure; NIV: noninvasive ventilation; PEEP: positive end-expiratory pressure)

The patient will show improvement in parameters if NIV is effective. ABG sample should be sent after 30 min–1 h after the application of NIV.

Manipulate the minute ventilation, the respiratory rate and tidal volume to control pH and pCO_2. So if pH is low or pCO_2 is high, increase IPAP in portable pressure ventilator to increase tidal volume or PS in ICU ventilator. If using pressure control ventilation, increase peak inspiratory pressure (PIP). To control pO_2, adjust the FiO_2 and the mean airway pressure (PEEP and PIP). Increasing the PEEP or EPAP is the most efficient way of increasing the MAP. One can also increase the I-time to increase the MAP (PC).

Look for air leaks, triggering and patient–ventilator interaction in ventilator settings.

Time on NIV should be maximized in the first 24 hours depending on patient acceptance and/or complications. NIV can be discontinued when there has been normalization of pH and pCO_2 and a general improvement in the patients' condition.

Troubleshooting

Monitor carefully for the deteriorating respiratory distress, sensorium, tachypnea, and deteriorating blood gases, and intervene early because delay in intubation is a common major complication of NIV. Most complications are can be managed easily, and so every attempt should be made to continue NIV **(Table 1)**.

Table 1: Troubleshooting of noninvasive ventilation.

Complications	Corrective action
➢ Mask discomfort ➢ Excessive leaks around mask ➢ Pressure sores	➢ Check mask for correct size and fit ➢ Minimize headgear tension ➢ Use spacers or change to a different mask ➢ Use wound care dressing over nasal bridge
➢ Nasal or oral dryness or nasal congestion	➢ Add or increase humidification ➢ Irrigate nasal passage with saline ➢ Apply topical decongestants ➢ Nasal topical glucocorticoids
➢ Aerophagia/gastric distension	➢ Use lowest effective pressure for adequate tidal volume ➢ Use simethicone agents
➢ Aspiration	➢ Make sure patients are able to protect the airway
➢ Mucus plugging	➢ Ensure adequate hydration ➢ Ensure adequate humidification ➢ Avoid excessive O_2 flow rates (>20 L/Min) ➢ Allow short breaks from NIV to permit directed coughing techniques
➢ Hypotension	➢ Avoid excessively high peak pressure (≥20 cm H_2O)

Mask discomfort is the most common problem encountered for individuals adapting to NIV. It is extremely important for the air seal to be tight. Ulceration and pressure necrosis related to local skin effects commonly occur at the bridge of the nose. Protective synthetic coverings may help prevent skin breakdown and ulceration on the bridge of the nose.

Air leaking through the mouth-leakage of air through the mouth is very common among users of nasal NIV, which can result in asynchrony. Most of the patients can still be ventilated despite such leakage, and no other measures are required. Pressure-limited ventilators are often capable to compensate for leaks by increasing airflow to maintain mask pressure. But leaks during volume-ventilation need an increase in tidal volume. An excessive increase in tidal volume can result in narrowing of the glottis, which will result in increase in the air leak or gastric insufflation and will not increase the effective ventilation.

Eye irritation and pain or congestion of the nasal sinuses due to airflow may occur. Put some decongestant nasal drops. Distension of the stomach can occur due to aerophagia and aspiration pneumonia can occur secondary to vomiting. A nasogastric tube can be used to relieve the gastric distension while still allowing the mask to seal. Bad hemodynamic effects from NIV are unusual, although preload reduction and hypotension may occur. Give intravenous fluids.

○ Noninvasive ventilation is also prescribed for home ventilation in chronic respiratory failure. Gas exchange improves within weeks of initiating NIV at home in chronic respiratory failure, if such improvement does not occur, adjustments in inspiratory pressure, tidal volume, ventilator rate, and duration of ventilator use may be helpful. Follow-up nocturnal monitoring in the sleep laboratory or at home is used to detect problems with untreated apneas and persistent air leaks.

Discontinuation of NIV

It is very important to know when to discontinue NIV and intubate and ventilate the patient. You should discontinue ventilation if NIV fails or patient does not tolerate. NIV failure is indicated by worsening mental status, deterioration of pH and $PaCO_2$ after 1–3 h of therapy

Chapter 8: Application of Noninvasive Ventilation: Algorithmic Approach...

and refractory hypoxemia, when even a brief discontinuation of NIV leads to significant fall in oxygen saturation. One should also discontinue NIV, if patient becomes hemodynamic unstable or has copious secretions.

Weaning

Initially, give NIV continuously as long as possible. Once the patient is tolerating periods off NIV, start discontinuing for brief periods during daytime and give continuously during nighttime. In 2–3 days, the patient can be weaned off the NIV.

A brief outline of the application of NIV is shown in **Flowchart 1**.

Flowchart 1: Application of noninvasive ventilation (NIV).

```
Acute respiratory distress
Tachypnea RR >25/min
Respiratory failure
PaCO₂>45, and/or pH <7.35
          ↓
Check for underlying disease ──────────────────────────┐
          ↓                                            ↓
Level of evidence A, B for NIV            Level of evidence C for NIV
Refer to Box 2                            Refer to Box 2
          ↓                                            ↓
                                          Assess for use of NIV
Need for ventilatory requirement ←────────────┤         ↓
   No        Yes                                  Poor candidate for NIV
   ↓          ↓
Supportive   Good candidate
medical      for NIV
therapy        ↓
         Check for contraindications      Yes
         Refer to Box 3 ─────────────────────────┐
              No ↓                               │
         Start NIV with use of appropriate       │
         facemask and oxygen                     │
         Use pressure support or CPAP mode    Intubate
              ↓                                  ↑
         1–2 hour check point         No         │
         • Improve gas exchange ──────────────────┤
         • Patient tolerance        Yes          │
              ↓                                  │
                                         Consider NIV
                                         for extubation in
                                         selected cases
         Improvement in respiratory failure and
         primary disease, O₂ saturation >90%
         on 6 lit/min O₂
              ↑
              └──────────── Continue NIV
              ↓
         Start intermittent      Patient remains stable      Discontinue
         discontinuation of NIV  No respiratory distress     NIV
```

Flowchart 1: Application of noninvasive ventilation (NIV).

CONCLUSION

Noninvasive ventilation can be used in a large number of diseases, if there is no obvious contraindication. NIV should only be considered, if there is sufficient evidence of its effectiveness in that particular disease condition. NIV has been proven to be most effective in COPD and cardiogenic pulmonary edema. Monitor for the deteriorating respiratory distress, worsening sensorium, tachypnea, and deteriorating blood gases, and take action early because delay in intubation is a common major complication of NIV. It is important to coordinate the patient selection, interface, and ventilator for the success of NIV. The application of NIV should be discontinued when endotracheal intubation is clearly indicated.

KEY POINTS

- Before application of NIV, it is important to assess the need of NIV.
- NIV should only be applied, if there is evidence of its effectiveness in that particular condition and there is no contraindication.
- Current guidelines recommend NIV can be used for patients with ARF due to COPD cardiogenic pulmonary, postoperative ARF, palliation in the setting of advanced cancer or other terminal conditions, and chest trauma with ARF and to prevent postextubation respiratory failure in high-risk patients.
- For successful NIV, it is important to coordinate the patient, interface, and ventilator. NIV can be delivered via the standard ICU type of ventilator found in most ICUs or a portable pressure ventilator.
- Pressure modes are preferred because there are many advantages of pressure-targeted modes like pressure delivered is constant and pressure-targeted ventilation compensates for air leak
- Manipulate the minute ventilation, the respiratory rate, and tidal volume to control pH and pCO_2. So if pH is low or pCO_2 is high, increase IPAP in portable pressure ventilator to increase tidal volume or PS in ICU ventilator. If using pressure control ventilation, increase PIP.
- To control pO_2, adjust the FiO_2 and the mean airway pressure (PEEP and PIP). Increasing the PEEP or EPAP is the most efficient way of increasing the MAP. One can also increase the I-time to increase the MAP (PC).
- Monitor carefully the patient on NIV for the worsening respiratory distress, sensorium, tachypnea, and deteriorating blood gases, and intervene early because delay in intubation is a common major complication of NIV.
- Most complications are minor that can be managed easily, and so every attempt should be made to continue NIV.

SUGGESTED READING

1. Ambrosino N, Vagheggini G. Noninvasive positive pressure ventilation in the acute care setting: where are we? Eur Respir J. 2008;31(4):874-86.
2. Confalonieri M, Garuti G, Cattaruzza MS, Osborn JF, Antonelli M, Conti G, et al. A chart of failure risk for noninvasive ventilation in patients with COPD exacerbation. Eur Respir J. 2005;25(2): 348-55.

3. Davidson AC, Banham S, Elliott M, Kennedy D, Gelder C, Glossop A, et al. BTS/ICS guideline for the ventilatory management of acute hypercapnic respiratory failure in adults. Thorax. 2016;71:ii1–ii35.
4. Faverio P, Stainer A, De Giacomi F, Messinesi G, Paolini V, Monzani A, et al. Noninvasive ventilation weaning in acute hypercapnic respiratory failure due to COPD exacerbation: A real-life observational study. Can Respir J. 2019;2019:3478968.
5. Lindenauer PK, Stefan MS, Shieh MS, Pekow PS, Rothberg MB, Hill NS. Outcomes associated with invasive and noninvasive ventilation among patients hospitalized with exacerbations of chronic obstructive pulmonary disease. JAMA Intern Med. 2014;174:1982-93.
6. Majid A, Hill NS. Noninvasive ventilation for acute respiratory failure. Curr Opin Crit Care. 2005;11(1):77-81.
7. Navalesi P, Costa R, Ceriana P, Carlucci A, Prinianakis G, Antonelli M, et al. Non-invasive ventilation in chronic obstructive pulmonary disease patients: helmet versus facial mask. Intensive Care Med. 2007;33:74-81.
8. Rochwerg B, Brochard L, Elliott MW, Hess D, Hill NS, Nava S, et al. Official ERS/ATS clinical practice guidelines: noninvasive ventilation for acute respiratory failure. Eur Respir J. 2017;50: 1602426.

Chapter 9

Physiology of Type I and Type II Respiratory Failure

Khalid Ismail Khatib, Subhal Bhalchandra Dixit

INTRODUCTION

Respiratory failure refers to severe abnormality in the function of the gas-exchange part of the respiratory system, leading to either reduction in oxygenation or problems of the ventilator pump leading to an accumulation of carbon dioxide. Hence, respiratory failure can denote either the gas-exchanging organ is functioning suboptimally (lung failure) or there is some abnormality of the ventilator pump (pump failure), i.e. the chest wall (rib cage including the respiratory muscles), the respiratory centers in the brain and the spinal and peripheral nerves that connect the respiratory muscles to the respiratory centers in the brain.

Respiratory failure is defined as a PaO_2 of ≤ 60 mm Hg, a $PaCO_2$ of ≥ 45 mm Hg or both. In general, lung failure caused due to a variety of lung diseases (e.g. pneumonia, emphysema and interstitial lung disease, etc.,) leads to hypoxemia with or without abnormalities of the CO_2 levels. This is known as hypoxemic or type I respiratory failure. On the other hand, failure of the pump (due to drug overdose, congenital or acquired respiratory muscle weakness, etc.) results in alveolar hypoventilation and increases in the CO_2 levels. This is known as hypercapnic or type II respiratory failure. Although there may be associated hypoxemia, the real hallmark of pump or ventilatory failure is the increase in the $PaCO_2$.

PATHOPHYSIOLOGY

Type I Respiratory Failure[1]

It can occur due to the following mechanisms:
- *Ventilation/perfusion inequality (V/Q mismatch):* It is the most common mechanism of type I respiratory failure. It occurs when normally ventilated lungs receive inadequate or no blood supply or when adequately perfused areas of the lung have reduced or absent ventilation. Administration of 100% oxygen reduces or eliminates hypoxia caused due to V/Q mismatch. The low V/Q ratio occurs due to a decrease in ventilation secondary to airway or interstitial lung disease. The high V/Q ratio may occur in case of pulmonary embolism, as ventilation is wasted in the areas without blood supply due to obstruction secondary to embolism.
- *Increased shunt:* Deoxygenated mixed venous blood bypasses the ventilated alveoli due to a shunt in the heart (intracardiac) or the lungs (intrapulmonary) leading to hypoxemia. Administration of 100% oxygen will not lead to improvement in patients with significant

shunt. Atrial septal defect, ventricular septal defect, and patent ductus arteriosus are examples of intracardiac shunts. Arteriovenous malformation in the lungs is example of intrapulmonary shunts.
- *Diffusion abnormality:* Diseases that reduce the pulmonary capillary surface area or reduce the time that blood remains in the pulmonary capillaries prevent adequate gas exchange. This leads to hypoxemia.
- Alveolar hypoventilation

The causes of type I respiratory failure are enumerated in **Table 1**.

Table 1: Causes of type I respiratory failure.	
Mechanisms	Causes
Lung abnormality (airway and lung parenchyma)	➢ COPD ➢ Pneumonia ➢ Pulmonary edema ➢ Pulmonary fibrosis ➢ Asthma ➢ Bronchiectasis ➢ Pneumoconiosis ➢ Granulomatous lung diseases ➢ Acute respiratory distress syndrome (ARDS)
Pleural cavity abnormality	Pneumothorax
Pulmonary vasculature abnormality	➢ Pulmonary embolism ➢ Fat embolism syndrome ➢ Pulmonary arterial hypertension

Type II Respiratory Failure[2]

It can occur due to the following mechanisms:
- *Decreased respiratory drive:* It may be due to anesthesia, drug overdose, or diseases of the medulla.
- *Diseases of the respiratory muscle/nerves/anterior horn cell:* There may be an abnormality of the chest wall due to a mechanical defect (flail chest) or kyphoscoliosis, diseases of the nerves such as demyelination (Guillain-Barré syndrome) or of anterior horn cells (poliomyelitis), or diseases of the respiratory muscles themselves (myopathies).
- Sometimes an excessive inspiratory load on the respiratory muscles leads to fatigue of the inspiratory muscles, due to which they become unable to generate negative pressure in the pleural cavity despite a normal respiratory center/drive and a normal chest wall.

The various causes of acute onset of type II respiratory failure are enumerated in **Table 2**. The various causes of chronic type II respiratory failure are enumerated in **Table 3**.

Table 2: Causes of acute onset type II respiratory failure.	
Mechanism	Causes
Decreased central drive	➢ Drugs (sedatives) ➢ CNS diseases (encephalitis, stroke, and trauma)
Altered neural and neuromuscular transmission	➢ Spinal cord trauma ➢ Transverse myelitis ➢ Tetanus

Contd...

Contd...

Mechanism	Causes
	➢ Amyotrophic lateral sclerosis ➢ Poliomyelitis ➢ Guillain-Barré syndrome ➢ Myasthenia gravis ➢ Organophosphate poisoning ➢ Botulism
Muscle abnormalities	➢ Muscular dystrophy ➢ Disuse atrophy ➢ Prematurity
Chest wall and pleural abnormalities	Chest wall trauma (flail chest, diaphragmatic rupture).
Lung and airways diseases	➢ Acute asthma ➢ Acute exacerbation of chronic obstructive pulmonary disease ➢ Cardiogenic and noncardiogenic pulmonary edema ➢ Pneumonia ➢ Upper airways obstruction ➢ Bronchiectasis
Other	➢ Sepsis ➢ Circulatory shock.

Table 3: Causes of chronic type II respiratory failure.

Mechanism	Causes
Lung and airways diseases	Chronic obstructive airway disease (bronchitis, emphysema, and bronchiectasis)
Chest wall abnormalities	➢ Kyphoscoliosis ➢ Thoracoplasty ➢ Obesity ➢ Pleural effusion ➢ Neuromuscular disorders
Lung and chest wall diseases	➢ Scleroderma ➢ Polymyositis ➢ Systemic lupus erythematosus
Central nervous system abnormalities	Primary alveolar hypoventilation (Ondine's curse)
Other	➢ Electrolyte abnormalities ➢ Malnutrition ➢ Endocrine disorders

CONCLUSION

Abnormalities of delivery of oxygen and removal of carbon dioxide lead to type I and type II respiratory failure. Failure of the gas exchange part of the respiratory system usually leads to type I respiratory failure while failure of the ventilator pump to type II respiratory failure. An understanding of the difference in the mechanisms and causes of the two types of respiratory failure helps us to properly classify the patient who presents with respiratory failure. This will lead to institution of the correct therapy for the respiratory failure.

REFERENCES

1. Hall JB, Schmidt GA, Wood LD. Acute hypoxemic respiratory failure. In: Murray JF, Nadel JA, (eds). Textbook of Respiratory Medicine. Philadelphia, PA, Saunders, 2000; pp.2413-42.
2. Roussos C, Macklem PR. The respiratory muscles. N Engl J Med. 1982;307:786-97.

Section 2

Noninvasive Ventilation: Disease Specific

10. Practical Approach to Use of Noninvasive Ventilation in Acute Hypercapnic Respiratory Failure
11. Noninvasive Ventilation in Acute Exacerbation of COPD: Rationale, Indications, and Factors for Failure
12. Noninvasive Ventilation in Hypoxemic Respiratory Failure: Rationale, Indications, and Outcomes
13. Noninvasive Ventilation in Cardiogenic Pulmonary Edema
14. Noninvasive Ventilation in Acute Respiratory Distress Syndrome
15. Role of Noninvasive Ventilation in Postoperative Cases
16. Noninvasive Ventilation in Obstructive Sleep Apnea
17. Noninvasive Ventilation in Neuromuscular Disease
18. Noninvasive Ventilation in Chest Wall Deformities and Chest Trauma
19. Noninvasive Ventilation in Immunocompromised Patients and Patients on Palliative Care
20. Noninvasive Ventilation in Pneumonia

Chapter 10

Practical Approach to Use of Noninvasive Ventilation in Acute Hypercapnic Respiratory Failure

Vivek Kumar, Abha Mahashur, Ashish Shukla

INTRODUCTION

Noninvasive ventilation (NIV) is delivery of mechanical ventilation without an artificial airway (endotracheal or tracheostomy tube). Use of NIV in acute respiratory failure has been a well-known fact now. NIV has emerged as a key component in management of an acute hypercapnic respiratory failure, the prototype being exacerbation of chronic obstructive pulmonary disease (COPD). Understanding the mechanism of NIV in different types of acute hypercapnic respiratory failure helps in titrating the ventilator settings to provide effective ventilation with minimal discomfort and dyssynchrony. This article is limited to the use of NIV in the intensive care unit (ICU). Goal of therapy is to prevent the occurrence of impending respiratory failure, prevent further physiological embarrassment, and wean a patient from invasive mechanical ventilation (IMV) support to complement the healing process and as palliative care where IMV is not preferred. Physiological gain with NIV centers around the improvement in gas exchange primarily due to increased tidal volume, ensuring improved alveolar ventilation. Augmentation in tidal volume thereby improves respiratory system compliance by recruiting the collapsed under ventilated alveoli and reduces work of breathing by reducing the intensity and duration of inspiratory muscle contraction.

WHAT IS ACUTE HYPERCAPNIC RESPIRATORY FAILURE?

Acute hypercapnic respiratory failure is defined as acute retention of carbon dioxide typically in less than 48 hours. It usually occurs in a setting of chronic type 2 respiratory failure as in patients of chronic obstructive airway disease. It can also occur in patients with acute severe asthma, neuromuscular disorders, and bronchiectasis.

WHAT ARE COMMON CAUSES OF ACUTE HYPERCAPNIC RESPIRATORY FAILURE?

Common causes include:
- COPD
- Postextubation respiratory failure
- Kyphoscoliosis and chest wall deformity (CWD)
- Obesity
- Neuromuscular disease (NMD)

WHAT IS THE PATHOPHYSIOLOGY OF ACUTE RESPIRATORY FAILURE IN COPD?

Work of breathing is remarkably increased in state of acute exacerbations. This happens because of bronchospasm causing increased resistive load, incomplete expiration leading to air trapping followed by dynamic hyperinflation causing generation of an intrinsic positive end-expiratory pressure (PEEP) and hemodynamic compromise. Diaphragm is pushed down to a further disadvantageous position leading to mechanical embarrassment. Gas exchange abnormalities and ventilation perfusion mismatch worsens the state of breathing.[1] There can be additional disorders like *concurrent infection or bronchiectasis* resulting in airway secretions, *obstructive sleep apnea* producing varying respiratory rate and frequency, and *malnourishment* along with an underlying frail body habitus producing early fatigue. All these contribute to an increased ventilatory load which results in respiratory muscle fatigue producing acute/acute on chronic hypercapnic respiratory failure.[1] Eventually, all these factors related to poor ventilatory function lead to pump failure and retention of carbon dioxide.

HOW DOES NONINVASIVE VENTILATION WORK IN THIS SITUATION?

Noninvasive ventilation has different mechanisms in different pathologies.

Chronic Obstructive Pulmonary Disease

Noninvasive ventilation helps by forcing the airways to open in both inspiration and expiration, increasing the tidal volume, decreasing the respiratory rate, offsetting intrinsic PEEP, facilitating effective triggering, improving efficiency of diaphragm, recruiting atelectatic alveoli, and thereby improving ventilation perfusion mismatch.[2] Difference in inspiratory positive airway pressure (IPAP) and expiratory positive airway pressure (EPAP) leads to increase in alveolar ventilation which helps in reduction of partial pressures of carbon dioxide.[2] EPAP stabilizes the upper airway, recruits the alveoli, and counters the intrinsic PEEP. This leads to an improvement in dyspnea, increase in tidal volume, reduction in respiratory rate, and reduction in partial pressures of carbon dioxide.[2]

How to Use NIV in Acute Hypercapnic Failure due to COPD?

The preferred mode is bilevel positive airway pressure (BPAP) using either pressure control (PC) or pressure support (PS) mode.[2] Prerequisite of NIV support is that patient should be able to initiate the breathing cycle (also known as triggering) wherein each breath initiated gets supported by NIV eventually. The PS or difference in IPAP and EPAP is set to provide adequate tidal volume. Tidal volume generated is titrated by the magnitude of difference between IPAP and EPAP. Adequacy of tidal volume is assessed by looking at the patient and seeing if the tidal volume delivered abrogates his air hunger. PEEP or EPAP is titrated to produce effective triggering, such that every respiratory effort of patient is supported by a ventilator breath.[3]

The use of NIV reduces the rate of intubation, length of hospital stay, mortality in these patients. These benefits are most marked in patients with severe COPD.[3-5]

Indications

Exacerbations of COPD that are complicated by hypercapnic acidosis [arterial carbon dioxide tension ($PaCO_2$) >45 mm Hg or pH <7.35].[4,6]

Other indications for NIV trial in exacerbations COPD are:[6]
- Moderate to severe dyspnea, accessory muscle use, paradoxical breathing, and respiratory rate >25 breaths/min
- Moderate to severe hypoxemia [partial pressure of oxygen (PaO_2) <60 mm Hg, PaO_2/fraction of inspired oxygen (FiO_2) <200]

Noninvasive ventilation should be undertaken as a therapeutic trial in most of the patients who are not candidates for emergent intubation, if they meet the indication and contraindication criteria.[6]

Contraindications[7]

Absolute contraindications are:
- Need for immediate intubation or respiratory arrest
- Severe hemodynamic instability
- Facial trauma/burns/abnormalities/inability to fit mask
- Fixed upper airway obstruction
- Severe vomiting
- Acute severe asthma
- Pneumothorax (unless chest drain inserted)
- Patient refusal

Relative contraindications:
- Impaired consciousness
- Confusion/agitation
- Inability to protect airway
- Hemodynamic instability/ongoing arrhythmia
- Excessive respiratory secretions or inability to clear secretions
- Bowel obstruction
- Recent esophageal anastomosis or upper airway surgery

Impaired consciousness secondary to hypercapnia with anticipation of reversibility by NIV is not considered as a contraindication now. Patients with hypercapnic encephalopathy should be monitored closely for improvement or any deterioration in consciousness level. An arterial blood gas (ABG) analysis should be repeated to titrate the settings.

A physician/intensivist may override exclusion criteria on individual case basis considering risk benefits ratio.

Choice of Interface

Choice of interface is a major determinant of NIV success or failure, mainly because the interface strongly affects patient comfort and decides compliance.[7] Available interfaces from least facial contact to maximum facial contact are as follows:
- *Mouthpiece*: Placed between the patients lips and held in place by lip seal.
- *Nasal pillows*: Plugs inserted into each nostril.
- *Nasal mask*: Covers only nose.
- *Oronasal*: Covers the nose and mouth. Commonly called as face mask. It is the most commonly used and preferable interface in acute settings.[7]

- *Full-face*: Covers the mouth, nose, and eyes and causes claustrophobia.
- *Helmet*: Covers the whole head and all or part of the neck; no contact with the face or head.

Generally, the straps to hold mask, should be tight enough to allow only two fingers to pass between the face and the strap. A small leak is acceptable, and a bilevel ventilator compensates for leak. Strapping the mask too tightly decreases patient tolerance and increases the risk of facial skin breakdown. When a nasal mask or prongs are used, it should be ensured that mouth remained closed either voluntarily or by chin straps.[8] Most patients with acute respiratory failure are mouth breathers; therefore, NIV delivered by a nasal mask or prongs (pillows) may result in a large air leak through the mouth and lead to failure of NIV trial in an acute setting.[8] Therefore, oronasal mask has emerged as the first choice in acute settings.

Along with the choice of interface, heating and humidification may be needed to prevent adverse effects from cool dry gas. Heated humidifier provides better CO_2 clearance and lower work of breathing than heat and moisture exchanger (HME) because heated humidifier adds less dead space than HME.[9] Interface introduction is an art and should be first done by expert. First, the head strap should be placed and fixed. Then an appropriate size mask covering the nasal (nasal mask) with or without oral orifice (oronasal mask) should be selected as patient's facial features. Mask should be placed on face gently and acceptance from patient as well as synchronized chest excursions should be ensured before fixing. Lastly, the straps should be secured. Skin peel at nasal bridge and contact area on face should always be checked.

Choice of Mode

Pressure support ventilation (PSV) is the most common mode chosen by clinicians who want to maximize patient comfort and improve synchrony. If patient needs a higher level of support use PC mode. The comfort and synchrony are less as compared to PS. The patient should be monitored very closely on controlled modes as sometimes they paradoxically retain carbon dioxide. If ventilator has a dual control mode like average volume-assured pressure support (AVAPS), this also is a good starting option. AVAPS have an added advantage of better patient comfort and compliance due to titrated breath delivery. The alarms should be monitored closely while using AVAPS so that the patient does not remain under supported just because the IPAP variables are insufficient to deliver the set target volume. Evidence for benefit of AVAPS is limited at this moment.

Initiation of Therapy

Initiation of therapy should be strictly done by an alert and empathic expert (intensivist/trained nurse). Start with lower settings and titrate to levels that reduce work of breathing and allow a reduction in FiO_2. This will improve patient tolerance and cooperation.

Steps to set NIV are as follows:
- Explain the therapy to the patient and provide reassurance.
- Keep head of bed raised >30°.
- *Start with EPAP/PEEP*: 4–8 cm H_2O, ensure the level at which patient triggers the machine best with least discomfort.
- Next IPAP should be set at least 4 cm H_2O above EPAP/PEEP and increase in increments of 2 cm H_2O every 10–15 minutes till patient looks comfortable, is breathing well, not sucking

Chapter 10: Practical Approach to Use of Noninvasive Ventilation...

for more air, and nor being disturbed by the gush of air. The target tidal volume generated should be 6-7 mL/kg. Check for leaks and adjust straps accordingly. This is especially important in edentulous patients and those with beards.
- IPAP should not exceed 25 cm H_2O to prevent gastric insufflation.
- Keep FiO_2 around 40% if severe hypoxemia is not an issue. Titrate FiO_2 to maintain peripheral capillary oxygen saturation (SpO_2) >92%.
- If available set the flow cycling to match the expiratory time of patient. The expiratory trigger sensitivity (ETS) percent is the percentage of peak flow at which the ventilator cycles into expiration. In COPD, we prefer to have the ventilator cycle early, e.g., at 60% of peak flow so ETS is set at 60%, so as to prolong expiratory time.
- In PSV mode, backup rate should always be kept below the patient's normal breath rate to avoid any desynchrony eventually.
- In case of PC, set the respiratory rate just below patient's own respiratory rate; as patient becomes comfortable and his respiratory rate reduces, reduce the set respiratory rate till a baseline of 12-16 breaths per minute is reached.
- In case of AVAPS, check that the set tidal volume is delivered by the IPAP.

Titration of Therapy

- To improve ventilation, increase IPAP in increments of 2 cm H_2O every 10-15 minutes until the patient looks comfortable with synchronized chest rise, or a target tidal volume of 6-7 mL/kg ideal body weight is reached or a maximum inspiratory pressure of 25 cm H_2O is reached.
- To improve oxygenation, increase EPAP in increments of 2 cm H_2O until a maximum of 12 is reached. Whenever EPAP is increased, the IPAP is also increased by same amount of pressure to maintain the same level of PS (difference between IPAP and EPAP). If a patient does not improve by increasing EPAP then it can be reduced back to 4-5 cm H_2O.
- Adjust rise time to patient's air hunger. Usually at time of initiation the rise time is kept short—that is the pressure delivered increases rapidly from baseline to peak pressure. The rise time can be prolonged if the patient is uncomfortable with the rapid burst of air.
- Adjust FiO_2 to achieve desired SpO_2, preferably 88-92% in a setting of COPD.
- In case of a dual control mode like AVAPS keep checking the upper and lower levels of IPAP to ensure that patient gets the set tidal volume. The levels will have to be adjusted as ventilation improves as bronchospasm resolves or worsens. Monitor alarms closely.
- Monitor for synchrony—look at patient's breathing and the ventilator waveform. See that the ventilator matches patient's respiratory cycle—machine delivers a breath when patient is in inspiration and machine cycles to expiration at the same time when patient expires. Check that every inspiratory effort of patient is translated by ventilator into a breath—monitor for ineffective triggering. A simple inspection will detect desynchrony of all types—trigger, limit, and cycling.
- Keep checking for mask tolerance, leaks, and patient comfort. The patient may need to be counseled repeatedly to successfully tolerate NIV.
- Can use short boluses of fentanyl or an infusion of dexmedetomidine to facilitate tolerance of NIV in some selected cases with caution and close monitoring.

Monitoring of Therapy

Continuous: Pulse oximetry, respiratory rate, heart rate, cardiac rhythm, and blood pressure.

Intermittent:
- Patient comfort—patient should look comfortable and not be using accessory muscles.
- Patient synchrony—check for trigger, limit, and cycling synchrony.
- Mask issues—check for tight and comfortable fit of mask. Check for leaks and adjust mask appropriately.
- Arterial blood gases—do serial ABGs, starting 30 minutes postinitiation, then at 60 and 120 minutes, thereafter as required.

At every step, assess the need for intubation to avoid delay, if needed. Also, ventilatory graphics should be given due importance to identify breath stacking, obstructive event, etc., timely.

Issues during Use
- Claustrophobia
- Agitation
- Intolerance
- Leaks
- Dry mouth
- Excessive secretions
- Drying up of secretions
- Worsening aspiration
- Persistent encephalopathy
- Development of acute respiratory distress syndrome (ARDS) due primary disease warranting increased support
- Pressure sores on face

Fate of Noninvasive Ventilation

Noninvasive ventilation failure: Noninvasive ventilation failure has been defined as clinical deterioration warranting endotracheal intubation or death. The effectiveness of NIV is often established in the first 1–2 hours. If patient fails to show clinical and physiologic improvement (no reduction in respiratory rate, no improvement in acidosis, or no improvement in CO_2 clearance) in 1–2 hours postinitiation; or shows signs of worsening of respiratory symptoms, signs, blood gases, develops hemodynamic instability; patient should be immediately intubated and mechanical ventilation should be commenced.[6] NIV failure can be categorized as early and late. Early failure is due to mask fit or lack of adequate time for medical therapy to work. Late failure is mostly due to disease progression.

Prognostic factors to be considered prior to initiating NIV in acute hypercapnic respiratory failure are:
- *Contributors of acute hypercapnic failure:* Cardiac failure with left ventricular (LV) or right ventricular (RV) dysfunction, obstructive sleep apnea, pulmonary fibrosis, cor pulmonale, pneumothorax or pneumonia. As extrapulmonary restriction has favorable prognosis while pulmonary fibrosis and pneumonia do not.

- *Premorbid and comorbid state*: Poor performance status—increased mortality, high comorbidity burden, and low body mass index have unfavorable outcome.
- *ABG abnormalities*: Late development of acute hypercapnic respiratory failure after admission—increased mortality; coexistent metabolic acidosis or low base excess, severe academia (pH <7.25)—unfavorable outcome.
- *Organ dysfunction*: Glasgow Coma Scale (GCS) <11, fluid unresponsive hypotension, pneumonia, liver or kidney involvement, hypoalbuminemia, elevated blood urea, and eosinopenia (<50 cells per microliter)—unfavorable outcome.
- Inability to clear secretions—unfavorable outcome.

Weaning and transition to homecare: Weaning should be considered when underlying acute cause has resolved and patient is distress free for 24 hours. Weaning from NIV may be accomplished by gradual lowering of PS and PEEP or IPAP and EPAP. Once IPAP comes down below 16 and respiratory rate <25, patient should be disconnected from the NIV intermittently and progressively for gradually increasing durations.[6] The basic disease pathology should be under control and specific pharmacotherapy optimized.

How to Use NIV in other Causes of Acute/Acute on Chronic Hypercapnic Failure?

Obesity Hypoventilation Syndrome

Obesity hypoventilation syndrome (OHS) is defined as presence of daytime hypercapnia in an obese patient [body mass index (BMI) > 30 kg/m²] with an evidence of obstructive sleep apnea hypopnea syndrome (OSAHS) or sleep hypoxemia on polysomnography, in absence of known causes of hypoventilation. Obese patients are admitted to ICUs for acute on chronic hypercapnic respiratory failure or cor pulmonale secondary to OHS, lower respiratory tract infection/pneumonia, congestive cardiac failure, and pulmonary embolism concomitant with OHS. The physiological rationale of using NIV in OHS is to overcome upper respiratory tract obstruction resulting in a high resistive respiratory muscle load, thereby increasing the work of breathing[10-12] and to correct hypoventilation.

Noninvasive ventilation settings in OHS:
- *EPAP*: 8–10 cm H_2O targeting SpO_2 ≥92% or patient's baseline SpO_2 (EPAP requirements are higher than COPD). Ideally, if they have a sleep study (titration analysis) available bedside, then EPAP should be comparable to the optimum pressure titrated to overcome obstructive events.
- *IPAP*: 18–24 cm H_2O targeting tidal volume 7–8 mL/kg of ideal body weight[10] (relatively higher as compared to settings for COPD).
- Inspiratory time limit 1.4 seconds. Monitor for desynchrony. The machine cycles into expiration by default. In case the patient has not completed his breath, the patient will be in inspiration while the machine will cycle into expiration. If there is a leak the target tidal volume will not be achieved and the machine may or may not cycle into expiration depending upon the make.
- *Respiratory rate*: 20–24 breaths per minute at initiation.

Postextubation Respiratory Failure

Pathophysiological changes related to extubation can be simplified as those that increase airway resistance and those that reduce pulmonary compliance. Factors increasing airway resistance postextubation include upper airway obstruction due to laryngeal edema, laryngospasm, and excessive tracheobronchial secretions. Reduction in lung compliance is primarily due to reduction in amount of aerated lung tissue. This increase in resistive and elastic work of breathing is coupled with a reduced patient effort precipitating acute respiratory failure with reduction in oxygenation, elevation in carbon dioxide levels, and metabolic acidosis. NIV support in the postextubation scenario targets multiple anatomical and physiological issues. In respiratory system, NIV reduces airway closure and collapse in end-expiration leading to alveolar recruitment. This increased aerated lung volume helps to reduce ventilation perfusion mismatch and improves hypoxemia and dyspnea. As in COPD, increasing PS increases tidal volume increases alveolar ventilation, improves gas exchange, reduces work of breathing, and reduces diaphragmatic effort manifested by reduction of transdiaphragmatic pressures. Increase of PEEP/EPAP reduces work of breathing by reducing inspiratory load threshold due dynamic hyperinflation and by improving lung compliance. The cardiovascular effects of NIV in this setting include reduction in LV preload and afterload, improved LV compliance, reduced LV transmural pressures thereby reducing extravascular lung water and helps reducing cardiogenic pulmonary edema. All these respiratory and cardiac effects put together result in improvement of pulmonary mechanics, gas exchange, reduction in work of breathing, optimization of left heart function, and reduction in heart rate thereby reducing the need for intubation and improving outcome.

The first part in postextubation scenario is identifying risk factors for postextubation failure. Common risk factors for postextubation failure include:

- Age >65 years, moderate or severe cardiorespiratory disease, body mass index >30.
- Neurological disease, airway patency problem, inability to deal with respiratory secretions, acute physiology and chronic health evaluation II (APACHE II) >12 on day of extubation, difficult or prolonged weaning, acute respiratory failure of cardiac origin, pneumonia as reason for intubation, and positive fluid balance.
- Respiratory rate >35, rapid shallow breathing index >105, maximum inspiratory pressure >−20 to −25 cm H_2O, peak expiratory flow rate <60 liters per minute, $P_{0.1}$ < 4.5 cm H_2O (airway occlusion pressure at 0.1 second), vital capacity (VC) <10 mL/kg.

Use of NIV in postextubation settings can be divided as follows:

- *Facilitative*: When used as an alternative to IMV to wean patients and facilitate extubation; thereby reducing duration and complications of invasive ventilation. This works well for hypercapnic patients like COPD. It also works well for patients who develop hypercapnia during spontaneous breathing trials despite failure of spontaneous breathing trial.
- *Prophylactic/preventive*: When used to prevent reintubation in extubated patients so as to prevent development of acute respiratory failure. This works well if there are risk factors for postextubation acute respiratory failure as listed above. NIV or continuous positive airway pressure (CPAP) is preferred for abdominal surgery while NIV or high-flow nasal cannula (HFNC) is preferred postcardiothoracic surgery.
- *Curative*: As a management strategy in patients who develop acute respiratory failure within 7 days postextubation. This strategy has not shown to be beneficial and may result in harm by delaying reintubation, resulting in increased morbidity and mortality. NIV is not recommended as a curative strategy in medical patients and intubation is preferred. In selected cases of COPD a trial of NIV may be given if close monitoring is feasible.[12,13]

Chapter 10: Practical Approach to Use of Noninvasive Ventilation...

Restrictive Thoracic Disorders (Obesity Excluded)

Neuromuscular disease and chest wall deformity/kyphoscoliosis: A trial of NIV is always given in acute respiratory failure with or without hypercapnia in NMD or CWD cases, especially when VC is less than 1L and respiratory rate >20. The trial should be given even if normocapnic. One should not wait for hypercapnic acidosis to develop. This is because this subset is difficult to wean once intubated and ventilated.[12,14] These patients are less likely to fail on NIV due to mask intolerance (early failure) or respiratory distress (late failure). Rather, bulbar dysfunction and inability to swallow oral secretions results in failure of NIV.[13] NIV should always be supplemented with active and passive physiotherapy.

Noninvasive ventilation settings in NMD and CWD:
- NMD usually require low levels of PS.
- CWD patients usually require higher levels of PS.
- PEEP 5–10 cm H_2O is usually needed to reduce basal atelectasis, increase residual lung volume, thereby improving oxygenation.

Acute Pneumothorax

The potential benefits of NIV in the ventilatory management of traumatic/nontraumatic pneumothorax patients have not been sufficiently investigated on a large scale. The risk of precipitating a tension pneumothorax overrides the gain of recruiting the collapsed lung. However, the same risk persists if the patient gets intubated and ventilated.

The following measures can be used to facilitate the trial of NIV in cases with acute pneumothorax.[14]
- Put intercostal chest drain with under water seal before initiating NIV.
- Use PC mode to limit the peak airway pressure.
- Use the lowest possible IPAP and EPAP pressure settings to avoid iatrogenic expansion of pneumothorax.
- Use analgesia and facilitate synchrony.

Exacerbation of Bronchial Asthma

Acute hypercapnia in acute exacerbation of bronchial asthma warrants immediate intubation and IMV. The use of NIV either early or late in the course of bronchial asthma is not recommended.[12]

COMPLICATIONS OF NONINVASIVE VENTILATION THERAPY

Major
- Aspiration pneumonia/nosocomial pneumonia
- Barotrauma
- Hemodynamic effects—hypotension and tachycardia (especially in state of desynchrony)

Minor
- Interface-related complications:
    - Facial skin lesions, i.e., erythema, abrasions, and pressure ulcers
    - Arm edema and deep venous thrombosis in those using helmet masks

- Rebreathing—resulting in CO_2 accumulation, especially in single limb circuits
- Claustrophobia
- Discomfort
- Patient—ventilator desynchrony
○ Air pressure and flow-related complications:
   - Air leaks
   - Nasal or oral dryness and nasal congestion
   - Airways dryness
   - Gastric insufflation

EVIDENCE FOR NIV USE IN ACUTE EXACERBATION OF CHRONIC OBSTRUCTIVE PULMONARY DISEASE

There is a consistent treatment benefit from use of NIV in acute exacerbation of COPD (AECOPD) with hypercapnic respiratory failure. NIV reduces the rate of intubation, mortality, complications, and length of stay in these cases. The benefit of NIV use is more in patients with more severe COPD exacerbations (initial pH <7.3). NIV decreased intubation rate by 28% (95% confidence interval 15-40%), inhospital mortality rate by 10% (95% confidence interval 5-15%), and absolute reduction in length of stay by 4.57 days (95% confidence interval 2.30-6.38 days). In patients with more severe COPD exacerbations NIV use decreased intubation rate by 34% (95% confidence interval 22-46%), inhospital mortality rate by 12% (95% confidence interval 6-18%), and absolute reduction in length of stay by 5.59 days (95% confidence interval 3.66-7.52 days).[15] NIV has shown to produce more improvement in respiratory acidosis and hypercapnia after 1 hour of treatment compared to standard medical therapy.[16] Patients with pH <7.25 and GCS <11 have varying outcomes at different centers, but are prone for NIV failure. They need close observation, but an improvement in first 1-2 hours is predictive of success.[17-19] NIV also reduces the rate of nosocomial infection by avoiding endotracheal intubation. There is a reduction in rate of nosocomial pneumonia from 20% in 1994 to 8% in 2001 in a retrospective study ($P = 0.04$).[20] The rates of nosocomial infections and of nosocomial pneumonia were also significantly lower in patients who received NIV than those treated with mechanical ventilation (18% vs 60% and 8% vs 22%; $P < 0.001$ and $P = 0.04$, respectively). The mean [standard deviation (SD)] duration of ventilation (6 [6] vs 10 [12] days; $P = 0.01$), mean (SD) length of ICU stay (9 [7] vs 15 [14] days; $P = 0.02$), and crude mortality (4% vs 26%; $P = 0.002$) were all lower among patients who received NIV than those treated with mechanical ventilation in this matched case-control study.[21] NIV is therefore superior to IMV as first-line therapy in AECOPD.[22,23]

WHAT DO THE GUIDELINES SAY?

European Respiratory Society/American Thoracic Society (ERS/ATS) has made the following recommendations for the use of noninvasive ventilation in acute respiratory Failure:[12]
○ The use of NIV in acute hypercapnic respiratory failure is restricted to prevent acute respiratory acidosis, i.e., when the $PaCO_2$ is normal or elevated but pH is normal; to prevent endotracheal intubation and IMV in patients with mild-to-moderate acidosis and respiratory distress, with the aim of preventing use of IMV; and as an alternative to invasive ventilation in patients with severe acidosis and more severe respiratory distress.

- ERS/ATS suggests NIV not be used in patients with hypercapnia who are not acidotic in the setting of a COPD exacerbation (conditional recommendation, low certainty of evidence). They recommend bilevel NIV for patients with acute respiratory failure leading to acute or acute-on-chronic respiratory acidosis (pH ≤7.35) due to COPD exacerbation (strong recommendation, high certainty of evidence). They recommend a trial of bilevel NIV in patients considered to require endotracheal intubation and mechanical ventilation, unless the patient is immediately deteriorating (strong recommendation, moderate certainty of evidence).
- ERS/ATS does offer a recommendation on the use of NIV for acute respiratory failure due to asthma.
- ERS/ATS suggests use of NIV for chest trauma patients with acute respiratory failure (conditional recommendation, moderate certainty of evidence).
- ERS/ATS suggests use of NIV for patients with postoperative acute respiratory failure (conditional recommendation, moderate certainty of evidence).
- ERS/ATS suggests use of NIV to prevent postextubation respiratory failure in high-risk patients (conditional recommendation, low certainty of evidence) and that NIV should not be used to prevent postextubation respiratory failure in nonhigh-risk patients (conditional recommendation, very low certainty of evidence). NIV should not be used in the treatment of patients with established postextubation respiratory failure (conditional recommendation, low certainty of evidence).
- ERS/ATS suggests NIV be used to facilitate weaning from mechanical ventilation in patients with hypercapnic respiratory failure.

CONCLUSION

Noninvasive ventilation has a pivotal role in acute hypercapnic respiratory failure, especially in patients with COPD. Use of NIV is successful if case selection is proper, therapy is initiated timely, monitored closely, and terminated timely. Both objective improvement with blood gas analysis, respiratory rate, oxygenation, and subjective improvement as per patient should be given importance. It warrants a continued care with troubleshooting at every step, to ensure compliance. Definitive therapy for underlying respiratory disease is utmost important for success or failure of NIV. In the right setting it helps to avoid intubation and its complications. However, a skilled team work is a must to monitor response carefully and to identify failure timely to avoid any delay in intubation in selected population.

REFERENCES

1. Stevenson NJ, Walker PP, Costello RW, Calverley PM. Lung mechanics and dyspnea during exacerbations of chronic obstructive pulmonary disease. Am J Respir Crit Care Med. 2005;172:1510-6.
2. Plant PK, Owen JL, Elliott MW. Early use of non-invasive ventilation for acute exacerbations of chronic obstructive pulmonary disease on general respiratory wards: a multicentre randomised controlled trial. Lancet. 2000;355:1931-5.
3. Kacmarek, RM. Characteristics of pressure-targeted ventilators used for noninvasive positive pressure ventilation. Respir Care. 1997;42:380.
4. Keenan SP, Kernerman PD, Cook DJ, Martin CM, McCormack D, Sibbald WJ. Effect of noninvasive positive pressure ventilation on mortality in patients admitted with acute respiratory failure: a meta-analysis. Crit Care Med. 1997;25:1685-92.

5. Peter JV, Moran JL, Phillips-Hughes J, Warn D. Noninvasive ventilation in acute respiratory failure: a meta-analysis update. Crit Care Med. 2002;30:555-62.
6. Nava S, Hill N. Non-invasive ventilation in acute respiratory failure. Lancet. 2009;374:250-59.
7. Girault C, Briel A, Benichou J, Hellot MF, Dachraoui F, Tamion F, et al. Interface strategy during noninvasive positive pressure ventilation for hypercapnic acute respiratory failure. Crit Care Med. 2009;37:124-31.
8. Soo Hoo GW, Santiago S, Williams AJ. Nasal mechanical ventilation for hypercapnic respiratory failure in chronic obstructive pulmonary disease: determinants of success and failure. Crit Care Med. 1994;22:1253-61.
9. Lellouche F, Maggiore SM, Lyazidi A, Deye N, Taillé S, Brochard L. Water content of delivered gases during non-invasive ventilation in healthy subjects. Intensive Care Med. 2009;35(6):987-95.
10. Rabec C, Rodenstein D, Leger P, Rouault S, Perrin C, Gonzalez-Bermejo J, et al. Ventilator modes and settings during non-invasive ventilation: effects on respiratory events and implications for their identification. 2011. Rev Mal Respir. 2013;30(10):818-31.
11. Cuvelier A, Muir JF. Acute and chronic respiratory failure in patients with obesity hypoventilation syndrome: a new challenge for noninvasive ventilation. Chest. 2005;128:483-5.
12. Rochwerg B, Brochard L, Elliott MW, Hess D, Hill NS, Nava S, et al. Official ERS/ATS clinical practice guidelines: noninvasive ventilation for acute respiratory failure. Eur Respir J. 2017;50:1602426.
13. Maggiore SM, Battilana M, Serano L, Petrini F. Ventilatory support after extubation in critically ill patients. Lancet Respir Med. 2018;6(12):948-62.
14. Hussein K. Noninvasive positive pressure ventilation in acute hypercapnic respiratory failure. Egypt J Bronchol. 2018;12(2):143-8.
15. Keenan SP, Sinuff T, Cook DJ, Hill NS. Which patients with acute exacerbation of chronic obstructive pulmonary disease benefit from noninvasive positive-pressure ventilation? A systematic review of the literature. Ann Intern Med. 2003;138(11):861-70.
16. Lightowler JV, Wedzicha JA, Elliott MW, Ram FS. Non-invasive positive pressure ventilation to treat respiratory failure resulting from exacerbations of chronic obstructive pulmonary disease: Cochrane systematic review and meta-analysis. BMJ. 2003;326(7382):185.
17. Diaz GG, Alcaraz AC, Talavera JC, Pérez PJ, Rodriguez AE, Cordoba FG, et al. Noninvasive positive-pressure ventilation to treat hypercapnic coma secondary to respiratory failure. Chest. 2005;127(3):952-60.
18. Confalonieri M, Garuti G, Cattaruzza MS, Osborn JF, Antonelli M, Conti G, et al. A chart of failure risk for noninvasive ventilation in patients with COPD exacerbation. Eur Respir J. 2005;25(2):348-55.
19. Scala R, Naldi M, Archinucci I, Coniglio G, Nava S. Noninvasive positive pressure ventilation in patients with acute exacerbations of COPD and varying levels of consciousness. Chest. 2005;128(3):1657-66.
20. Girou E, Brun Buisson C, Taille S, Lemaire F, Brochard L. Secular trends in nosocomial infections and mortality associated with noninvasive ventilation in patients with exacerbation of COPD and pulmonary edema. JAMA. 2003;290(22):2985-91.
21. Girou E, Schortgen F, Delclaux C, Brun-Buisson C, Blot F, Lefort Y, et al. Association of noninvasive ventilation with nosocomial infections and survival in critically ill patients. JAMA. 2000;284(18):2361-7.
22. Lindenauer PK, Stefan MS, Shieh MS, Pekow PS, Rothberg MB, Hill NS. Outcomes associated with invasive and noninvasive ventilation among patients hospitalized with exacerbations of chronic obstructive pulmonary disease. JAMA Intern Med. 2014;174(12):1982-93.
23. Stefan MS, Nathanson BH, Higgins TL, Steingrub JS, Lagu T, Rothberg MB, et al. Comparative Effectiveness of Noninvasive and Invasive Ventilation in Critically Ill Patients With Acute Exacerbation of Chronic Obstructive Pulmonary Disease. Crit Care Med. 2015;43(7):1386-94.

Chapter 11
Noninvasive Ventilation in Acute Exacerbation of COPD: Rationale, Indications, and Factors for Failure

Sumit Ray, Shivangi Khanna

INTRODUCTION

Chronic obstructive pulmonary disease (COPD) patients characteristically have intermittent periods of acute deterioration in the clinical condition, referred to as exacerbations, which can be marked by severe disabling symptoms of dyspnea, worsening of gas exchange, encephalopathy, or right ventricular failure. These exacerbations are a frequent cause of hospital admissions and can eventually lead to chronic hypercapnic respiratory failure (CHRF) and severe impairment of health related quality of life (HRQoL). Unfortunately, medical treatment alone has limited efficacy to reverse the respiratory failure.

Noninvasive ventilation has been shown to be beneficial in patients with acute hypercapnic respiratory failure and COPD since the mid-1990s, endorsed by evidence of reduction in mortality by some studies.[1] It is now the standard of practice in these patients[2,3] and has pushed endotracheal intubation and invasive mechanical ventilation as the second line of therapy in certain group of selected patients.[4,5] However, its use in other COPD scenarios is still controversial.

The use of NIV for management of CHRF as a long-term home noninvasive ventilation (LTH-NIV) therapy,[6,7] as an adjunct to exercise training in COPD patients[8] and as a palliative care therapy[9] in patients with advanced disease still lacks robust evidence.

RATIONALE OF NIV IN ACUTE EXACERBATIONS OF COPD

Exacerbations of COPD are associated with worsening of expiratory airflow limitation, leading to dynamic hyperinflation. This leads to increased load on the inspiratory muscles due to the mechanical disadvantage **(Figs. 1A and B)** and due to the rapid and shallow breathing.[10] The eventual rise of $PaCO_2$, respiratory acidosis and neuromechanical uncoupling lead to chemoreceptor and mechanoreceptor triggering of the ventilatory control center (VCC),[11,12] further worsening the tachypnea.

Application of positive pressure ventilation increases the tidal volume and minute ventilation[13] and offloads the inspiratory muscles, by reducing the required patient effort for maintenance of minute ventilation[14] leading to improved gas exchange. Consequent reduction in $PaCO_2$ and improvement in pH, along with reduced anxiety and muscle load reduces the ventilatory drive, thereby improving the tachypnea and work of breathing **(Flowchart 1)**.[15]

Thus, application of NIV in acute exacerbations of COPD has a multifaceted role in improving outcomes and reducing the need for invasive ventilatory support **(Flowchart 2)**.

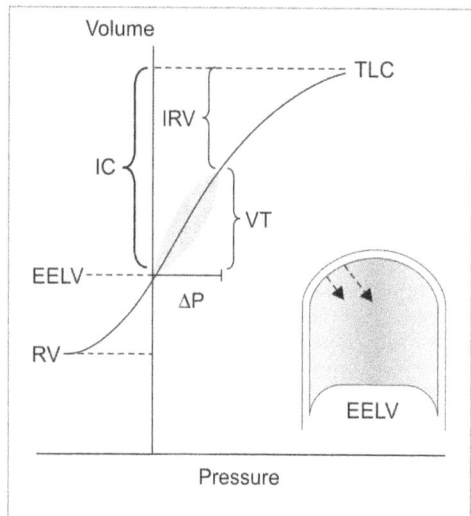 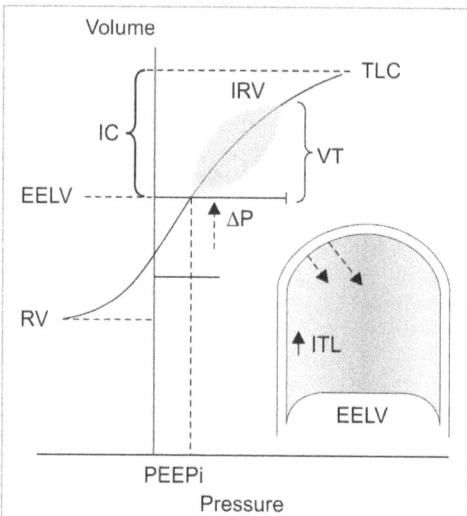

Figs. 1A and B: (A) Stable chronic obstructive pulmonary disease (COPD); (B) COPD exacerbation. During a COPD exacerbation, the tidal breathing shifts toward right, closer to the TLC on the PV loop, leading to the patient trying to breathe on the higher, flatter portion of the pressure volume (PV) loop, leading to decreased tidal volume, and poor dynamic compliance. Therefore, higher pressures have to be generated for maintenance of minute ventilation. The RV and EELV increase, while the IRC and IRV decrease. The intrapulmonary pressures might not return to zero during an exacerbation, due to intrinsic PEEP, leading to increased inspiratory threshold loading (ITL) of the respiratory muscles.

(ΔP: change in pleural pressure; EELV: end expiratory lung volume; IC: inspiratory capacity, IRV: inspiratory reserve volume, RV: residual volume; TLC: total lung capacity; Vt: tidal volume)

(*Source:* Bafadhel M, McKenna S, Terry P, Mistry V, Reid C, Haldar P, et al. Acute exacerbations of chronic obstructive pulmonary disease: identification of biologic clusters and their biomarkers. Am J Respir Crit Care Med. 2011;184(6):662-71.)

■ INDICATIONS OF NIV IN COPD

NIV can be considered in acute COPD exacerbations in the following conditions:

- In patients with mild-to-moderate acidosis and respiratory distress. To prevent endotracheal intubation. Patients with a pH of 7.25–7.35, in the absence of a metabolic cause for the acidosis, have the strongest evidence for use of NIV.[16,17] The improvement in respiratory rate or pH or both is considered as NIV success and is usually seen within 1–4 hours of starting treatment.[18] Bilevel NIV should be considered when the pH is ≤7.35, $PaCO_2$ is >45 mm Hg and the respiratory rate is >20–24 breaths/min^{-1} despite standard medical therapy.
- NIV can also be tried in patients requiring endotracheal intubation, if the patient is not immediately deteriorating.[4,5] It has shown to be associated with lesser incidences of VAP and has also been shown to be cost effective.[19] There is no lower limit of pH below which a trial of NIV is inappropriate; however, the lower the pH, the greater risk of failure, and patients must be very closely monitored with rapid access to endotracheal intubation and invasive ventilation if not improving.
- The use of NIV in COPD patients who are hypercapnic but are not acidotic is not recommended currently due to lack of consistent evidence of benefit.[17,20]

Flowchart 1: Noninvasive ventilation (NIV) has effects on the ventilatory control center (VCC) in the brainstem. The VCC has an intrinsic pattern generator with important inputs from gas exchange sensors and from mechanical load sensors. The output from the VCC controls ventilatory muscle inspiratory muscle intensity and timing. Importantly, this output can be modulated by cortical influences and drugs, an effect sometimes referred to as a loop gain. Positive-pressure NIV can affect the VCC in a variety of ways that include beneficial (and sometimes harmful) effects on gas exchange, ventilatory muscle loading, and even cortical influences that are affected by the sense of dyspnea/anxiety.

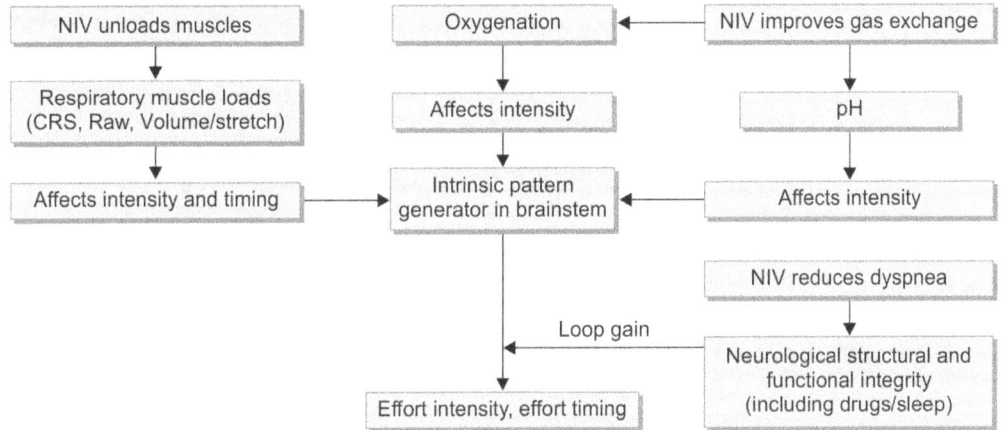

(CRS: compliance of the respiratory system; Raw: airway resistance)

- NIV can also be used as a sole method of ventilatory support in patients who are not willing for or are not candidates for invasive ventilation.
- NIV may also be used to prevent ARF in high-risk patients postextubation, especially COPD patients.[21]
- It can also be used as an aid in weaning of COPD patients from mechanical ventilation.[22]
- Long-term home NIV may be used in patients after a life-threatening hypercapnic respiratory failure episode, if the hypercapnia persists after the episode.[23]
- LTH-NIV may also be used in patients with chronic stable COPD.[24]

FAILURE OF NIV

Despite the use of NIV in experienced hands and proper selection of patients, its failure rate ranges between 5 and 60%, depending upon various factors.[25] It can be predicted by the presence of severe acidosis, hypercapnic encephalopathy, presence of comorbidities, and no improvement in blood gases within 1–2 hours of initial ventilation.[26] Early identification of NIV failure is imperative for avoiding unnecessary delay in initiation of invasive ventilation, which may be associated with increased mortality.

The type of underlying disease plays an important role in determination of NIV failure. Hypoxemic failure in patients without underlying respiratory or cardiac disease is less likely to respond to NIV therapy than hypercapnic respiratory failure in patients with an underlying COPD. The presence of community acquired pneumonia (CAP) with hypoxemic respiratory failure is associated with higher failure rates.[27] NIV has been shown to reduce intubation rates in patients with hypercapnic respiratory failure due to cardiogenic pulmonary edema.[28] The initial presence of severe acidosis (pH < 7.25), hypoxemia ($PaO_2/FiO_2 < 200$), signs of

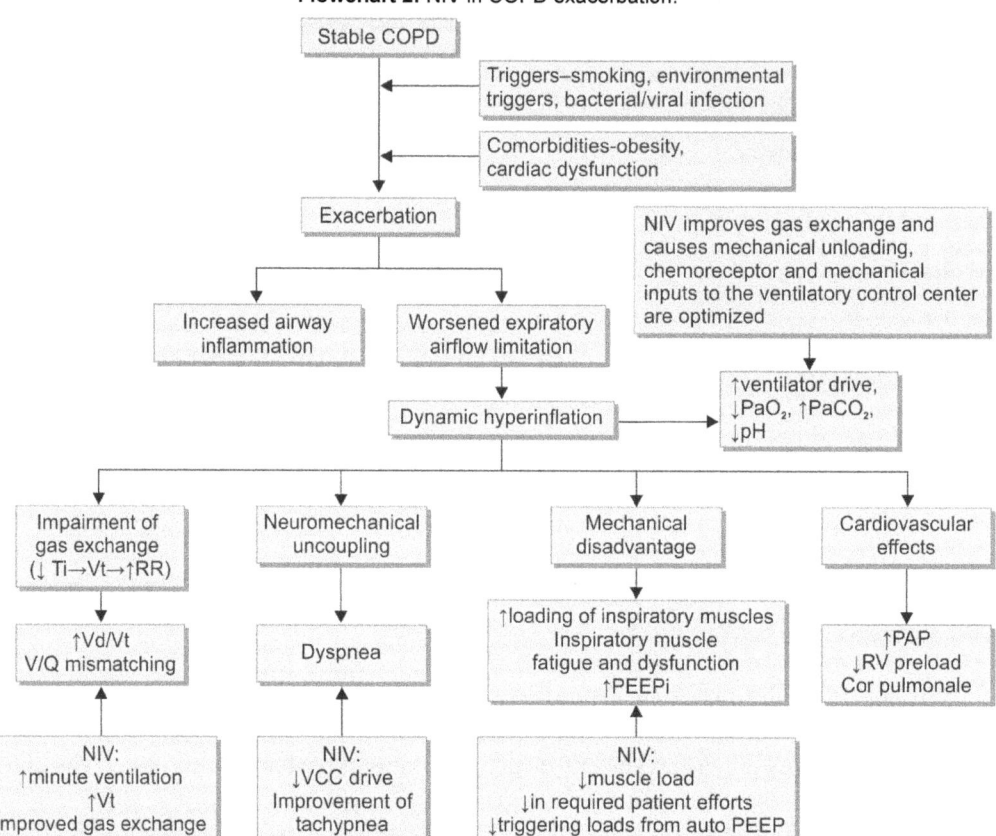

(NIV: noninvasive ventilation; PAP: pulmonary artery pressure; Vt: tidal volume; Vd: dead space ventilation; V/Q: ventilation, perfusion ratio; VCC: ventilatory control center)

respiratory distress (respiratory rate > 25 breaths/min) and nonpulmonary organ failure has been associated with greater failure rates.[29]

NIV failure can be classified according to the timing of occurrence into:

- *Immediate:* It occurs within minutes to 1 hour of initiation. It mostly occurs due to improper clearance of secretions, hypercapnic encephalopathy, and agitation of the patient or ventilator–patient asynchrony.
- *Early:* It occurs within 1–48 hours. It occurs due to high respiratory rate, muscle fatigue, or very severe acute illness
- *Late:* It occurs after 48 hours of ventilation initiation. It occurs after an initial favorable response to NIV. It is related to sleep disturbance and severe comorbidities.

Strategies to Reduce NIV Failure

- *NIV failure due to accumulation of secretions:* Use of "mini-invasive" integrated strategies:
  - In neuromuscular diseases, use of in-exsufflator or manual cough assistance devices could be used for airway clearance and avoiding intubation.[30]

- High-frequency chest wall oscillation and intrapulmonary percussive ventilation have also been tried in patients with acute COPD exacerbations. They have been shown to be successful in reducing intubations in these patients.[31]
- *NIV failure in altered consciousness*:
  - It can be tried with caution and in expert hands in patients with poor sensorium due to hypercapnic encephalopathy. It has been demonstrated to achieve rapid reduction in $PaCO_2$ and sensorium improvement, while being advantageous over invasive ventilation.[32]
  - In agitated or delirious patients, "safe sedation" can be tried with low-dose sedatives and short-acting drugs, but risk of oversedation and need for invasive ventilation should be kept in mind.
- Long sessions of NIV support can be better managed with the use of "interface rotational technology," where different types of interfaces like, total face, oronasal, helmets, nasal masks, nasal pillows, or mouthpieces can be applied alternately.[33]
- Other integrated strategies like $ECCO_2R$ with NIV have been tried in patients with COPD exacerbations leading to ARF. Although, it rapidly reduces the CO_2 level initially, it cannot be routinely recommended.[34]

CONCLUSION

Noninvasive ventilation remains in the frontline of managing COPD patients. It is an extremely useful modality for both acute exacerbation and for long-term management of these patients. The best candidates for the use of NIV in acute exacerbation are those with mild-moderate degree of acidosis with respiratory distress, who are not comatose. Responders to NIV usually show a response within 1–4 hours of initiation by a decline in distress and a reduction acidosis and dynamic hyperinflation. Careful observation and monitoring, along with appropriate timely interventions can prevent NIV failure and unnecessary intubations in these patients. However, intubation and invasive mechanical ventilation should not be delayed in patients who are critical, just in the hope of an improvement, as this increases mortality. A combination of continuous objective and subjective evaluation is essential for the successful use of NIV in the acute exacerbation of COPD.

REFERENCES

1. Brochard L, Mancebo J, Wysocki M, Lofaso F, Conti G, Rauss A, et al. Noninvasive ventilation for acute exacerbations of chronic obstructive pulmonary disease. N Engl J Med. 1995;333:817-22.
2. Davidson AC, Banham S, Elliott M, Kennedy D, Gelder C, Glossop A, et al. BTS/ICS guideline for the ventilatory management of acute hypercapnic respiratory failure in adults. Thorax. 2016;71 Suppl 2:ii1-35.
3. Wedzicha JAEC-C, Miravitlles M, Hurst JR, Calverley PM, Albert RK, Anzueto A, et al. Management of COPD exacerbations: a European Respiratory Society/American Thoracic Society guideline. Eur Respir J. 2017;49.pii:1600791.
4. Conti G, Antonelli M, Navalesi P, Rocco M, Bufi M, Spadetta G, et al. Noninvasive vs. conventional mechanical ventilation in patients with chronic obstructive pulmonary disease after failure of medical treatment in the ward: a randomized trial. Intensive Care Med. 2002;28:1701-7.
5. Jurjevic M, Matic I, Sakic-Zdravcevic K, Sakić S, Danić D, Buković D. Mechanical ventilation in chronic obstructive pulmonary disease patients, noninvasive vs. invasive method (randomized prospective study). Coll Antropol. 2009;33:791-7.

6. Köhnlein T, Windisch W, Köhler D, Drabik A, Geiseler J, Hartl S, et al. Non-invasive positive pressure ventilation for the treatment of severe stable chronic obstructive pulmonary disease: a prospective, multicentre, randomised, controlled clinical trial. Lancet Respir Med. 2014;2(9):698-705.
7. Struik FM, Sprooten RT, Kerstjens HA, Bladder G, Zijnen M, Asin J, et al. Nocturnal non-invasive ventilation in COPD patients with prolonged hypercapnia after ventilatory support for acute respiratory failure: a randomised, controlled, parallel-group study. Thorax. 2014;69(9):826-34.
8. Márquez-Martín E, Ruiz FO, Ramos PC, López-Campos JL, Azcona BV, Cortés EB. Randomized trial of non-invasive ventilation combined with exercise training in patients with chronic hypercapnic failure due to chronic obstructive pulmonary disease. Respir Med. 2014;108:1741-51.
9. Lanken PN, Terry PB, Delisser HM, Fahy BF, Hansen-Flaschen J, et al. An official American Thoracic Society clinical policy statement: palliative care for patients with respiratory diseases and critical illnesses. Am J Respir Crit Care Med. 2008;177:912-27.
10. Bellemare F, Grassino A. Effect of pressure and timing of contraction on human diaphragm fatigue. J Appl Physiol. 1982;53(5):1190-5.
11. Georgopoulos D, Roussos C. Control of breathing in mechanically ventilated patients. Eur Respir J. 1996;9(10):2151-60.
12. Mitrouska J, Xirouchaki N, Patakas D, Siafakas N, Georgopoulos D. Effects of chemical feedback on respiratory motor and ventilator output during different modes of assisted mechanical ventilation. Eur Respir J. 1999;13(4):873-82.
13. MacIntyre NR. Design features of modern mechanical ventilators. Clin Chest Med. 2016;37(4):607-14.
14. Banner MJ, Kirby RR, MacIntyre NR. Patient and ventilatory work of breathing and ventilatory muscle loads at different levels of pressure support ventilation. Chest. 1991;100(2):531-3.
15. MacIntyre NR. Physiologic effects of noninvasive ventilation. Respir Care. 2019;64(6):617-28.
16. Plant PK, Owen JL, Elliott MW. Early use of non-invasive ventilation for acute exacerbations of chronic obstructive pulmonary disease on general respiratory wards: a multicentre randomised controlled trial. Lancet. 2000;355:1931-5.
17. Keenan SP, Powers CE, McCormack DG. Noninvasive positive-pressure ventilation in patients with milder chronic obstructive pulmonary disease exacerbations: a randomized controlled trial. Respir Care. 2005;50:610-6.
18. Plant PK, Owen JL, Elliott MW. Non-invasive ventilation in acute exacerbations of chronic obstructive pulmonary disease: long term survival and predictors of in-hospital outcome. Thorax. 2001;56:708-71.
19. Keenan SP, Gregor J, Sibbald WJ, Cook D, Gafni A. Noninvasive positive pressure ventilation in the setting of severe, acute exacerbations of chronic obstructive pulmonary disease: more effective and less expensive. Crit Care Med. 2000;28:2094-102.
20. Barbe F, Togores B, Rubi M, Pons S, Maimó A, Agustí AG. Noninvasive ventilatory support does not facilitate recovery from acute respiratory failure in chronic obstructive pulmonary disease. Eur Respir J. 1996;9:1240-5.
21. Thille AW, Boissier F, Ben-Ghezala H, Razazi K, Mekontso-Dessap A, Brun-Buisson C, et al. Easily identified at-risk patients for extubation failure may benefit from noninvasive ventilation: a prospective before–after study. Crit Care. 2016;20:48.
22. Ornico SR, Lobo SM, Sanches HS, Deberaldini M, Tófoli LT, Vidal AM, et al. Noninvasive ventilation immediately after extubation improves weaning outcome after acute respiratory failure: a randomized controlled trial. Crit Care. 2013;17:R39.
23. Murphy PB, Rehal S, Arbane G, Bourke S, Calverley PMA, Crook AM, et al. Effect of home noninvasive ventilation with oxygen therapy vs oxygen therapy alone on hospital readmission or death after an acute COPD exacerbation: a randomized clinical trial. JAMA. 2017;317(21):2177-86.
24. Windisch W, Dreher M, Storre JH, Sorichter S. Nocturnal non-invasive positive pressure ventilation: physiological effects on spontaneous breathing. Respir Physiol Neurobiol. 2006;150(2-3):251-60.
25. Scala R, Latham M. How to start a patient on NIV. In: Elliott MW, Nava S, Schönhofer B (Eds). Principles and Practice of Non-Invasive Ventilation and Weaning. London, Hodder Arnold; 2010. pp. 70-83.

26. Elliott MW. Non-invasive ventilation in acute exacerbations of chronic obstructive pulmonary disease: a new gold standard? Intensive Care Med. 2002;28:1691-4.
27. Jolliet P, Abajo B, Pasquina P, Chevrolet JC. Non-invasive pressure support ventilation in severe community acquired neumonia. Intensive Care Med. 2001;27:812-21.
28. Nava S, Carbone G, DiBattista N, Bellone A, Baiardi P, Cosentini R, et al. Noninvasive ventilation in cardiogenic pulmonary edema. A multicenter, randomized trial. Am J Respir Crit Care Med. 2003;168:1-6.
29. Antonelli M, Conti G, Esquinas A, Montini L, Maggiore SM, Bello G, et al. A multiple-center survey on the use in clinical practice of noninvasive ventilation as a first-line intervention for acute respiratory distress syndrome. Crit Care Med. 2007;35:18-25.
30. Vianello A, Corrado A, Arcaro G, Gallan F, Ori C, Minuzzo M, et al. Mechanical insufflation-exsufflation improves outcomes for neuromuscular disease patients with respiratory tract infections. Am J Phys Med Rehabil. 2005;84:83-8.
31. al-Saady NM, Fernando SS, Petros AJ, Cummin AR, Sidhu VS, Bennett ED. External high frequency oscillation in normal subjects and in patients with acute respiratory failure. Anaesthesia. 1995;50:1031-5.
32. Scala R, Nava S, Conti G, Antonelli M, Naldi M, Archinucci I, et al. Noninvasive versus conventional ventilation to treat hypercapnic encephalopathy in chronic obstructive pulmonary disease. Intensive Care Med. 2007;33:2101-8.
33. Pisani L, Carlucci A, Nava S. Interfaces for noninvasive mechanical ventilation: technical aspects and efficiency. Minerva Anestesiol. 2012;78:1154-61.
34. Del Sorbo L, Pisani L, Filippini C, Fanelli V, Fasano L, Terragni P, et al. Extracorporeal CO_2 removal in hypercapnic patients at risk of non-invasive ventilation failure: a matched cohort study with historical control. Crit Care Med. 2015;43:120-7.

Chapter 12

Noninvasive Ventilation in Hypoxemic Respiratory Failure: Rationale, Indications, and Outcomes

Dhruva Chaudhry, Sateesh A

■ INTRODUCTION

Respiratory failure is characterized by impaired ability of the respiratory system for its normal gas exchange function. Hypoxemic respiratory failure is defined as partial pressure of oxygen in blood (PaO_2) less than 55 mm Hg when fraction of inspired oxygen (FiO_2) is ≥0.60. It can be acute, chronic or acute on chronic depending on the onset of illness. Acute hypoxemic respiratory failure is seen in various conditions like acute cardiogenic pulmonary edema, pneumonia, acute respiratory distress syndrome (ARDS), drug and toxin induced lung injury, blood transfusion-related reactions, blunt chest injury, and in postoperative setting. When the underlying disease is less severe or hypoxemia is mild it can be treated with standard oxygen therapy alone. More severe disease needs further management with endotracheal intubation and mechanical ventilator support. Sedatives, analgesics, and/or paralytics should be administered to facilitate invasive mechanical ventilation (IMV) support and to relieve patient discomfort. These drugs have several side effects including myocardial depression, hypotension, and can result in prolonged intensive care unit (ICU) stay. IMV itself is associated with various complications like volutrauma, barotrauma, atelectrauma, biotrauma, and myotrauma (diaphragmatic dysfunction) collectively known as ventilator-induced lung injury (VILI). Moreover, IMV is a risk factor for ventilator-associated pneumonia (VAP) resulting in increased mortality in patients admitted to ICU.

Noninvasive ventilation (NIV) is a method of ventilator support in which patient's ventilation is assisted noninvasively through application of a simple interface (e.g., face mask) between the patient and ventilator. It has now become a standard of care for patients with acute hypercapnic respiratory failure due to chronic obstructive pulmonary disease (COPD) and its role in the management of hypoxemic respiratory failure has been evolving in the recent times. NIV avoids endotracheal intubation, sedation, and their complications. When compared with IMV, NIV has several advantages including its simplicity, comfort to the patient, ease of application, and associated with less number of complications. Moreover, NIV is more economical and easily available. By avoiding endotracheal intubation it can decrease the incidence of nosocomial infections and their associated mortality.

■ RATIONALE OF NONINVASIVE VENTILATION IN HYPOXEMIC RESPIRATORY FAILURE

The physiological benefits of NIV are mainly due to its efficacy to improve oxygenation and alveolar ventilation **(Box 1)**. The applied positive end-expiratory pressure (PEEP) in NIV prevents alveolar collapse and helps in recruitment of already collapsed alveoli along with increased pulmonary compliance and functional residual capacity (FRC) **(Flowchart 1)**. Arterial oxygen tension improves due to availability of more surface area for gas exchange. PEEP improves ventilation perfusion inequalities.[1] It also prevents surfactant aggregation which can cause alveolar collapse. Positive-pressure ventilation decreases venous return to heart as a result of positive intrathoracic pressure. Left ventricular preload is decreased and at the same time it also decreases left ventricular afterload. In patients with concomitant left ventricular dysfunction ejection fraction is improved; hence, oxygen delivery to tissue enhanced. It also helps in clearance of alveolar and interstitial fluid. Inspiratory positive airway pressure (IPAP) or pressure support improves minute ventilation, decreases respiratory rate and work of breathing.[1]

Box 1: Physiological benefits of NIV.

Physiological benefits of CPAP/EPAP/PEEP
- Prevents alveolar collapse
- Opens already collapsed alveoli. Hence more surface area is available for oxygen exchange
- Prevents surfactant aggregation resulting in decreased alveolar collapse
- Lung compliance improved
- Function residual capacity increased
- Decreased ventilation perfusion mismatch
- Decreased work of breathing by improving respiratory mechanics
- In patients with concomitant LV dysfunction it improves LV systolic function by decreasing left ventricular preload and afterload. Hence oxygen delivery to tissue enhanced.
- Helps in clearance of alveolar and interstitial fluid

Physiological benefits of IPAP/PS
- Improved minute ventilation
- Decreased respiratory rate
- Offsets respiratory loading and decreases work of breathing

(CPAP: continuous positive airway pressure; EPAP: expiratory positive airway pressure; IPAP: inspiratory positive airway pressure; LV: Left ventricular; PEEP: positive end-expiratory pressure; PS: pressure support)

Flowchart 1: Physiological benefits of NIV.

(EPAP: expiratory positive airway pressure; FiO$_2$: fraction of inspired oxygen; FRC: functional residual capacity; IPAP: inspiratory positive airway pressure; NIV: noninvasive ventilation; V/Q: ventilation/perfusion).

NONINVASIVE VENTILATION APPLICATION IN HYPOXEMIC RESPIRATORY FAILURE WITH DIFFERENT CLINICAL SETTINGS

Cardiogenic Pulmonary Edema

Cardiogenic pulmonary edema is characterized by flooding of pulmonary interstitium and alveoli due to increased hydrostatic pressure resulting from failed left ventricle, which can be seen in various conditions especially in the setting of acute coronary syndrome. It can cause severe respiratory distress necessitating endotracheal intubation and ventilator support. The clinical benefit of NIV in acute cardiogenic pulmonary edema is due to decreased venous return resulting from increased intrathoracic pressure caused by positive-pressure ventilation that leads to reduced cardiac preload. Moreover, NIV reduces left ventricular after load resulting in improved left ventricular systolic function.[2] NIV helps in clearance of interstitial and alveolar fluid, prevents collapse of alveoli and also reduces the work of breathing.

Several studies showed the beneficial role of NIV in cardiogenic pulmonary edema. In a randomized trial, NIV showed rapid improvement in patient symptoms and metabolic disturbances, but without any short-term mortality benefit.[3] A recent meta-analysis of 24 studies involving patients with respiratory distress due to acute cardiogenic pulmonary edema, not requiring immediate mechanical ventilation, NIV was associated with decreased hospital mortality and reduced endotracheal intubation rates.[4] Early initiation of NIV in cardiogenic pulmonary edema can decrease the need for intubation and IMV support. When used in prehospital setup it is associated with decreased mortality. Its role in concomitant cardiogenic shock is not known since majority of studies excluded this category of patients.

Pneumonia

Overall, pneumonia is the sixth leading cause of death. The rationale for using NIV in patients with pneumonia is to overcome an episode of severe respiratory failure avoiding the need of IMV. Even though the use of NIV for pneumonia has increased many folds in recent times, its role in management of pneumonia still unclear. Studies showed that NIV was less effective and had poor outcome in treatment of acute respiratory failure (ARF) due to pneumonia when compared to COPD exacerbation and acute cardiogenic pulmonary edema.[5,6] The difference of success of NIV in comparison with acute cardiogenic pulmonary edema may be due to the requirement of long time for the effect of medical treatment on pneumonia. Also, the favorable effect of PEEP on oxygenation depends on the pattern of lung involvement with greater recruitment in interstitial involvement than in consolidation.

The role of NIV in patients with respiratory failure due to pneumonia can be summarized as follows: In patients without previous cardiac or pulmonary disease, defined as "de novo" respiratory failure, the use of NIV was associated with a high rates of NIV failure and consequently high intubation rates,[7] whereas, in patients with cardiac or pulmonary diseases (i.e., COPD), defined "comorbidities" group, the outcome is more favorable compared with those with "de novo" respiratory failure (74% vs 54%, respectively);[7] finally in patients with an impaired immune system, defined "immunodepressed" group, NIV may decrease intubation rate and improve outcome.

Acute Respiratory Distress Syndrome

Acute respiratory distress syndrome is characterized by rapidly progressive respiratory failure which is associated with high mortality. Majority of these patients requires invasive ventilator support. The rationale of applying NIV in ARDS is to improve oxygenation, to decrease dyspnea and the work of breathing and finally to avoid intubation.

In a study conducted by Antonelli et al., the failure rates of NIV was 30% with highest intubation rates observed in patients with ARDS and community-acquired pneumonia.[5] Reasons for high rates of failure in these patients might be due to the need for higher levels of PEEP or higher levels of pressure support to counter the increased compliance and to alleviate work of breathing. Another potential reason is that patients with ARDS often have high tidal volumes that are potentially injurious and difficult to control during NIV. Also, the inability to use high doses of sedation and analgesia or paralytics in these patients might lead to high failure rates.[6]

Several concerns exist regarding the use of NIV in patients with ARDS. It remains unclear which subgroup of ARDS patients will be most likely to benefit from NIV. Some studies show that NIV may best be reserved for patients with mild ARDS (i.e., patients with a PaO_2/FiO_2 ratio of 200–300 mm Hg).[8] The LUNG SAFE (Large observational study to UNderstand the Global impact of Severe Acute respiratory FailurE) study showed that NIV failure occurred in 22.2% of mild, 42.3% of moderate, and 47.1% of patients with severe ARDS and is associated with higher ICU mortality in patients with a PaO_2/FiO_2 less than 150 mm Hg.[9] This implies that use of initial NIV trail may be more hazardous in patients with more severe ARDS than proceeding directly to invasive mechanical ventilation. In patients who are being considered for NIV as an initial ventilatory strategy we should ensure the appropriate environment for NPPV delivery, i.e., either an ICU or high dependency unit, should use oronasal mask to minimize leaks, start with lower levels of PEEP and pressure support to improve patient comfort and titrate gradually to maintain a saturation of ≥94%. Patients should be regularly reassessed with arterial blood gases (ABGs) to look for any worsening of blood gases. It is necessary to maintain a low threshold for intubation in ARDS patients as delaying a necessary intubation may harm patients and increase mortality.[8]

Blunt Injury to Chest

Chest trauma composes 10–15% of all traumas and is responsible for 17–25% of all deaths caused by trauma.[10] Chest injury can result in pulmonary contusion, pneumothorax, hemothorax, rib fractures, and flail chest. It causes significant damage to alveolar capillary membrane resulting in exudation of fluid into the interstitium and alveoli. The main concern in patients with chest trauma is significant pain that results in decreased cough reflex and clearance of secretions. All these factors contribute to atelectasis of alveoli resulting in ventilation perfusion mismatch and hypoxemia. If the damage is severe enough it can even lead to ARDS.

The role of NIV in blunt chest trauma is controversial. Positive-pressure ventilation physiologically acts as an internal splint against unstable chest wall. It also decreases basal atelectasis and improves oxygenation. Challenges associated with NIV use in chest trauma include decreased level of consciousness due to associated head injuries; facial trauma prohibiting NIV use; decreased cough reflex and respiratory efforts due to pain; significant blood loss resulting in hemodynamic instability; diaphragmatic injuries; and reduced pulmonary compliance due to pneumothorax and hemothorax. Moreover, multiple blood transfusions in these patients can lead to acute lung injury resulting in further worsening of patient's oxygenation. Patients with pulmonary contusion, flail chest can receive a trail of NIV before going to endotracheal intubation. NIV when combined with adequate analgesia, chest physiotherapy, and mobilization helps in early recovery. Meta-analysis showed that early NIV in these patients reduced mortality, need for intubation and mechanical ventilator support without increase in complications.[11,12]

Perioperative Respiratory Failure

Hypoxia is a relatively common complication after major surgical procedure and it is associated with increased hospital length of stay, morbidity, and mortality. It is seen in up to 30–50% cases following upper abdominal surgery. Several factors contribute to respiratory failure in immediate postoperative period—impaired cough and mucociliary clearance; respiratory and diaphragmatic dysfunction due to sedatives; decreased FRC and lung volumes; and basal atelectasis due to prolonged immobilization. All these factors can contribute to pneumonia, causing further worsening of patient's condition. Preoperative risk factors like older age, smoking, alcohol intake, poor nutritional status, underlying respiratory disorders (COPD), and obstructive sleep apnea (OSA) can contribute to respiratory failure after surgery.

Acute hypoxemia following major surgical procedure can be treated with standard oxygen therapy; however, in some cases it can progress to ARF requiring IMV support. There is a recent trend towards increased NIV utilization in these populations to avoid endotracheal intubation and its complications. NIV can be applied prophylactically when respiratory failure is anticipated or it can be therapeutic once patient develops respiratory failure. NIV prevents basal atelectasis, increases FRC, and decreases work of breathing, resulting in improvement in patient's oxygenation and relief of dyspnea. The applied PEEP also maintains the patency of upper airway. Jaber et al. showed that NIV use in patients with ARF following abdominal surgery was associated with decreased reintubation rates [33.1% in NIV group vs 45.5% in the standard oxygen group with absolute difference of −12.4%; 95% confidence interval (CI), −23.5% to −1.3%, P = 0.03%). NIV use was associated with significant more invasive ventilation free days compared to standard oxygen therapy and reduced incidence of hospital acquired infections.[13] Although NIV was associated with decreased mortality, the difference was not statistically significant. The decreased mortality associated with NIV can be attributed to decreased incidence of nosocomial infections by avoiding endotracheal intubation and IMV support. A meta-analysis showed that in patients with ARF following upper abdominal surgery, NIV compared to oxygen therapy, reduced intubation rates, and IMV support. It also reduced the length of stay in ICU. However, the mortality rate and the mean length of stay in the hospital were similar in the two groups.[14] NIV is considered as a relative contraindication for respiratory failure following esophageal and stomach surgery as positive-pressure ventilation can cause abdominal distention and anastomotic leak.

Immunocompromised Patients

Over the past decades, the overall survival of immunocompromised patients has been gradually increasing owing to highly effective retroviral treatment in patients with acquired immunodeficiency syndrome (AIDS), advances in chemotherapy in cancer patients, and better outcomes of allogeneic hematopoietic cell transplantations. Immunocompromised patients are at increased risk of acquiring infections due to their inadequate immune response. These patients are at high risk of a number of life-threatening complications like opportunistic infections, pulmonary involvement secondary to malignancy, and drug-related pulmonary toxicity. All these conditions can lead to ARF leading to repeated hospital admissions. NIV can be used as an initial management strategy in these patients to avoid intubation as IMV has increased mortality in these patients.

In a study conducted by Huang et al., early use of NIV significantly reduced short-term mortality and intubation rate when compared with oxygen therapy alone. In addition, early NIV was associated with a shorter length of ICU stay but not long-term mortality.[15] In contrast, Lemiale V et al., who conducted a randomized trial among 374 critically ill immunocompromised patients, of whom 317 (84.7%) were receiving treatment for hematologic malignancies or solid tumors reported that immunocompromised patients admitted to the ICU with hypoxemic ARF, early NIV compared with oxygen therapy alone did not reduce 28-day mortality.[16] Also, in an observational study of 99 patients with hematologic malignancy and ARF, by Adda M et al., approximately one-half of patients failed a trial of NIV and required endotracheal intubation.[17] The independent predictors of NIV failure include an elevated respiratory rate during NIV, need for vasopressors, and an increased duration between admission and the initiation of NIV.

■ NONINVASIVE VENTILATION SETUP IN HYPOXEMIC RESPIRATORY FAILURE

Initial step in the management of NIV is proper selection of a patient. Even though NIV seems to be an attractive modality when managing a patient with acute hypoxemic respiratory failure, the risk benefit ratio must be carefully weighed before choosing this modality. Very few patients with acute hypoxemic respiratory failure are initially suitable for NIV after careful consideration of contraindications **(Box 2)**. The next step is to select ventilator type, mask type, and appropriate mode. NIV can be delivered via the standard ICU ventilators used for invasive mechanical ventilation or dedicated noninvasive ventilators. The standard ICU ventilators have advantages like precise and high concentration of FiO_2, better patient monitoring, and alarm features. The inspiratory and expiratory limbs in these ventilators prevent rebreathing of carbon dioxide which is a problem in portable NIV ventilators. Continuous positive airway pressure (CPAP), bilevel positive airway pressure (BPAP), and conventional ventilatory modes used in standard ICU ventilators can be used for this purpose. Different types of masks (helmet mask, full-face mask, oronasal mask, nasal mask, and nasal pillows) are available and treating physician can chose any one of them depending on patient's characteristics and preference. Oronasal masks are generally preferred to other masks. In a meta-analysis comparing helmet mask with other types of masks, helmet mask was associated with lower mortality, intubation rates, and complications compared to other types of interfaces. However, there were no significant differences in the gas exchange and length of ICU stay. It also included patients with acute exacerbation of COPD but on subgroup analysis the reduced mortality benefit was found in hypoxemic respiratory failure patients.[18]

Box 2: Contraindications for noninvasive ventilation (NIV).

Contraindications for NIV
- Severe respiratory distress
- Unable to protect the airway or clear the secretions
- High risk of aspiration
- Impaired consciousness
- Cardiac or respiratory arrest
- Noncooperative patients
- Hemodynamic instability and arrhythmias
- Facial trauma
- Upper airway obstruction

After starting NIV patient should be monitored for mask leaks which is a challenging problem. Complications include local tissue injury, abdominal distension, and increased chance of aspiration. It can cause dryness of mucus membranes which can be avoided with proper humidification. Patient's mental status and vitals should be monitored carefully. It is difficult to use NIV in patients with claustrophobia and uncooperative patients. Facilities for immediate endotracheal intubation and invasive ventilator support should be available if patient's clinical condition worsens or patient is not able to tolerate NIV. Once the patient's clinical condition improves and/or underlying disease resolves he/she should be gradually weaned off from NIV support. Most common reasons for NIV failure include severity of underlying disease, uncooperative patients, issues with mask fitting, and leak. Proper selection of patients and careful monitoring can decrease the risk of NIV failure. Management of patient presenting with hypoxemic respiratory failure summarized in **Flowchart 2**.

Flowchart 2: NIV management of patient presenting with hypoxemic respiratory failure.

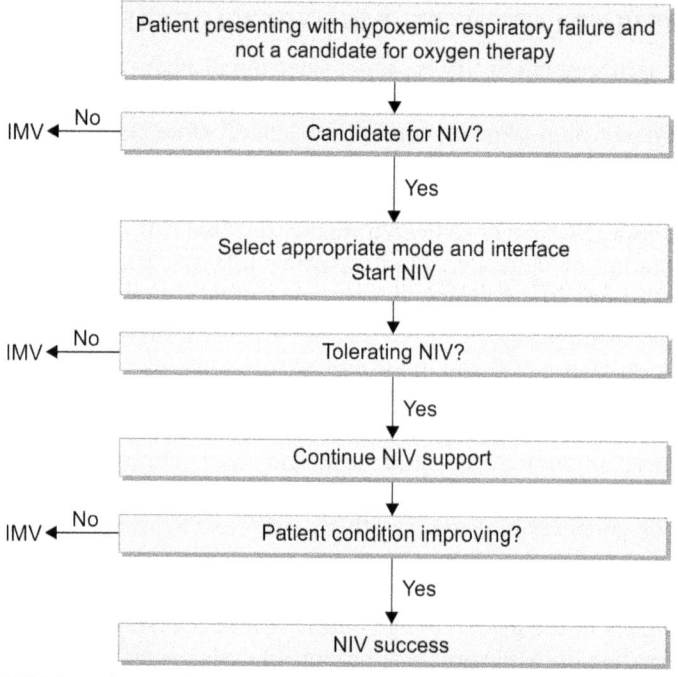

(IMV: invasive mechanical ventilation, NIV: noninvasive ventilation)

In summary NIV is a good initial choice for patients presenting with hypoxemic respiratory failure. The rational is to avoid endotracheal intubation and its complications. By preventing alveolar collapse NIV improves oxygenation and relieves dyspnea. It also decreases the work of breathing and gives rest to respiratory muscles. It can decrease mortality in carefully selected patients with hypoxemic respiratory failure. More randomized controlled trials with larger sample size are required to confirm the efficacy and clinical benefits of NIV compared to invasive ventilator support.

KEY POINTS

- The role of NIV in hypoxemic respiratory failure is still evolving and its benefit depends on the underlying cause of acute hypoxemic respiratory failure.
- The rationale of NIV in acute hypoxemic respiratory failure is due to its capacity to improve oxygenation by recruiting collapsed alveoli and prevention of collapse of normal alveoli. It also improves minute ventilation and decreases the work of breathing.
- In acute cardiogenic pulmonary edema, NIV, by decreasing preload and afterload of left ventricle, improves cardiac output and decreases edema fluid formation.
- NIV failure rates are very high in patients with ARDS. Hence, it is necessary to maintain a low threshold for intubation in these groups of patients.
- In patients with blunt trauma chest, NIV by acting as an internal splint against unstable chest wall improves oxygenation through recruitment of collapsed alveoli.
- NIV can be applied prophylactically when respiratory failure is anticipated or it can be therapeutic once patient develops respiratory failure in patients undergoing major surgery.
- All patients receiving NIV should be carefully monitored for mask fitting, leaks, asynchrony, and regularly assessed for patient's mental status as these factors are responsible for NIV failure.
- Proper selection of patients is a key to successful NIV. It should be kept in mind that in patients with severe disease, NIV may actually worsen patient's condition and contribute to increased mortality.
- In carefully selected patients NIV decreases mortality. The mortality benefit is attributed to decreased incidence of nosocomial infections by avoiding endotracheal intubation.

REFERENCES

1. MacIntyre NR. Physiologic effects of mechanical ventilation. Respiratory Care. 2019;64(6):617-28.
2. Pinsky MR. Cardiopulmonary interactions: physiologic basis and clinical applications. Ann Am Thorac Soc. 2018;15:S45-8.
3. Gray A, Goodacre S, Newby DE, Masson M, Sampson F, Nicholl J, et al. Noninvasive ventilation in acute cardiogenic pulmonary edema. N Engl J Med. 2008;359:142-51.
4. Berbenetz N, Wang Y, Brown J, Godfrey C, Ahmad M, Vital FMR, et al. Non-invasive positive pressure ventilation (CPAP or bilevel NPPV) for cardiogenic pulmonary oedema. Cochrane Database Syst Rev. 2019;(4):CD005351.
5. Antonelli M, Conti G, Moro ML, Esquinas A, Gonzalez-Diaz G, Confalonieri M, et al. Predictors of failure of noninvasive positive pressure ventilation in patients with acute respiratory failure: a multi-center study. Intensive Care Med. 2001;27:1718-28.

6. Carteaux G, Millan-Guillarte T, De Prost N, Razazi K, Abid S, Thille AW, et al. Failure of noninvasive ventilation for de novo acute hypoxemic respiratory failure: role of tidal volume. Crit Care Med. 2016;44:282-90.
7. Risom MB, Kjaer BN, Risom E, Guldager H. Non-invasive ventilation is less efficient in pneumonia than in chronic obstructive pulmonary disease exacerbation. Dan Med J. 2014;61:A4799.
8. Antonelli M, Conti G, Esquinas A, Montini L, Maggiore SM, Bello G, et al. A multiple-center survey on the use in clinical practice of noninvasive ventilation as a first-line intervention for acute respiratory distress syndrome. Crit Care Med. 2007;35:18-25.
9. Bellani G, Laffey JG, Pham T, Madotto F, Fan E, Brochard L, et al. Noninvasive ventilation of patients with acute respiratory distress syndrome. Insights form the LUNG SAFE study. AM J Respir Crit Care Med. 2017;195:67-77.
10. Veysi VT, Nikolau VS, Paliobeis C, Efstathopoulos N, Giannoudis PV. Prevalence of chest trauma, associated injuries and mortality: a level I trauma centre experience. Int Orthop. 2009;33:1425-33.
11. Roberts S, Skinner D, Biccardi B, Rodseth RN. The role of noninvasive ventilation in blunt chest trauma: systematic review and meta-analysis. Eur J Trauma Emerg Surg. 2014;40:553-9.
12. Duggal A, Perez P, Golan E, Tremblay L, Sinuff T. Safety and efficacy of noninvasive ventilation in patients with blunt chest trauma: a systematic review. Crit Care. 2013;17:R142.
13. Jaber S, Lescot T, Futier E, Paugam-Burtz C, Seguin P, Ferrandiere M, et al. Effect of noninvasive ventilation on tracheal reintubation among patients with hypoxemic respiratory failure following abdominal surgery: a randomized clinical trial. JAMA. 2016;315:1345-53.
14. Faria DA, da Silva EM, Atallah AN, Vital FM. Noninvasive positive pressure ventilation for acute respiratory failure following upper abdominal surgery. Cochrane Database Syst Rev. 2015;10: CD009134.
15. Huang HB, Xu B, Liu GY, Lin JD, Du B. Use of noninvasive ventilation in immunocompromised patients with acute respiratory failure: a systematic review and meta-analysis. Crit Care. 2017; 21(1):4.
16. Lemiale V, Mokart D, Resche-Rigon M, et al. Effect of noninvasive ventilation vs oxygen therapy on mortality among immunocompromised patients with acute respiratory failure: A randomized clinical trial. JAMA. 2015;314(16):1711-9.
17. Adda M, Coquet I, Darmon M, Thiery G, Schlemmer B, Azoulay E. Predictors of noninvasive ventilation failure in patients with hematologic malignancy and acute respiratory failure. Crit Care Med. 2008;36(10):2766-72.
18. Liu Q, Gao Y, Chen R, Cheng Z. Noninvasive ventilation with helmet versus control strategy in patients with acute respiratory failure: a systematic review and meta-analysis of controlled studies. Critical Care. 2016;20:265.

Chapter 13

Noninvasive Ventilation in Cardiogenic Pulmonary Edema

Rajesh Chandra Mishra, Sharmili Sinha, Gopal Raval, K Swarna Deepak

■ INTRODUCTION

Cardiogenic pulmonary edema (CPE) is reflection of increasing left ventricular end-diastolic pressure (LVEDP) which is initially interstitial then floods the alveoli depending upon cause, type, and time frame of left ventricle (LV) dysfunction development. This LV dysfunction can be systolic, diastolic or both. Increasing LVEDP and LV dysfunction increases intracardiac pressure, which leads to increased cardiac transmural pressure. This increased transmural pressure further complicates pulmonary edema leading to breathing difficulty and hypoxemia. Isolated diastolic dysfunction in patients of chronic hypertension, diabetes or chronic kidney failure causing pulmonary edema and hypoxemia is the most common missed diagnosis. Diagnosis here can be established by clinical suspicion in appropriate patients, echocardiography, Doppler, lung ultrasound, and high N-terminal pro-brain natriuretic peptide (NT pro BNP).

Noninvasive ventilation (NIV) in form of continuous positive airway pressure (CPAP) off loads the LV by increasing alveolar and pericardial pressure which decreases transmural pressure, in turn improves cardiac function and oxygenation.[1] This helps in improving the outcome in reversible causes of acute LV dysfunction.[2] On the other hand NIV as bilevel positive airway pressure (BiPAP) may not replicate same results in isolated CPE as it will cyclically change the intrathoracic pressure, cardiac output, alveolar pressure, and oxygen delivery. So this chapter will focus on pathophysiology of CPE without shock, heart lung interaction during NIV/CPAP and how CPAP (NIV) helps in reversing these physiological changes; available clinical evidence in favor of using CPAP/NIV in CPE.

■ PATHOPHYSIOLOGY OF CARDIOGENIC PULMONARY EDEMA

Cardiogenic pulmonary edema is an episode of sudden heart failure leading to severe respiratory failure and oxygen saturation <90% on room air.[3] The pathogenesis of CPE is complex interplay of increasing LVEDP, decreasing systolic function and increasing systemic vascular resistance, leading to exudation of fluid from the intravascular compartment into the lung interstitium and alveoli. This process initiates a vicious cycle of hypoxemia, tissue ischemia leading to increasing systemic and pulmonary vascular resistance which further increase afterload causing increase oxygen demand. This vicious cycle is further propagated by increasing myocardial transmural pressure, failing ventricular interdependence mechanism perpetuating right ventricular failure. This complex vicious cycle is further axed by impending lactic acid induced metabolic acidosis.[4]

Mechanical effect of pulmonary interstitial edema reduces lung compliance, decreases diffusion capacity further perpetuating arterial hypoxemia and myocardial suppression. Vicious cycle of interstitial edema progress to alveolar flooding and airway edema, which causes air trapping, dynamic hyperinflation, increased airway resistance, and CO_2 retention. CO_2 retention in CPE is bad sign of respiratory muscle mechanical failure.[5,6] The fatigued respiratory muscle have to generate large negative pleural swings to increase inspiratory flow to meet the demand of adequate ventilation.[7] This increase in negative intrathoracic pressure aggravates pulmonary edema by increasing both preload and afterload. One always need to remember that while managing these patients the respiratory distress and dyspnea are not related to hypoxemia only, so cannot be reversed with oxygen administration alone.[8]

HEART–LUNG INTERACTION DURING CPAP AND HOW CPAP (NIV) HELPS IN REVERSING THESE PHYSIOLOGICAL CHANGES

Interaction of Heart and Lungs during Spontaneous Respiration

During spontaneous respiration, pleural pressure (P_{pl}) is lowered during phase of inspiration as thoracic cavity expands. This reduces the extramural pressure in pericardium (P_{ex}) of the heart. Thus venous return increases to ventricles but impedes ejection to small extent. **Figure 1** depicts various pressures in thoracic cavity during different phases of respiration.

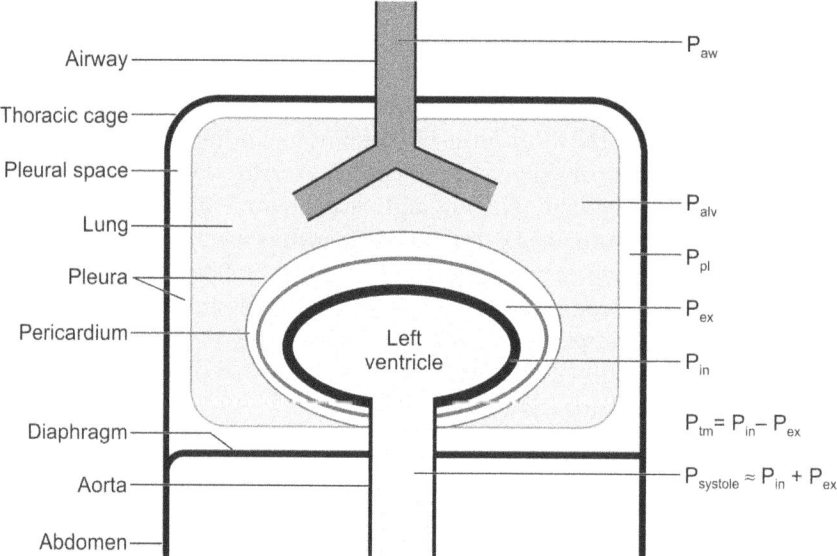

Fig. 1: Schematic representation of cardiorespiratory relationship. (P_{alv}: alveolar pressure; P_{aw}: airway pressure; P_{ex}: extramural stress; P_{in}: intramural stress; P_{pl}: intrathoracic pleural pressure; $P_{systole}$: aortic blood pressure; P_{tm}: transmural pressure)
(*Source*: Duke GJ. Cardiovascular effects of mechanical ventilation. Crit Care Resusc. 1999;1:388-99.)

The thoracic cage contains heart and the great vessels and the lungs with pulmonary vessels. Their close anatomical juxtaposition and functional interplay is responsible for the dynamics of pressure change during phases of respiration, especially positive pressure ventilation.

During inspiration due to expansion of lungs, there occurs nonuniform compression of the ventricles of varying magnitude depending on cardiac muscle elastance and volume. The right ventricle (RV) and LV are in series, the output of RV provides the input (venous return) for the LV.

Ventricular interdependence is important to understand as LV and RV share a common pericardial sac and a common interventricular septum. Ideally septum is part of LV in systole. As afterload on RV increases septum no longer contract with LV and this further increases afterload and cardiac output.[9,10]

Cardiovascular Effects of Spontaneous Respiration

In healthy individuals, spontaneous breathing is associated with a slight fall in systolic blood pressure up to 10 mm Hg. This phenomenon is due to increase in LV afterload, decrease in LV venous return, ventricular interdependence, and transmission of reduced intrathoracic aortic P_{ex} to extrathoracic vessels.

Figure 2 summarizes cardiovascular pressure changes during spontaneous respiration.

With the onset of inspiration P_{pl} fall as well P_{ex}. This increases P_{tm} which facilitates filling of the RV and higher right ventricular end-diastolic volume (RVEDV).[11] As a consequence pulmonary vascular flow increases and results in higher left ventricular end-diastolic volume (LVEDV) after one to two breaths. So blood pressure tends to rise to small extent in expiration.

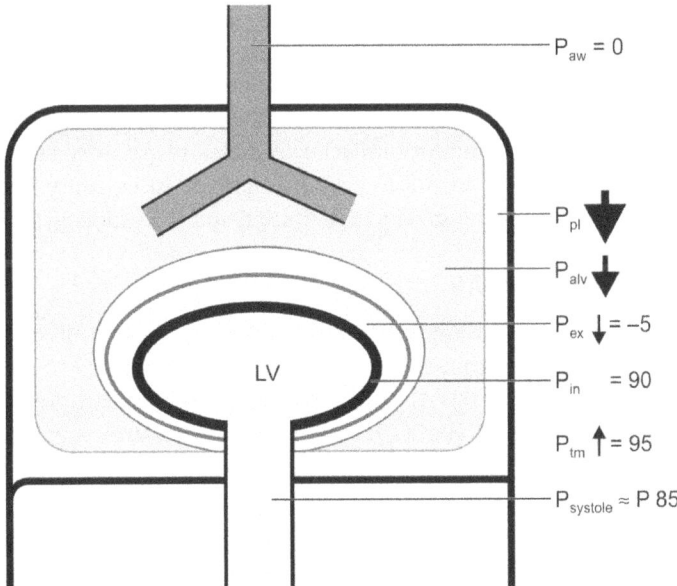

Fig. 2: Schematic representation of cardiorespiratory interaction during spontaneous inspiration and cardiac systole. Arrows depict direction of change. Spontaneous inspiration increases P_{tm} and reduces $P_{systole}$. (LV: left ventricle; P_{alv}: alveolar pressure; P_{aw}: airway pressure; P_{ex}: extramural stress; P_{in}: intramural stress; P_{pl}: intrathoracic pleural pressure; $P_{systole}$: aortic blood pressure; P_{tm}: transmural pressure)
(*Source*: Duke GJ. Cardiovascular effects of mechanical ventilation. Crit Care Resusc. 1999;1:388-99.)

Heart Lung Interaction during NIV (CPAP)

Continuous positive airway pressure had been known to be an effective therapy to unresponsive CPE to medical treatment since 1936.[12] CPAP therapy in patients with CPE improves respiratory and hemodynamic mechanics.[13] CPAP improves the inspiratory and expiratory flow and pressure, unloading the inspiratory muscles.[14] CPAP improves ventilation perfusion mismatch, alveolar ventilation, re-expands flooded alveoli, and counteracts intrinsic positive end-expiratory pressure (PEEP).

The cardiac transmural pressure (P_{tm}) is the pressure difference between pressure inside the heart and intrathoracic pressure (pleural/pericardial). This cardiac transmural pressure varies cyclically during inspiration and expiration and is responsible for effective filling (preload) and emptying (afterload) of the pump (myocardium). The amplitude of inspiratory swings is greater in patients with CPE and leads to an increase in P_{tm} in patients with CPE.[15] The more positive the P_{tm} is during diastole, the greater the filling of the heart (preload). The more positive the P_{tm} is during systole, the higher the workload is for the heart (afterload). During systole, CPAP induced increase in intrathoracic pressure reduces the venous return, decreasing the right and left ventricular preload, thereby improving mechanics in an overloaded ventricle, whereas in diastole, CPAP increases pericardial pressure, reduces transmural pressure, and thus decreases afterload.[16] Thus increasing cardiac index in patients with CPE.[17]

Treatment with NIV (CPAP) in CPE is more beneficial in patients with systolic dysfunction.

HOW DOES BILEVEL POSITIVE AIRWAY PRESSURE WORK?

Bilevel positive airway pressure works by two different pressures—inspiratory positive airway pressure (IPAP) and expiratory positive airway pressure (EPAP). BiPAP decreases inspiratory work of breathing, and can improve diaphragmatic function better than CPAP alone.[18] Recent studies shows BiPAP has similar cardiac and hemodynamic effect as CPAP in patients with CPE. BiPAP also unloads the respiratory muscles, reduces respiratory effort, and increases tidal volume before any changes in pulmonary mechanics. In contrary CPAP requires the pulmonary mechanics to change before any benefits of respiratory muscle unloading are seen.

CPAP COMPARED WITH BIPAP

Four randomized trials that have attempted to answer whether BiPAP is better than CPAP in CPE.

Mehta et al.[19] randomized patients to receive either nasal CPAP (10 cm H_2O) or BiPAP (IPAP 15 cm H_2O/EPAP 5 cm H_2O). Although the BiPAP group had greater reductions in partial pressure of carbon dioxide ($PaCO_2$), systolic blood pressure, mean arterial pressure, and hypercapnia than did the CPAP group, myocardial infarction rates were higher in the BiPAP group (71%) than in the CPAP group (31%) and the study was stopped prematurely after the enrolment of 27 patients. While this difference could have been attributable to unequal randomization as more patients in the BiPAP group presented with chest pain, the results none the less raised concerns about the safety of the ventilatory techniques used to treat CPE.

Park et al.[20] and Bellone et al.[21] showed that BiPAP was as effective as CPAP in the treatment of CPE and both methods improved ventilation and vital signs in patients with acute CPE. No significant differences were found in hospital mortality and acute myocardial infarction rates in patients with acute CPE in comparison with CPAP alone.

Crane et al.[22] randomized 60 patients presenting with acute CPE to receive conventional oxygen therapy, CPAP (10 cm H_2O), or bilevel ventilation (IPAP 15 cm H_2O, EPAP 5 cm H_2O). Although treatment success (respiratory rate <23 breaths/min, oxygen saturation >90%, pH >7.35 occurred in three patients in the control group, seven in the CPAP group, and nine in the BiPAP group ($p = 0.116$), 14 of the control group patients survived to hospital discharge, compared with 20 in the CPAP group and 15 in the bilevel group ($p = 0.029$).

There are also concerns in pooled data analysis that BiPAP may increase intubation rate and overall hospital mortality.

PRACTICAL ASPECTS OF NONINVASIVE VENTILATION IN CARDIOGENIC PULMONARY EDEMA

Where These Patients are Best Treated?

Patients with severe CPE requiring NIV need to be triaged to an environment with round the clock medical care, adequate nurse-patient ratio, and continuous electrocardiographic and pulse oximetry monitoring facilities, facility to intubate and if needed revascularization.

Do All Patients with CPE Require NIV?

Noninvasive ventilation benefits more in patients with more severe forms of CPE without shock who are not responding to medical therapy. NIV can be useful support to patients who are not candidates for intubation, due to poor prognosis related to an underlying disease. Better approach is to give NIV (CPAP) trials to all case of CPE without shock and look for response for 30 minutes.[23]

How should NIV be Applied Initially?

The application of NIV is an art of medicine. All physicians using NIV should personally apply NIV to actually understand what the patient is experiencing. You should not order a specific pressure level for a given patient without first applying NIV and assessing the patient's tolerance to the device. Initial application of NIV requires careful instruction of the patient, with a goal to gain the patient's confidence and acceptance of NIV. You must start with low pressures and the mask should be held and not strapped to the patient's face. As the patient accepts the NIV, pressures are increased to reach the gas exchange goal, but generally should not exceed 20–25 cm H_2O to minimize gastric distension and the risk of vomiting.[24] Although time consuming, the cost savings are large compared with the alternative, i.e., invasive ventilation.

What should be the Interface?

The masks most commonly used for short-term applications of NIV include nasal or oronasal (also called full face) masks. Although the nasal mask is theoretically more comfortable for the patient as it is less claustrophobic, has lower dead space volume, permits speech and eating, and better mobilization of secretions; oronasal masks achieve better control of mouth leak in mouth breathers (common feature during acute respiratory failure) and result in better quality of ventilation, in terms of improved minute ventilation and blood gas pressures.[25]

In a study of 70 patients with acute respiratory failure randomized to receive a nasal or oronasal mask, both the masks performed similarly with regard to improvements in gas exchange and avoidance of intubation; however, the nasal mask was less well tolerated because of excessive mouth leaks probably because mouth leaks with nasal CPAP lead to high unidirectional nasal airflow and increased nasal resistance. From the available evidence it cannot be said that any interface is clearly superior to another in terms of important outcomes such as intubation rate or mortality. Thus, a sensible approach would be to start with an oronasal mask for most patients with acute respiratory failure, and switch to a nasal mask if prolonged use is contemplated. Whichever mask is chosen, a comfortable fit is of paramount importance, and thus using a mask of proper size, not strapping the headgear too tightly, and using wound care tape on the bridge of the nose are important considerations to avoid pressure ulcers.

Does the Type of Ventilator Make any Difference?

Noninvasive ventilation can be delivered through ventilators designed for invasive mechanical ventilation ("critical care ventilators") and portable devices. Critical care ventilators are less leak tolerant and are thus likely to sound alarms more inappropriately. But the monitoring capabilities and presence of oxygen blenders make it superior to portable devices. On the other hand, the portable ventilators are more leak tolerant and less likely to sound alarms inappropriately than the critical care ventilators. However, they may promote rebreathing by virtue of their single inspiratory and expiratory tubing minimized by assuring adequate expiratory pressure[26,27] and expiratory ports over the nasal bridge[28] also, most of the portable ventilators do not have an oxygen blender and supplemental oxygen is usually given by adding it into the mask or the circuit. Thus continuous pulse oximetry is required to monitor oxygenation when using this device in patients with CPE. However, comparisons of the two devices show that the portable device performs as well as the critical care ventilators. Recently, ventilators that deliver either invasive ventilation or NIV have been designed. When in the non-invasive mode, they are more leak tolerant and use only the alarms essential for the operation of NIV. On the other hand, newer portable devices with graphic monitors, oxygen blenders, and sophisticated alarms have also become available for use in the acute setting.

CONCLUSION

There is a strong evidence for the use of CPAP by facemask in patients with CPE, and CPAP decreases the need for endotracheal intubation and improves survival. However, there is insufficient evidence to recommend the use of BiPAP, probably the exception being patients with hypercapnic CPE. Although evidence suggests that patients presenting with CPE are more likely to survive to hospital discharge if treated with CPAP, rather than with BiPAP, and probably there is no relation between early physiological changes and hospital survival, the evidence is not strong so as to completely exclude BiPAP, and more studies are required to elucidate the role of BiPAP in CPE.

REFERENCES

1. Brochard L, Mancebo J, Elliott MW. Noninvasive ventilation for acute respiratory failure. Eur Respir J. 2002;19(4):712-21.

2. Chadda K, Annane D, Hart N, Gajdos P, Raphaël JC, Lofaso F. Cardiac and respiratory effects of continuous positive airway pressure and noninvasive ventilation in acute cardiogenic pulmonary edema. Crit Care Med. 2002;30(11):2457-61.
3. Cotter G, Moshkovitz Y, Milovanov O, Salah A, Blatt A, Krakover R, et al. Acute heart failure: a novel approach to its pathogenesis and treatment. Eur J Heart Fail. 2002;4(3):227-34.
4. Atherton JJ, Moore TD, Lele SS, Thomson HL, Galbraith AJ, Belenkie I, et al. Diastolic ventricular interaction in chronic heart failure. Lancet. 1997;349(9067):1720-4.
5. Sharp JT, Griffith GT, Bunnell IL, Greene DG. Ventilatory mechanics in pulmonary edema in man. J Clin Invest. 1958;37(1):111-17.
6. Aberman A, Fulop M. The metabolic and respiratory acidosis of acute pulmonary edema. Ann Intern Med. 1972;76(2):173-84.
7. Aubier M, Trippenbach T, Roussos C. Respiratory muscle fatigue during cardiogenic shock. J Appl Physiol. 1981;51(2):499-508.
8. Taylor RR, Covell JW, Sonnenblick EH, Ross J Jr. Dependence of ventricular distensibility on filling of the opposite ventricle. Am J Physiol. 1967;213(3):711-8.
9. Maughan WL, Kallman CH, Shoukas A. The effect of right ventricular filling on the pressure-volume relationship of the ejecting canine left ventricle. Circ Res. 1981;49(2):382-8.
10. Scharf SM, Brown R, Tow DE, Parisi AF. Cardiac effects of increased lung volume and decreased pleural pressure in man. J Appl Physiol. 1984;47(2):1237-45.
11. Aisanen IT, Rasanen J. Continuous positive airway pressure and supplemental oxygen in the treatment of cardiogenic pulmonary edema. Chest. 1987;92(3):481-5.
12. Poulton EP, Oxon DM. Left-sided heart failure with pulmonary edema: its treatment with the "pulmonary plus pressure machine". Lancet. 1936;6(18):981-3.
13. Bradley TD, Holloway RM, McLaughlin PR, Ross BL, Walters J, Liu PP. Cardiac output responses to continuous positive airway pressure in congestive heart failure. Am Rev Respir Dis. 1992;145: 377-82.
14. Hess DR. The evidence for noninvasive positive-pressure ventilation in the care of patients in acute respiratory failure: a systematic review of the literature. Respir Care. 2004;49(7):810-29.
15. Naughton MT, Rahman MA, Hara K, Floras JS, Bradley TD. Effect of continuous positive airway pressure on intrathoracic and left ventricular transmural pressures in patients with congestive heart failure. Circulation. 1995;91(6):1725-31.
16. Fessler HE, Brower RG, Wise RA, Permutt S. Mechanism of reduced LV afterload by systolic and diastolic pleural pressure. J Appl Physiol. 1988;65(3):1244-50.
17. Lenique F, Habis M, Lofaso F, Dubois-Randé JL, Harf A, Brochard L. Ventilatory and hemodynamic effects of continuous positive airway pressure in left heart failure. Am J Respir Crit Care Med. 1997;155(2):500-5.
18. Mehta S, Hill NS. Noninvasive ventilation. Am J Respir Crit Care Med. 2001;163(2):540-77.
19. Mehta S, Jay GD, Woolard RH, Hipona RA, Connolly EM, Cimini DM, et al. Randomized, prospective trial of bilevel versus continuous positive airway pressure in acute pulmonary edema. Crit Care Med. 1997;25(4):620-8.
20. Park M, Sangean MC, Volpe MDS, Feltrim MI, Nozawa E, Leite PF, et al. Randomized, prospective trial of oxygen, continuous positive airway pressure, and bilevel positive airway pressure by face mask in acute cardiogenic pulmonary edema. Crit Care Med. 2004;32(12):2407-15.
21. Bellone A, Monari A, Cortellaro F, Vettorello M, Arlati S, Coen D. Myocardial infarction rate in acute pulmonary edema: Noninvasive pressure support ventilation versus continuous positive airway pressure. Crit Care Med. 2004;32(9):1860-5.
22. Crane SD, Elliott MW, Gilligan P, Richards K, Gray AJ. Randomized controlled comparison of continuous positive airways pressure, bilevel non-invasive ventilation, and standard treatment in emergency department patients with acute cardiogenic pulmonary edema. Emerg Med J. 2004;21(2):155-61.

23. Poponick J, Renston J, Bennett R, Emerman CL. Use of a ventilatory support system (BiPAP) for acute respiratory failure in the emergency department. Chest. 1999;116(1):166-71.
24. Hess DR. The evidence for noninvasive positive-pressure ventilation in the care of patients in acute respiratory failure: a systematic review of the literature. Respir Care. 2004;49(7):810-29.
25. Navalesi P, Fanfulla F, Frigerio P, Gregoretti C, Nava S. Physiologic evaluation of noninvasive mechanical ventilation delivered with three types of masks in patients with chronic hypercapnic respiratory failure. Crit Care Med. 2000;28(6):1785-90.
26. Ferguson GT, Gilmartin M. CO_2 rebreathing during BiPAP ventilatory assistance. Am J Respir Crit Care Med. 1995;151(4):1126-35.
27. Lofaso F, Brochard L, Hang T, Lorino H, Harf A, Isabey D. Home versus intensive care pressure support devices. Experimental and clinical comparison. Am J Respir Crit Care Med. 1996;153(5):1591-9.
28. Saatci E, Miller DM, Stell IM, Lee KC, Moxham J. Dynamic dead space in face masks used with non-invasive ventilators: a lung model study. Eur Respir J. 2003;23(1):129-35.

Chapter 14

Noninvasive Ventilation in Acute Respiratory Distress Syndrome

Praveen Kumar G, Deepak Govil

■ INTRODUCTION

Conventional invasive mechanical ventilation is lifesaving intervention in patients with acute hypoxemic respiratory failure. Despite being lifesaving, it exposes the patient to multiple complications like ventilator-associated pneumonia, ventilator-induced lung injury, diaphragmatic dysfunction, thereby prolonging stay in the intensive care and adversely affecting outcomes. The use of noninvasive positive pressure ventilation (NIPPV) has improved clinical outcomes over the years, especially in patients of chronic obstructive pulmonary disease (COPD) with hypercapnic respiratory failure,[1] pulmonary edema of cardiac origin,[2] and in immunosuppressed patients.[3] The major impact of noninvasive ventilation (NIV) is avoidance of invasive mechanical ventilation and thereby preventing the complications. Albeit, the role of NIV in these settings is well established, its use in acute hypoxemic respiratory failure of noncardiac origin and acute respiratory distress syndrome (ARDS) has not been studied extensively. This is also reflected in the LUNG SAFE study, which showed that only 18% patients with ARDS were treated with NIV across the world.[4]

■ NONINVASIVE VENTILATION IN ACUTE RESPIRATORY DISTRESS SYNDROME

Application of positive pressure ventilation opens the collapsed alveoli and thereby increases the functional residual capacity. This increases the area of membrane for gas exchange. Also, positive pressure ventilation with positive end expiratory pressure (PEEP) prevents the collapse of recruited alveoli, thereby improving gas transfer. The potential benefits of NIV in patients with ARDS are described in **Box 1**.

> **Box 1:** Potential benefits of NIV in ARDS.
> ➢ Alveolar recruitment by positive end expiratory pressure (PEEP)
> ➢ Improve gas exchange and hypoxemia by positive pressure ventilation
> ➢ Unload the respiratory muscles, reduce work of breathing and relieve dyspnea
> ➢ Avoid endotracheal intubation, invasive ventilation, and associated complications

Noninvasive Ventilation in Acute Respiratory Distress Syndrome: Interface and Settings

Multiple interfaces are available for use with NIV. Face mask, nasal mask, and helmet are the most commonly used in the clinical practice. Use of face mask as an interface to deliver NIV has been associated with pressure ulcers, intolerance, and air leaks, thereby treatment failure. In a study comparing the efficacy of NIV delivered by helmet and facemask, Patel and his colleagues showed a significant reduction in need for intubation in helmet group. Patients in helmet group also had better outcomes in terms of ventilator-free days and mortality.[5] Authors of the study attributed the results to better tolerance in the helmet group. But a closer look into the study parameters shows that a significantly higher PEEP was set in helmet group and the driving pressure was less in the helmet group, emphasizing the usefulness of lung protective ventilation even with NIV. Albeit the use of helmet over face mask is associated with better tolerance, use of helmet is associated with higher dead space ventilation, and carbon dioxide rebreathing. Thus, while helmet is used, higher alveolar recruitment is needed to overcome rebreathing and dead space ventilation.

The use continuous positive airway pressure (CPAP) has been shown to reduce shunting and improve gas exchange in cardiogenic pulmonary edema. This has been associated with reduced work of breathing. Patients with ARDS have extremely high inspiratory drive which cannot be supported by noninvasive CPAP alone.[6] In patients with high inspiratory drive, if there is no reduction in work of breathing, it can lead to extremely high swings in transpulmonary pressure, thereby aggravating lung injury. Addition of pressure support above the CPAP helps in reducing the respiratory drive and unload the respiratory muscles. Caution should be exercised in using high levels of pressure support as it may increase the leaks around the interface and cause NIV failure.[6] In patients on NIV, pressure support should be appropriately adjusted to target a tidal volume of 6–8 mL/kg of predicted body weight (PBW). Higher tidal volumes of >9.5 mL/kg have been shown to be an independent predictor of impending NIV failure.[7] Lung protective ventilation with low tidal volume should be the preferred strategy in patients with ARDS, irrespective of mode of ventilation. **Box 2** summarizes the settings to be used in NIV in patients with ARDS.

Box 2: NIV in ARDS: Settings.

- *Interface*: Helmet is better tolerated than face mask.
- *CPAP with pressure support*: Plain CPAP should not be used. Appropriate pressure support to unload respiratory muscles.
- *Tidal volume*: Adjust pressure support to achieve a tidal volume of 6–8 mL/kg
- *PEEP*: Higher PEEP strategy, especially in patients using helmet as interface

Noninvasive Ventilation to Prevent Intubation in Acute Respiratory Distress Syndrome

Case reports and studies on successful use of CPAP in ARDS dates back to 1977,[8] but there were no uniform criteria in defining severity until 1994, when the American European Consensus Conference defined various categories of ARDS. In one of the earliest pilot studies on use of NIV in acute lung injury (ALI) and ARDS, Rocker et al.[9] showed that early use of NIV was associated with over 25% improvement in oxygenation levels. Use of NIV also prevented the need for endotracheal intubation in 6 out of 12 occasions. The authors also showed that this improvement was sustained only in those patients who had limited extrapulmonary organ failure (one or no extrapulmonary organ failure) at the time of initiation of NIV. Patients with multiorgan failure at the time of onset did not benefit from NIV. In a randomized controlled trial, comparing use of NIV with high oxygen by face mask for patients with acute hypoxemic respiratory failure, Ferrer et al. showed that use of NIV was associated with reduced rates of intubation and better outcomes in patients with hypoxemic respiratory failure. But in the subgroup of patients of ARDS, use of NIV did not reduce the rates of intubation and was associated with poorer outcomes.[10] In a multicenter trial, comparing the use of NIPPV, high flow nasal oxygen, and standard oxygen therapy in ARDS, the use of NIPPV was associated with higher needs for rescue intubation and invasive ventilation (50% in NIPPV group vs. 38% in high flow oxygen group and 47% in standard group), though it did not reach statistical significance. The trend for higher intubation rates persisted irrespective of severity of hypoxemia at enrolment.[11] In a meta-analysis of 540 patients, Agarwal et al. showed that use of NIV was associated with 50% success rate in terms of preventing intubation. Though the studies included in the meta-analysis did not have publication bias, there was significant heterogeneity in data, causing a shadow on the end result.[12] In a recent meta-analysis involving 128 patients of acute lung injury and ARDS, use of NIV reduced the incidence of endotracheal intubation in patients with mild-to-moderate ARDS, without any improvement in mortality outcomes. This meta-analysis did not include any study with severe ARDS.[13]

The current evidence does not support the routine use of NIV as a treatment strategy to prevent invasive ventilation in ARDS. It can be considered in highly selective patients, in centers experienced with use of NIV and with continuous and close monitoring. Invasive ventilation should not be delayed, if NIV fails to improve respiratory distress.

Severity of Acute Respiratory Distress Syndrome and Use of Noninvasive Ventilation

Noninvasive positive pressure ventilation has been successfully used in patients with mild ARDS. In a randomized trial of patients with mild ARDS, early use of NIPPV has been shown to reduce the progression to more severe forms of ARDS and thereby reducing the need for intubation and progression to multiple organ failures.[14] Patients with moderate-to-severe ARDS have extremely high inspiratory drive and use of NIV in this settings can cause high transpulmonary driving pressures, aggravating lung injury. There is no randomized control trial using NIV in patients with severe ARDS. In patients with moderate ARDS, lower ratio of blood oxygen to inspired oxygen ratio (P/F), <150 mm Hg, has been associated with higher chances of NIV failure and increased mortality (36.2% in NIV group vs. 24.7% in invasive ventilation group).[4]

The current data does not support the use of NIV in severe ARDS. NIV can be used in patients with mild ARDS, with close monitoring for progression and need for intubation.

Noninvasive Ventilation in Immunocompromised Host with De Novo Acute Respiratory Distress Syndrome

With advancements in medical therapies, more and more immunocompromised patients are admitted to intensive care units. The use of invasive ventilation has been associated with increased mortality in this subset. In a pooled meta-analysis of 592 patients with de novo hypoxemic respiratory failure, use of NIV was associated with reduced need for intubation, length of stay in hospital, and short-term mortality.[15] Three of the studies included in meta-analysis included patients with moderate ARDS and were associated with better outcomes when compared to conventional oxygen therapy. In the secondary analysis of LUNG SAFE study of immunocompromised patients, use of NIV was higher as a first-line respiratory support.[16] The major cause for improved outcomes was due to avoidance of endotracheal intubation and invasive ventilation.

The current evidence supports the use of NIV as first-line respiratory support in immunocompromised patients with mild-to-moderate ARDS.

Predictors of Noninvasive Ventilation Failure in Acute Respiratory Distress Syndrome

The main risk of using NIV in ARDS is the delay in recognition of failure of NIV and thereby delay in intubation and initiation of invasive ventilation. Limited evidence exist in predicting failure of NIV in ARDS. In a multivariate analysis, Antonelli et al.[17] identified community-acquired pneumonia, ARDS, persistent hypoxemia after 1 hour of NIV (P/F ratio <146), age >40 years, and high organ failure scores (Simplified Acute Physiology Score II of >35) as independent predictors of NIV failure in patients presenting with acute hypoxemic respiratory failure. Patients with hemodynamic instability and multiorgan failure were not included in the study. In an observational study involving 54 patients with ARDS, use of NIPPV was associated with failure in over two-thirds of the patients. Severity of hypoxemia, hemodynamic instability, and presence of metabolic acidosis were identified as independent predictors of treatment failure. Patients who failed NIV had longer stay in intensive care unit and had higher mortality.[18] In a small observational cohort, presence of bacteremia and sepsis with positive blood cultures was shown to be associated with higher incidence of NIV failure.[19] NIV failure has been associated with higher mortality in patients with ARDS. Various factors which are associated with failure of NIV in ARDS are summarized in **Box 3**.

Box 3: Predictors of NIV failure in ARDS.
- Hemodynamic instability
- Severity of hypoxemia (Moderate and severe ARDS)
- Persistent hypoxia after 1 hour of NIPPV (P/F ratio <150)
- Tidal volume of >9.5 mL/kg
- More than one extrapulmonary organ failure
- Severity of the disease (Higher organ dysfunction scores)
- Bacteremia
- Metabolic acidosis
- Age >40 years

Noninvasive Ventilation in Acute Respiratory Distress Syndrome: Stepwise Approach

A simplified algorithm-based approach for use of NIV in ARDS is described in **Flowchart 1**.

■ CONCLUSION

The primary goal of using NIV in ARDS is to improve oxygenation and relieve dyspnea. Though NIV can be considered as a modality in mild-to-moderate ARDS, to avoid invasive ventilation and associated complications, evidence in the literature is inconclusive and needs large randomized control trials in the future.

Chapter 14: Noninvasive Ventilation in Acute Respiratory Distress Syndrome

Flowchart 1: Simplified approach for use of noninvasive ventilation (NIV) in acute respiratory distress syndrome (ARDS).

```
Patient with ARDS and hypoxemic respiratory failure
                        ↓
        Conventional contraindications for NIV
                        │
                        │  → Low Glasgow Coma Score
                        │    Severe hemodynamic instability
                        │    High risk of aspiration
                        │    Uncooperative patient
                        │
            No                        Yes
             ↓                         ↓
```

- P/F ratio <150 mm Hg at onset
- More than one extra pulmonary organ failure
- Severe metabolic acidosis
- Hemodynamic instability

→ Yes → Invasive ventilation

No ↓

If any of these is present

Can consider NIV with following settings
- PSV (pressure support ventilation) with high PEEP
- Pressure support to target TV of 6 to 8 mL/kg

Reassess after 1 hour of NIV

- Improved oxygenation
- Respiratory rate (RR) <25/min
- Tidal volume 6 to 8 mL/kg

↓

Continue noninvasive ventilation with close monitoring for features of NIV failure

- P/F ratio <150 mm Hg
- New organ failures
- No unloading of respiratory muscles (RR >25/min)
- Hemodynamic instability
- Tidal volume >9 mL/kg

The treating team should always be ready to initiate invasive mechanical ventilation and it should not be delayed under any circumstances

REFERENCES

1. Ram F, Picot J, Lightowler J, Wedzicha J. Noninvasive positive pressure ventilation for treatment of respiratory failure due to exacerbations of chronic obstructive pulmonary disease. Cochrane Database Syst Rev. 2004;(1):CD004104.
2. Vital FM, Saconato H, Ladeira MT, Sen A, Hawkes CA, Soares B, et al. Noninvasive positive pressure ventilation (CPAP or bilevel NPPV) for cardiogenic pulmonary edema. Cochrane Database Syst Rev. 2008;(3):CD005351.
3. Hilbert G, Gruson D, Vargas F, Valentino R, Gbikpi-Benissan G, Dupon M, et al. Noninvasive ventilation in immunosuppressed patients with pulmonary infiltrates, fever, and acute respiratory failure. N Engl J Med. 2001;344(7):481-7.

4. Bellani G, Laffey JG, Pham T, Madotto F, Fan E, Brochard L, et al. Noninvasive Ventilation of Patients with Acute Respiratory Distress Syndrome: Insights from the LUNG SAFE Study. Am J Respir Crit Care Med. 2017;195(1):67-77.
5. Patel BK, Wolfe KS, Pohlman AS, Hall JB, Kress JP. Effect of noninvasive ventilation delivered by helmet vs face mask on the rate of endotracheal intubation in patients with acute respiratory distress syndrome a randomized clinical trial. JAMA. 2016;315(22):2435-41.
6. L'Her E, Deye N, Lellouche F, Taille S, Demoule A, Fraticelli A, et al. Physiologic effects of noninvasive ventilation during acute lung injury. Am J Respir Crit Care Med. 2005;172(9):1112-8.
7. Carteaux G, Millán-Guilarte T, De Prost N, Razazi K, Abid S, Thille AW, et al. Failure of noninvasive ventilation for de novo acute hypoxemic respiratory failure: role of tidal volume. Crit Care Med. 2016;44(2):282-90.
8. Shah DM, Newell JC, Dutton RE, Powers SR. Continuous positive airway pressure versus positive end-expiratory pressure in respiratory distress syndrome. J Thorac Cardiovasc Surg. 1977;74(4):557-62.
9. Rocker GM, Mackenzie MG, Williams B, Logan PM. Noninvasive positive pressure ventilation. Successful outcome in patients with acute lung injury/ARDS. Chest. 1999;115(1):173-7.
10. Ferrer M, Esquinas A, Leon M, Gonzalez G, Alarcon A, Torres A. Noninvasive Ventilation in Severe Hypoxemic Respiratory Failure. Am J Respir Crit Care Med. 2003;168(12):1438-44.
11. Frat JP, Thille AW, Mercat A, Girault C, Ragot S, Perbet S, et al. High-flow oxygen through nasal cannula in acute hypoxemic respiratory failure. N Engl J Med. 2015;372(23):2185-96.
12. Agarwal R, Aggarwal AN, Gupta D. Role of noninvasive ventilation in acute lung injury/acute respiratory distress syndrome: a proportion meta-analysis. Respir Care. 2010;55(12):1653-60.
13. Luo J, Wang MY, Zhu H, Liang BM, Liu D, Peng XY, et al. Can non-invasive positive pressure ventilation prevent endotracheal intubation in acute lung injury/acute respiratory distress syndrome? A meta-analysis. Respirology. 2014;19(8):1149-57.
14. Zhan Q, Sun B, Liang L, Yan X, Zhang L, Yang J, et al. Early use of noninvasive positive pressure ventilation for acute lung injury: a multicenter randomized controlled trial. Crit Care Med. 2012;40(2):455-60.
15. Huang H Bin, Xu B, Liu GY, Lin JD, Du B. Use of noninvasive ventilation in immunocompromised patients with acute respiratory failure: a systematic review and meta-analysis. Crit Care. 2017;21(1).
16. Cortegiani A, Madotto F, Gregoretti C, Bellani G, Laffey JG, Pham T, et al. Immunocompromised patients with acute respiratory distress syndrome: secondary analysis of the LUNG SAFE database. Crit Care. 2018;22(1).
17. Antonelli M, Conti G, Moro M, Esquinas A, Gonzalez-Diaz G, Confalonieri M, et al. Predictors of failure of noninvasive positive pressure ventilation in patients with acute hypoxemic respiratory failure: a multi-center study. Intensive Care Med. 2001;27(11):1718-28.
18. Rana S, Jenad H, Gay PC, Buck CF, Hubmayr RD, Gajic O. Failure of non-invasive ventilation in patients with acute lung injury: observational cohort study. Crit Care. 2006;10(3).
19. Domenighetti G, Moccia A, Gayer R. Observational case-control study of non-invasive ventilation in patients with ARDS. Monaldi Arch Chest Dis - Pulm Ser. 2008;69(1):5-10.

Chapter 15

Role of Noninvasive Ventilation in Postoperative Cases

Prasad Padwal, Rahul Pandit

BACKGROUND

Postoperative respiratory failure due to any surgery is a result of anesthesia, postoperative pain with diaphragmatic dysfunction associated with both thoracic and abdominal surgeries.

Hypoxemic respiratory failure is a result of lung volume reduction and atelectasis, and hypercapnic respiratory failure is due to muscle fatigue.[1]

Both continuous positive airway pressure (CPAP) and bilevel noninvasive positive pressure ventilation (NPPV) play important role in postoperative period post extubation for respiratory failure, which further prevents intubation and eventually shortens time on mechanical ventilation, prevents nosocomial infections, and significant morbidity and mortality after surgery.[2]

Noninvasive ventilation (NIV) is suggested for patients with postoperative acute respiratory failure.

Explanation

Noninvasive ventilation is a tool which acts against pathophysiological mechanisms leading to respiratory failure especially for thoracic and abdominal surgeries more than cardiac surgeries. Cumulative analysis explains that NIV reduces reintubation (RR 0.27, 95% CI 0.12–0.61; low certainty), decreases mortality (RR 0.28, 95% CI 0.009–0.84; moderate certainty), and reduces possibility of nosocomial pneumonia (RR 0.20, 95% CI 0.004–0.88; very low certainty) in postoperative respiratory failure condition.

ROLE OF NIV IN ABDOMINAL SURGERY

Multicenter randomized controlled trial (RCT) published by Jaber et al. included 298 patients with hypoxemic respiratory failure post-abdominal surgery, compared use of NIV versus standard oxygen therapy, and explained reduced risk of ventilator associated pneumonia (31% vs 49%; $p = 0.003$) and reduced risk of reintubation within 7 days (46% vs 33%; $p = 0.03$) with NIV use.[3]

An another prospective observational study by Jaber et al. explained avoiding reintubation in 67% and improving mortality by reducing hospital stay.[4] Antonelli et al. explained improving oxygenation with use of NIV and reduced reintubation compared with conventional therapy in solid organ transplant patients.[5]

This recommends use of NIV in post-abdominal surgeries with acute respiratory failure (Low quality evidence).

ROLE OF NIV IN BARIATRIC SURGERY

Obesity is a significant risk factor for developing obstructive sleep apnea (OSA). Approximately 27–70% of patients undergoing bariatric surgery show coexistence of OSA.[6-8]

Kaw et al. explained that patients with obesity hypoventilation syndrome with or without OSA are more likely to develop postoperative complications including respiratory failure. Resulting into increasing use of NIV in postoperative condition to overcome OSA or obesity hypoventilation syndrome.

Both Gaszynski et al.[9] and Pessoa et al.[10] have shown that NIV improves oxygenation in postoperative obese patients. Wongetal et al.[11] compared the use of the CPAP mask with the standard air-entrainment mask and found improving oxygenation but no difference in postoperative %FEV_1 and %FVC.

In this large observational study by Mihaela S Stefan et al., of more than 5,000 patients with OSA and planned for bariatric surgery, one out of five patients received NIV on the day of or the day after surgery. Early use of NIV in postoperative period does not improve outcomes, including chances of reintubation, mortality, and hospital length of stay.[12]

Two single-center retrospective cohort studies presented one of patients undergoing Roux-en-Y bypass and the other patients undergoing gastric banding surgeries and did not show any benefit of NIV in postoperative period.[13,14]

Systemic review of literature by Tong S et al. explained there is no increased anastomotic dehiscence risk when NIV is administered during immediate post-bariatric surgery.[15]

This recommends use of NIV in post-bariatric surgery patients with pre-existent OSA or obesity hypoventilation syndrome.

ROLE OF NIV IN SPINAL SURGERY

Noninvasive ventilation is widely used in the treatment of acute respiratory failure secondary to neuromuscular disease,[16] thoracoplasty, and scoliosis[17] with benefits including improved oxygenation, improved quality of life, and decreased hospital stay.[18,19] Acute respiratory failure can develop following corrective surgery for scoliosis, especially in those patients with poor preoperative pulmonary function.

In patients undergoing surgery for neuromuscular weakness or scoliosis, use of postoperative NIV facilitate pulmonary rehabilitation.[20]

This recommends use of NIV in post-spinal surgery patients for acute respiratory failure also for facilitation of respiratory outcome.

ROLE OF NIV IN THORACIC SURGERY

In cardiothoracic surgeries, deterioration of pulmonary function is a frequent postoperative complication and remains a significant cause of postoperative mortality.[21] Impaired oxygenation is primarily attributed to a decrease in functional residual capacity in about 70% of patients post-thoracotomy.[22]

In case of postoperative lung resection, NIV significantly reduced need of reintubation and reduced mortality demonstrated in RCT of Auriant I et al.[23]

Post-cardiothoracic surgery, among 830 patients with or at risk for respiratory failures, use of high flow nasal cannula therapy compared with intermittent NIV did not result in worse rate of treatment failure defined as need for reintubation in Stéphan et al. study.[24]

Meta-analysis of 14 trials by Guangfa Zhu et al. included 1,740 patients explained that NIV had no significant effect in the treatment of patients after cardiothoracic surgery. But NIV improved oxygenation and reduced chances of reintubation.[25]

Noninvasive ventilation in early esophageal surgery is a relative contraindication for application of positive pressure at high level[26] with and risk of loss of integrity esophageal sutures.[27]

In cardiothoracic surgeries, use of NIV is recommended post operatively for acute respiratory failure to improve oxygenation and reduce chance of reintubation.

ROLE OF NIV IN POST-LUNG TRANSPLANT

During postoperative period of lung transplant graft- and recipient-related respiratory difficulty requiring mechanical ventilation is common scenario which can present in hours to days. Prolonged intubation in these immunocompromised patients is one of the main predisposing factors for developing nosocomial pneumonia, leading to prolonged ICU stay with significant morbidity and mortality. Noninvasive mechanical ventilation is recommended for shorten weaning time and to avoid reintubation following lung transplantation.

Rapid extubation plus prompt NIV application is a useful strategy for lung recipients who do not completely fulfil the criteria for safe extubation.

Noninvasive mechanical ventilation is recommended for shorten weaning time and to avoid reintubation following lung transplantation.[28]

ROLE OF NIV IN ATELECTASIS

Most common postoperative lung condition is atelectasis, affecting oxygenation.

Atelectasis is mainly due to postoperative diaphragmatic dysfunction and diminished surfactant activity. After induction of anesthesia, atelectasis increases by 1–11% of total lung volume. CPAP is often used to prevent or treat postoperative atelectasis.

In postoperative condition, postextubation bilevel NIV significantly improves oxygenation without affecting hemodynamic by reducing atelectasis.[1]

Significant atelectasis is with radiological score ≥2 after tracheal extubation.

The Radiological Atelectasis Score was defined according to Richter et al.:[29]

0, clear lung field; 1, plate-like atelectasis or slight infiltration; 2, partial atelectasis; 3, lobar atelectasis; and 4, bilateral lobar atelectasis.

Reinius et al. study demonstrated that combined use of recruitment with positive end expiratory pressure reduced atelectasis to 3–4%, with improving oxygenation.[30]

Role of NIV postoperatively is recommended to treat atelectasis and improve oxygenation.

REFERENCES

1. Jaber S, Chanques G, Jung B. Postoperative noninvasive ventilation. Anaesthesiology. 2010;112(2):453-61.
2. Rochwerg B, Brochard L, Elliott MW, Hess D, Hill NS, Nava S, et al. Official ERS/ATS clinical practice guidelines: noninvasive ventilation for acute respiratory failure. Eur Respir J. 2017;50(2):1602426.
3. Jaber S, Lescot T, Futier E, Paugam-Burtz C, Seguin P, Ferrandiere M, et al. Effect of noninvasive ventilation on tracheal reintubation among patients with hypoxemic respiratory failure following abdominal surgery; randomised clinical trial. JAMA. 2016;315(13):1345-53.
4. Jaber S, Delay JM, Chanques G, Sebbane M, Jacquet E, Souche B, et al. Outcome of patients with acute respiratory failure after abdominal surgery treated with non-invasive positive pressure ventilation. Chest. 2005;128(4):2688-2695.

5. Antonelli M, Conti G, Bufi M, Costa MG, Lappa A, Rocco M, et al. Noninvasive ventilation for treatment of acute respiratory failure in patients undergoing solid organ transplantation: a randomized trial. JAMA. 2000;283(2):235-41.
6. Romero-Corral A, Caples SM, Lopez-Jimenez F, Somers VK. Interactions between obesity and obstructive sleep apnea: implications for treatment. Chest. 2010;137(3):711-9.
7. Lopez PP, Stefan B, Schulman CI, Byers PM. Prevalence of sleep apnea in morbidly obese patients who presented for weight loss surgery evaluation: more evidence for routine screening for obstructive sleep apnea before weight loss surgery. Am Surg. 2008;74(9):834-8.
8. Sareli AE, Cantor CR, Williams NN, Korus G, Raper SE, Pien G, et al. Obstructive sleep apnea in patients undergoing bariatric surgery—a tertiary center experience. Obes Surg. 2011;21(3):316-27.
9. Gaszynski T, Tokarz A, Piotrowski D, Machala W. Boussignac CPAP in the postoperative period in morbidly obese patients. Obes Surg. 2007;17(4):452-6.
10. Pessoa KC, Araujo GF, Pinheiro AN, Ramos MR, Maia SC. Noninvasive ventilation in the immediate postoperative of gastrojejunal derivation with Roux-en-Y gastric bypass. Rev Bras Fisioter. 2010;14(4):290-5.
11. Wong DT, Adly E, Ip HY, Thapar S, Maxted GR, Chung FF. A comparison between the Boussignac continuous positive airway pressure mask and the venturi mask in terms of improvement in the $PaO_2/F(I)O_2$ ratio in morbidly obese patients undergoing bariatric surgery: a randomized controlled trial. Can J Anaesth. 2011;58(6):532-9
12. Stefan MS, Hill NS, Raghunathan K, Liu X, Pekow PS, Memtsoudis SG, et al. Outcomes associated with early postoperative non-invasive ventilation in bariatric surgical patients with sleep apnea. J Clin Sleep Med. 2016;12(11):1507-16.
13. Jensen C, Tejirian T, Lewis C, Yadegar J, Dutson E, Mehran A. Postoperative CPAP and BiPAP use can be safely omitted after laparoscopic Roux-en-Y gastric bypass. Surg Obes Relat Dis. 2008;4(4):512-4.
14. Kurrek MM, Cobourn C, Wojtasik Z, Kiss A, Dain SL. Morbidity in patients with or at high risk for obstructive sleep apnea after ambulatory laparoscopic gastric banding. Obes Surg. 2011;21(10):1494-8.
15. Tong S, Gower J, Morgan A, Gadbois K, Wisbach G. Noninvasive positive pressure ventilation in the immediate post-bariatric surgery care of patients with obstructive sleep apnea: a systematic review. Surg Obes Relat Dis. 2017;13(7):1227-33.
16. Ellis ER, Bye PT, Bruderer JW, Sullivan CE. Treatment of respiratory failure during sleep in patients with neuromuscular disease. Am Rev Respir Dis. 1987;135(1):148-52.
17. Ellis ER, Grunstein RR, Chan S, Bye PT, Sullivan CE. Noninvasive ventilatory support during sleep improves respiratory failure in kyphoscoliosis. Chest. 1988;94(4):811-5.
18. Leger P, Bedicam JM, Cornette A, Reybet-Degat O, Langevin B, Polu JM, et al. Nasal intermittent positive pressure ventilation; Long term follow up in patients with severe chronic respiratory insufficiency. Chest. 1994;105(1):100-5.
19. Simmonds AK, Elliott MW. Outcome of domiciliary nasal intermittent positive pressure ventilation in restrictive and obstructive disorders. Thorax. 1995;50(6):604-9.
20. Khirani S, Bersanini C, Aubertin G, Bachy M, Vialle R, Fauroux B. Non-invasive positive pressure ventilation to facilitate the post-operative respiratory outcome of spine surgery in neuromuscular children. Eur Spine J. 2014;23 Suppl 4:S406-11.
21. Weiss YG, Merin G, Koganov E, Ribo A, Oppenheim-Eden A, Medalion B, et al. Postcardiopulmonary bypass hypoxemia: a prospective study on incidence, risk factors, and clinical significance. J Cardiothorac Vasc Anesth. 2000;14(5):506-13.
22. Tenling A, Hachenberg T, Tydén H, Wegenius G, Hedenstierna G. Atelectasis and gas exchange after cardiac surgery. Anesthesiology. 1998;89(2):371-8.
23. Auriant I, Jallot A, Hervé P, Cerrina J, Le Roy Ladurie F, Fournier JL, et al. Noninvasive ventilation reduces mortality in acute respiratory failure after lung resection. Am J Respir Crit Med. 2001;164(7):1231-5.
24. Stéphan F, Barrucand B, Petit P, Rézaiguia-Delclaux S, Médard A, Delannoy B, et al High flow nasal oxygen vs noninvasive positive pressure in hypoxemic patients after cardiothoracic surgery: a randomised clinical trial. JAMA. 2015;313(23):2331-9.

25. Zhu G, Huang Y, Wei D, Shi Y. Efficacy and safety of noninvasive ventilation in patients after cardiothoracic surgery. Medicine (Baltimore). 2016;95(38):e4734.
26. Jean-Lavaleur M, Perrier V, Roze H, Sarrabay P, Fleureau C, Janvier G. Stomach rupture associated with noninvasive ventilation. Ann Fr Anesth Reanim. 2009;28(6):588-91.
27. Van de Louw A, Brocas E, Boiteau R, Perrin-Gachadoat D, Tenaillon A. Esophageal perforation associated with noninvasive ventilation: a case report. Chest. 2002;122(5):1857-8.
28. Feltracco P, Serra E, Barbieri S, Milevoj M, Furnari M, Rizzi S, et al. Noninvasive ventilation in postoperative care of lung transplant recipients. Transplant Proc. 2009;41(4):1339-44.
29. Richter Larsen K, Ingwersen U, Thode S, Jakobsen S. Mask physiotherapy in patients after heart surgery: a controlled study. Intensive Care Med. 1995;21(6):469-74.
30. Reinius H, Jonsson L, Gustafsson S, Sundbom M, Duvernoy O, Pelosi P, et al. Prevention of atelectasis in morbidly obese patients during general anesthesia and paralysis: a computerized tomography study. Anesthesiology. 2009;111(5):979-87.

Chapter 16

Noninvasive Ventilation in Obstructive Sleep Apnea

Kapil Zirpe, Kapil S Borawake

OBSTRUCTIVE SLEEP APNEA

Obstructive sleep apnea (OSA) is a disorder associated with sleep characterized by impaired ventilation during sleep and disruption of sleep. The apnea and hypopnea episodes are feature of OSA, which is due to collapse of upper airway. This leads to excessive daytime sleepiness impair daytime function, increased insulin resistance which may cause type II diabetes mellitus (DM), impaired glucose tolerance, and dyslipidemia. It increases the risk for cardiovascular events, chronic kidney disease, and mortality.[1]

Symptoms and signs do not predict severity in OSA but this is done by objective assessment of breathing during sleep. The gold standard is overnight polysomnography (PSG).[1,2]

Following things are seen in sleep study **(Table 1)**:
- Measurement of breathing (Changes in airflow, respiratory excursions)
- Oxygenation
- Body position
- Cardiac rhythm

Table 1: Symptoms and signs of obstructive sleep apnea.	
AHI (apnea–hypopnea index)	Number of apneas and hypopneas episodes in 1 hour of sleep.
RERA (respiratory effort-related arousals)	Partially obstructed breaths.
RDI (respiratory disturbance index)	Number of apnea, hypopneas, and RERA per hour sleep.

Classification (Table 2)

Table 2: Classification of OSA.	
Mild OSA	Apnea hypopnea 5–14 in 1 hour duration sleep
Moderate OSA	Apnea hypopnea 15–29 in 1 hour duration sleep
Severe OSA—AHI	>30 apnea hypopnea events in 1 hour duration sleep

(AHI: apnea–hypopnea index; OSA; obstructive sleep apnea)

Goals of Management

OSA is chronic disease that requires long-term multidisciplinary management.

Chapter 16: Noninvasive Ventilation in Obstructive Sleep Apnea

The goals of OSA therapy are resolution of signs and symptoms of OSA leading to following:
- Sleep quality improvement
- To reduce apnea–hypopnea index (AHI) to near normal, i.e., less than 5
- Oxyhemoglobin saturation levels improvement to near normal[1]
- To reduce the cardiovascular events which ultimately will the cost or treatment and burden on healthcare system.

In All the patients with confirmed OSA, positive airway pressure (PAP) as initial therapy is recommended as per guidelines from various societies.[1,2]

POSITIVE AIRWAY PRESSURE THERAPY

The gold standard therapy for adults with OSA is PAP therapy.

The continuous positive airway pressure (CPAP) is responsible for maintaining positive pharyngeal transmural pressure, which ultimately increases intramural pressure as compared to surrounding pressure. The increase in end-expiratory lung volume by CPAP stabilizes the upper airway. This helps to prevent upper airway collapse and apneas and hypopneas episodes.[3]

Efficacy

The randomized trials and meta-analyses, which has high-quality evidence proven that PAP therapy reduces the frequency of apneas hypopneas during sleep, reduction in daytime sleepiness, reduction in blood pressure (BP), lessens erectile dysfunction, and improves quality of life.

It also improves symptoms of gastroesophageal reflux, heart failure incidences, and reduction in nocturnal arrhythmias and recurrent atrial fibrillation.[4]

CPAP is effective than MADs (mandibular advancement devices) and is most effective at reducing AHI. It is also more effective in total reduction of respiratory events and its severity in sleep. It is also better in reducing oxyhemoglobin desaturations episodes during sleep.

Even after multiple observational studies, no mortality benefit from PAP therapy. The impact of CPAP on body weight is not very clear.[5,6]

Indications

Indications of OSA are given in **Table 3**.

Table 3: Indications of OSA.	
1	Patients with AHI > 5 events per hour of sleep and one or more clinical or physiologic effects which are due to OSA.
2	Patients with AHI ≥ 15 event per hour of sleep even if patient is asymptomatic
3	The workers like drivers on bus or truck, pilots, and airport controllers (responsible for life of many)—AHI between 5 and 15 events per hour of sleep without even clinical or physiological symptoms due to OSA
4	AHI is ≤ 5 events per hour sleep and patient has excessive daytime sleepiness with RERAs > 10 per hour.

(AHI: apnea–hypopnea index; OSA: obstructive sleep apnea; RERA: respiratory effort-related arousal)

Modes of Administration

Modes of administration of OSA are given in **Table 4**. CPAP is recommended as therapy to begin with by most studies.

Table 4: Modes of administration of OSA.	
1	CPAP means continuous positive airway pressure
2	BIPAP means bilevel positive airway pressure
3	APAP means auto-titrating positive airway pressure
CPAP	In this machine delivers positive airway pressure which remains *constant* through the respiratory cycle. It is most used and the most extensively evaluated by studies. It also has the most clinical experience and is the simplest.
BIPAP	In this machine delivers a *preset* inspiratory positive airway pressure (IPAP) and expiratory positive airway pressure (EPAP). The difference between the IPAP and EPAP is responsible amount of tidal volume and degree of pressure support.
APAP	Variable degree of positive airway pressure (increases or decreases) depending on change in flow of air, a change in pressure of the circuit, or change in upper airway resistance like snore
Adaptive servo ventilation (ASV)	In this machine provides a low level of CPAP with a *varying amount of inspiratory pressure*. Is if of help for patients with associated central apneas, patients on long-acting sedatives and patients who have had renal or cerebrovascular disease.

Initiation of Positive Airway Pressure Therapy

The selection of a mode of PAP, device setting(s), and a patient-device interface is required for initiation of therapy.[7]

■ MODES OF POSITIVE AIRWAY PRESSURE

Continuous positive airway pressure and bilevel positive airway pressure (BIPAP) are the modalities most frequently used.

CPAP simplest, cheap, and most studied, and is preferred for most patients. Both of these have fixed or auto-titrating technology.[8]

Selecting the Mode

Fixed CPAP—initial treatment as its efficacy is established and supported by extensive clinical studies. In-home auto-titrating CPAP (APAP) is useful for uncomplicated OSA patients. Its efficacy is comparable but it is more expensive.

BIPAP is rarely indicated as first-line therapy. The patients who may benefit from a trial of BIPAP include patients with coexisting OSA and chronic hypersonic respiratory failure (obesity hypoventilation syndrome who are unresponsive to CPAP therapy), with neuromuscular disorder leading to hypoventilation and chronic opioid users. OSA plus central sleep apnea (CSA; including those with OSA and treatment-emergent CSA) may respond spontaneous-timed (S-T) BIPAP.

Auto-titrating BIPAP is useful for OSA patients, who do not tolerate fixed or APAP. Due to technical considerations concerning auto-titrating these complicated devices to used only after confirming efficacy during an overnight PSG. Auto-titrating BPAP in uncomplicated OSA has very less value.[9,10]

Continuous Positive Airway Pressure

Fixed CPAP

It delivers PAP level that remains relatively constant (within 1–2 cm of H_2O) through entire respiratory cycle. The upper airways are splinted and kept open by PAP thus preventing upper airway collapse or narrowing during sleep. Patients must initiate every breath and additional pressure above the level of CPAP is not provided. The optimal amount of PAP delivered by a fixed CPAP device must be determined by titration. There are various methods like manually done in the sleep laboratory, as part of a full night or split-night study, or at home using an APAP device.[10,11]

Auto-titrating CPAP

In this variable amount of PAP is delivered during night. The variation is dependent on event detection software algorithms.

In response to flow changes, the pressure gradually increased up to level till adequate patency is achieved. It leads to period where sustained upper airway patency is kept. After this, the delivered level of pressure gradually decreases and reaches to the point where the algorithm again identifies recurrent upper airway obstruction. On identification point, the delivered pressure again increased. That is the reason the lowest pressure required to keep airway patency varies.[11,12]

The event detection algorithms used vary considerably among manufacturers and successive production versions of a given device. This leads to changes in performance of the APAP devices making it is highly variable.

APAP does not function properly, if a significant leak exists as leak causes changes in airflow. Newer fixed or auto-titrating flow generators (both CPAP and BIPAP) will estimate the AHI

APAP has being suggested in three different situations:
1. As a pressure-relief strategy for patients who are unable to tolerate the CPAP required to prevent apnea and hypopnea events in all sleep positions and all sleep stages. The device delivers higher pressures in supine and/or in rapid eye movement (REM) sleep and otherwise low pressure.
2. Patients who have nasal congestion from allergies or nasal obstruction due to infections in upper respiratory tract. Patients with high-body weight, in REM sleep and in supine position.
3. Patients in whom CPAP titration is difficult due to some reason or delayed.

Choosing between Fixed and Auto-titrating CPAP

There is little difference in the use of fixed or APAP in comparison with efficacy or adherence in patients with OSA particularly moderate to severe OSA and are uncomplicated.

Patients with suspected or proven comorbid sleep disorders (e.g., narcolepsy, severe insomnia, parasomnia, and movement disorders to be cautiously used).

The patients who has moderate to severe OSA (uncomplicated) can be effectively treated with APAP after a diagnosis of OSA is made by home sleep apnea testing (HSAT). Patients who do not improve clinically after initiation of APAP without a titration study should undergo careful reevaluation with consideration of an attended PAP titration.[12]

Bi-level Positive Airway Pressure

In this, PAP is delivered during inspiration and expiration at different levels.

Inspiratory positive airway pressure (IPAP) is amount of pressure delivered during inspiration and expiratory positive airway pressure (EPAP) is pressure delivered during expiration.

BIPAP splints the upper airway open by the same way as by CPAP, with the exception that the EPAP component is thought to be effective in suppressing frank obstructive apneas but IPAP primarily acts to prevent obstructive hypopneas, respiratory effort related arousals, and snoring.

BIPAP additionally provides pressure support (PS) through the pressure difference between EPAP and IPAP.

In the spontaneous mode BIPAP (BPAP-S), breaths are provided only in response to patient inspiratory efforts.
- "Spontaneous" (S) mode—backup rate is not set in only S mode
- S-T mode—when both patient-initiated and backup breaths are possible
- "Timed" (T) mode—only preset back up breaths are delivered.

BIPAP in S-T mode is not a mode for OSA patients except when associated with CSA. Timed mode is for patients with hypoventilation and or with CSA like congenital central hypoventilation syndrome. It is useful in patients with neuromuscular disease or neurological disease leading to altered ventilation.

BIPAP has been considered as a "pressure-relief" therapy in patients who are unable to tolerate fixed CPAP.[13]

How to Determine the Amount of Positive Airway Pressure?

Optimal pressure means the amount of PAP that is acceptable to patient and which will prevent the recurrent upper airway obstruction in sleep. The pressure will be responsible to maintain sleep quality with improved oxyhemoglobin saturation.

Selecting the Pressure Settings

CPAP and BIPAP require engaging expiratory pressure relief and selecting the level of pressure relief. The use of BPAP devices has additional choices of mode (spontaneous or timed), inspiratory rise time and related timings (these relate to patient comfort when receiving a breath), and backup rate.

In an auto-titrating device, pressure range(s) must be chosen. If an auto-titrating BPAP flow generator of the adaptive servo ventilation (ASV) type is required for a patient with complex combinations of OSA and CSA, additional decision-making will be necessary in terms of whether to target peak inspiratory flow or minute ventilation (varies by device manufacturer) and fixed backup rate versus automatic setting of backup rate.[1,10,14]

Fixed CPAP

The optimal settings for fixed CPAP after laboratory PSG with the patient wearing their device.

It is recommended to start at a low level (4 cm H_2O), the amount of CPAP is serially increased (usually in increments of 1–2 cm H_2O) until evidence of upper airway obstruction is eliminated, allowing at least 5 minutes at each pressure. The minimal amount of CPAP that consistently prevents upper airway obstruction becomes the fixed CPAP setting. Clinical evidence of upper airway obstruction is signified by episodes of snoring, apneas, hypopneas, respiratory effort related arousals, and/or episodic oxyhemoglobin desaturation.

The optimal titration pressure is one which reduces frequency of respiratory events to <5 per hour for minimum 15 minutes and which includes supine (REM sleep, with few or no spontaneous arousals, or awakenings.

For adults the recommended maximum level of PAP is 20 cm H_2O.

Auto-titrating CPAP

Patients who are prescribed APAP as their initial mode of ongoing therapy may not need to undergo formal laboratory titration.

BIPAP

In BIPAP, two levels of PAP need to be set—EPAP and IPAP.

In a patient not previously titrated on PAP, initial IPAP is to be 8 cm of water and EPAP is set at 4 cm water. Both then serially increased by 1–2 cm H_2O, with at least 5 minutes at each pressure. PAP alone is titrated after that to in the same manner until obstructive hypopneas, respiratory effort related arousals, and snoring are eliminated.

In a patient previously titrated on CPAP, the starting EPAP can be set to the CPAP value that eliminated obstructive apneas during the previous use and the IPAP is set to a level 4 cm H_2O higher. In uncomplicated OSA, the minimum recommended IPAP-EPAP differential is 4 cm H_2O and the maximum difference is 10 cm H_2O.

After partial and complete upper airway obstruction is eliminated, the IPAP alone is increased, if additional ventilation is required. The recommended maximum IPAP level is 30 cm H_2O for adults.[1,10,13]

Titration Modality

During laboratory, PSG manual titration of fixed CPAP and BIPAP is performed incorporating all of the physiologic monitoring necessary to identify apneas (including recognition of obstructive versus central mechanisms), hypopneas, and respiration effort related wake up and snore episodes.

For the fixed CPAP titration, the sleep study is can be done at sleep lab as full-night PSG or as split-night PSG, or at home titration using APAP. BPAP titration is more complex and should never be guided by unattended, in-home portable monitoring.[1,7,10]

Full-night Studies

The gold standard approach for the initiation of CPAP and BPAP is PSG which is done full-night attended in sleep laboratory.

Split-night Studies

The split night study to be valid as recommended by American Academy of Sleep Medicine (AASM) must be done for at least a 2-hour diagnostic phase and a minimum AHI indicative of quite severe OSA (AHI ≥ 40/hour) before doing PAP titration.[2]

AASM guideline advocates that a split-night study may be performed based on "clinical judgment" like repetitive long obstructions and major desaturations when AHIs are between 20 and 40/hour.

For titrating fixed CPAP split-night, attended, in-laboratory PSG is advised.
- Advantages—it is less costly, reduces the delay in prescribing treatment, and is more convenient for patients than titration during full-night studies.
- Drawbacks—it does not allow enough time for an optimal CPAP titration or for transitioning to BPAP if that becomes necessary.
    - The risk of OSA is highest (i.e., during REM sleep in the supine position) the possibility of observation is reduced, thus underestimating true severity.
    - This leads to fewer opportunities for patient education, and a higher degree of technologist skill is required.[10]

In-home Titration

The patient is given APAP containing event detection software which provides REIs that reflect estimates of the AHI, hours of use, and presence or absence of a mask leak. The usually a minimum of 5 cm H_2O and maximum of 20 cm H_2O will be the pressure requirements of most patients. The level of pressure that eliminates all evidence of upper airway obstruction for more than 90% or 95% of the time (depending on the device model) becomes the fixed CPAP setting.

Guidelines for scoring respiratory events include the presence of ox hemoglobin desaturations and/or arousal from sleep and the auto-titrating devices do not measure them.

The primary advantage of in-home titration is the elimination of a separate stay in the sleep laboratory. This strategy may reduce both the costs and any delay until titration can be performed, depending upon the time necessary to access sleep laboratory services in any given location. In-home titration may also extend care to patients in areas that lack sleep laboratories.

The major disadvantage of in-home titration is the absence of a technologist or clinician. Additional disadvantages of in-home titration include the inability to determine the effect of positional changes (ideally, titration should encompass supine and nonsupine sleep), the need for a pressure-relief setting, and the effect of humidification.

BIPAP titration is more complex and should never be guided by unattended, in-home portable monitoring.[7,8,12]

PATIENT-DEVICE INTERFACE

The interface that offers the best mix of comfort and efficacy is ideal. As a properly fitting interface optimizes efficacy by ensuring delivery of the target airway pressure and adherence by optimizing patient comfort and convenience.

The most comfortable mask is not always the best-fitting and the best-fitting mask is not always the most comfortable so try several different interfaces at the same. The various options include nasal masks, nasal pillows, full facemasks (i.e., or nasal masks), and oral interfaces. The best interface is "the one the patient will use."

The common problems to consider when selecting an interface include:
- Claustrophobia—claustrophobic patients may find nasal pillows more acceptable than other interfaces. Desensitization to a nasal mask can be tried by asking the patient to wear mask throughout day.
- Nasal congestion—precipitated by PAP therapy. It causes higher Airflow resistance, which impairs comfortable breathing through the nose and negatively impact adherence. It may reduce the transmission of enough PAP to the upper airway leading to upper airway collapse during sleep.
- The solution is to use topical nasal glucocorticoids, nasal antihistamines or ipratropium, or oral antihistamines and use a facemask that covers both the nose.
- Mouth breathing—oral breathers while asleep or who are unable to keep their mouth closed against the PAP develop a mouth leak when PAP therapy is initiated through a nasal interface. A chin strap that holds the mouth closed is sufficient to tackle a mouth leak.
- Facial hair—mustache or beard may causes excessive leakage with nasal masks or full facemasks in this case nasal pillows can be employed.
- Cosmetic issues—the interface headgear disturbs their hair style.
- Reading or watching television in bed——as it interferes with vision.
- Headgear placement—nasal pillows are often the easiest to take on and off. Always instruct patients to simply disconnect the distal end of the tubing from the PAP device instead of trying to remove and replace the interface.
- Nasal pillows—If CPAP or IPAP is below 12 cm H_2O causes no discomfort. The pressure above 12 cm causes excessive airflow against the nasal mucosa so patient won't tolerate nasal pillows.
- Oral interfaces—In situations, if nasal or nasal interfaces cannot be tolerated.[1,3,6,10]

ACCESSORY FEATURES

- *Pressure relief*—expiratory pressure relief briefly lowers the delivered PAP. In CPAP, the pressure is lowered during early expiration and in BIPAP it is lowered at end-inspiration and early expiration. It helps to improve compliance by reducing the uncomfortable feeling of breathing against very high pressure.[10,12]
- *Humidification*—the nasal dries causing increase nasal resistance. Heated humidification decreases the nasal resistance significantly by more than half. But cold humidification has almost no impact as it does little to increase relative humidity.
    - The heated humidification is mandatory in dry climates and in patients with allergic rhinitis and also in patients who have undergone uvulopalatopharyngoplasty.
    - Tube condensation called as "rain-out," occur because of temperature differences between the environment and the tubing. It causes excess water droplets in the tubing, which could even reach to the interface reducing adherence. External insulation of PAP tubing is required.[8,10,14]

- *Pressure ramp*—this is where the PAP delivery at a low level initially (usually 4–5 cm H_2O) and then gradually increased to the PAP to the prescribed level over a duration designated by the clinician (usually 5–45 minutes). It helps as a comfort measure which allows the patient to fall asleep before reaching the higher pressures that might interfere with sleep onset.
    - Ramp abuse is repeated activation of the ramp feature, which diminishes the effectiveness of therapy. Tackled by increasing the starting pressure to a level just below the therapeutic pressure or disabling the ramp function or changing from a nasal mask to a facemask.
- *Altitude compensation*—the generations of PAP devices at lower altitudes may decrease significantly than at higher altitudes compensation is always confirmed.[12]

ASSESSING ADEQUACY OF PAP SETTINGS

The goal of PAP titration is to deliver the minimal pressure required to resolve all episodes of apneas and or hypopneas, snoring, and arousals from sleep in all positions and stages of sleep. This is best evaluated in an attended in-laboratory setting with polysomnographic monitoring.
- Goal is met; no further titration is necessary and starts on therapy.
- Goal is not met perform or repeat an attended in-laboratory PAP titration.

Once patients are started on PAP therapy, the response should be assessed clinically, for the first time in 1–8 weeks.

Adherence

The average nightly usage of CPAP is around 4 hours (240 minutes). The increased adherence will increase the benefits of CPAP therapy. It is estimated less than 40 patients use regularly. There are varieties of educational, behavioral, and troubleshooting interventions that can help promote CPAP use.[12]

Follow-up

Patients need frequent evaluation particularly in the first few weeks of therapy. It can be through frequent telephone calls and meet face-to-face with a clinician. This will quickly identify and manage any side as it is directly related adherence.[1,8]

REFERENCES

1. Jordan AS, McSharry DG, Malhotra A. Adult obstructive sleep apnoea. Lancet. 2014;383:736-47.
2. Jonas DE, Amick HR, Filner C, Weber RP, Arvanitis M, Stine A, et al. Screening for obstructive sleep apnea in adults: evidence report and systematic review for the US Preventive Services Task Force. JAMA. 2017;317:415.
3. McDaid C, Dupree KH, Griffin SC, Weatherly HL, Stradling JR, Davies RJ, et al. A systematic review of continuous positive airway pressure for obstructive sleep apnoea-hyperpnoea syndrome. Sleep Med Rev. 2009;13:427-36.
4. Martínez-García MÁ, Chimer E, Hernandez L, Cortes JP, Catalán P, Ponce S, et al. Obstructive sleep apnoea in the elderly: role of continuous positive airway pressure treatment. Euro Respire J. 2015;46:142-51.
5. Tamanna S, Campbell D, Warren R, Ulla MI. Effect of CPAP therapy on symptoms of nocturnal gastro esophageal reflux among patients with obstructive sleep apnea. J Clin Sleep Med. 2016;12:1257-61.

6. Campos-Rodriguez F, Martinez-Garcia MA, de la Cruz-Moron I, Almeida-Gonzalez C, Catalan-Serra P, Montserrat JM. Cardiovascular mortality in women with obstructive sleep apnea with or without continuous positive airway pressure treatment: a cohort study. Ann Intern Med. 2012;156:115-22.
7. Epstein LJ, Kris D, Stroll PJ Jr, Friedman N, Malhotra A, Patil SP, et al. Clinical guideline for the evaluation, management and long-term care of obstructive sleep apnea in adults. J Clin Sleep Med. 2009;5:263-76.
8. Reeves-Hoché MK, Hudgel DW, Meck R, Witteman R, Ross A, Zwillich CW. Continuous versus bilevel positive airway pressure for obstructive sleep apnea. Am J Respire Crit Care Med. 1995;151:443-9.
9. Cowie MR, Wohler H, Wegscheider K, Angermann C, d'Ortho MP, Erdmann E, et al. Adaptive servo-ventilation for central sleep apnea in systolic heart failure. N Engle J Med. 2015;373:1095-105.
10. Patil SP, Ayappa IA, Cables SM, Kimoff RJ, Patel SR, Harrod CG. Treatment of Adult obstructive sleep apnea with positive airway pressure: An American Academy of Sleep Medicine Clinical Practice Guideline. J Clin Sleep Med. 2019;15:335-43.
11. Kunisaki KM, Greer N, Khalil W, Koffel E, Koeller E, MacDonald R, et al. Provider types and outcomes in obstructive sleep apnea case finding and treatment: A systematic review. Ann Intern Med. 2018;168:195-202.
12. Bloch KE, Huber F, Farina M, Latshang TD, Lo Cascio CM, Nussbaumer-Ochsner Y, et al. Auto adjusted versus fixed CPAP for obstructive sleep apnoea: a multicentre, randomized equivalence trial. Thorax. 2018;73:174-84.
13. Kushida CA, Chugiak A, Berry RB, Brown LK, Gozal D, Iber C, et al. Clinical guidelines for the manual titration of positive airway pressure in patients with obstructive sleep apnea. J Clin Sleep Med. 2008;4:157-71.
14. Wiest GH, Hirsch IA, Fuchs FS, Kitzbichler S, Bogner K, Brueckl WM, et al. Initiation of CPAP therapy for OSA: does prophylactic humidification during CPAP pressure titration improve initial patient acceptance and comfort? Respiration. 2002;69:406-12.

Chapter 17

Noninvasive Ventilation in Neuromuscular Disease

Raymond Dominic Savio, Pratheema Ramachandran, Babu Abraham

■ INTRODUCTION

Neuromuscular diseases consist of a large array of clinical conditions of varying pathophysiologies that eventually cause weakness of the muscles, including respiratory muscles, leading to respiratory failure. The role and mode of respiratory support in each of these cases can vary. This chapter will explore the evidence and role for the use of noninvasive ventilation (NIV) in these conditions. For the ease of discussion, these pathologies have been classified as myopathies, diseases that affect the neuromuscular junctions, and quadriplegia/tetraplegia.

■ MYOPATHIES

Duchenne's muscular dystrophy (DMD) and Becker's muscular dystrophy (BMD) are two similar forms of progressive degenerative myopathies with the latter being less severe and having a later onset of symptoms. These are inherited as X-linked recessive disorders and therefore manifest in boys born to carrier mothers. A defect in the gene encoding for the protein dystrophin has been implicated in progressive degeneration of skeletal muscles and therefore weakness, beginning with the girdles and finally involving the respiratory and cardiac muscles. DMD was first reported as "pseudohypertrophic muscular paralysis" in the original case series by Guillaume-Benjamin-Amand Duchenne in 1868. Increasing muscle load and loss of endurance are the hallmark of the disease which ultimately results in profound respiratory failure. Molecular genetic testing has rendered diagnosis easy and has obverted the need for muscle biopsy. While survival never extended into adolescence in earlier times, it is not uncommon to encounter a young adult in 30s or early 40s with one of the dystrophinopathies these days, given the advancements in respiratory support.

There is quite often a delay in the identification of DMD which starts manifesting very early in childhood. Respiratory problems begin in early adolescence as a consequence of gradually waning vital capacity (VC) and muscle tolerance to workload.[1] In due course, compensatory mechanisms fail and hypercapnia ensues. Nocturnal hypercapnia is the first to occur when VC diminishes below 40% of the predicted figure.[2] Diurnal hypercapnia proceeds in the following few months with further deterioration in muscle endurance, unless treated. In due course, there is a substantial increase in work of breathing culminating in respiratory fatigue and failure. Additionally, impaired cough may predispose to atelectasis and infections. Many a times, the compensatory mechanisms such as rapid and labored breathing are not perceived by the patient leading to undue delay in presentation. As a result, one of the aforesaid complications is often the presenting manifestation on diagnosis.

In those patients diagnosed early, the role of periodic spirometry and monitoring for gas exchange and adequacy of cough cannot be stressed enough in attempting to retard disease progression.

Role of Noninvasive Ventilation

In addition to respiratory muscle strain and fatigue, a high incidence of sleep disordered breathing has been reported in patients with DMD. This includes hypopnea arising from either central or obstructive sleep apnea (CSA or OSA) resulting in hypoxia. NIV using bilevel positive airway pressure (BiPAP) can therefore assist in both off-loading the respiratory muscles as well as mitigating sleep apnea. Pure continuous positive airway pressure (CPAP) is unlikely to be of benefit in patients with DMD as it fails to mitigate muscle fatigue. Negative pressure ventilators have also been tried in this setting but fraught with the risk of upper airway obstruction due to asynchrony between the assisted respiratory cycle and vocal cord opening.

During early phase of the disease, it may suffice to initiate the patient on nasal nocturnal NIV (nNIV) allowing for daytime unassisted breathing. This has been shown to improve quality of sleep, daytime respiratory performance, and survival[3] as a result of slower rate of decline in respiratory function.[4] Titration of inspiratory positive airway pressure (IPAP) and expiratory positive airway pressure (EPAP) needs to be based on sleep laboratory assessment and careful bedside observation. It needs to be stressed that despite respiratory support, lung functions deteriorate albeit slower and periodic reassessment of positive pressure assistance is mandatory.[5] Likewise, over time, there could be a change in preference and performance of the NIV interface. As the disease progresses, intermittent diurnal NIV (dNIV) and eventually 24-hour NIV may be needed.

Daytime or diurnal NIV is recommended when the waking up pCO_2 is in excess of 50 mm Hg or when SpO_2 is less than 92% during awake hours. The initial approach can consist of intermittent dNIV for a few hours at a time and allowing for unassisted breathing as per tolerance. Needless to say, gas exchange and respiratory dynamics need to be closely observed for deterioration and the number of hours on dNIV be gradually extended. Patients with extremely low VC may require 24-hour NIV support and may rapidly progress to needing invasive ventilatory assistance. The use of 24-hour NIV may defer the need for invasive mechanical ventilation.[6]

The disadvantages of using NIV are similar as for any other setting including irritation of eyes, nasal stuffiness, mask associated pressure ulcer, inadvertent mask/circuit disconnection and fatal hypoxia, gastric insufflation and regurgitation of contents etc. Careful attention to humidification, mask fit, patient training, battery back-up, and the use of appropriate pressure assistance can help lessen the problems associated with NIV.

Long-term home NIV and ambulatory NIV are quite feasible in this population of patients with muscle dystrophy and many home-care organizations currently specialize in the delivery of the same.

Novel Noninvasive Approaches

Patients requiring continuous ventilatory assistance may benefit from novel methods such as mouthpiece intermittent positive pressure ventilation, glossopharyngeal breathing (GPB), and intermittent abdominal pressure ventilation. It may be difficult to derive any evidence-based guidelines regarding their use, considering the rarity of the disease. The mouthpiece ventilation is perhaps a more commonly used option in comparison to the other methods and is also available commercially (or can be custom made). It involves the patient breathing through a mouthpiece placed between his lips and connected to a portable ventilator which can be mounted on his wheelchair. The patient can intermittently take an assist-controlled breath. The main advantage of this method is that it does not compromise eating or speech and therefore is better accepted. Case series have documented the successful use of this technique in patients with DMD and a mean VC of 0.6 L for prolonged period of time.[7]

The GPB is an unassisted breathing where the patient is trained to take small gulps or boluses of air into the lungs. A few gulps may together contribute one tidal volume (Vt) and this comes in handy especially during a ventilator failure. The intermittent abdominal pressure ventilator uses an inflatable bladder applied over the abdomen and operated by a portable ventilator. A forced exhalation induced by bladder inflation is followed by passive inhalation that happens from a downward descent of the diaphragm and probably chest wall recoil.

Goals of Care

The role and prospects of long-term NIV and perhaps later on invasive ventilation need to be discussed with the family and preferably with the patient himself unless too immature. It is paramount that the clinician is open for a wider perspective as often there is an under-rating of the quality of life of a patient requiring long-term respiratory assistance. Decisions also need to be based on various social, religious, and legal factors. Patients deciding against long-term ventilatory assistance shall be provided with appropriate palliative care.

■ DISEASES THAT AFFECT THE NEUROMUSCULAR JUNCTION

Myasthenia gravis (MG) is perhaps a relatively common disorder that affects the neuromuscular junction with a prevalence of 70–320 per million population. This autoimmune disorder involves T cell-mediated damage to acetylcholine receptors and other receptor-associated proteins on the postsynaptic membrane at the neuromuscular (NM) junction. While MG can occur at any age, it often follows a bimodal distribution, presenting at the second to third decades (female preponderance) and sixth to eight decades (male preponderance). Fluctuating degree and variable combinations (ocular, bulbar, limb, respiratory) of skeletal muscle weakness with true fatigue are the characteristic presentations of MG. Respiratory system involvement is marked by a gradual reduction in VC, impaired cough, and ultimately resulting in gas exchange abnormalities. This muscle weakness additionally has a diurnal variability and is typically more, later during the evenings and following exercise. It is possible that in a section of patients with MG and advancing age, there could be a significant reduction in symptom-free period despite medication. The severity of MG can be classified using the modified Osserman system **(Table 1)**. Neonatal and congenital MG are other distinct entities and their discussion is beyond the scope of this chapter.

Table 1: Modified Osserman classification.

Class I	Patients with ocular involvement alone
Class II	Mild muscular weakness, not incapacitating
Class III	Moderate muscular weakness, not incapacitating, including oropharyngeal and respiratory muscle weakness
Class IV	Incapacitating weakness of any muscle system, including oropharyngeal and respiratory muscle weakness
Class V	Life-threatening respiratory insufficiency requiring ventilatory assistance (crisis)

Role of NIV

Patients with MG class III to V are the ones who present with varying need for respiratory assistance. Invasive positive pressure ventilation (IPPV) has dramatically changed the outlook for these patients and has tremendously improved survival over the recent few decades. However, the associated morbidity (infectious and non-infectious) and higher cost of care have always been a concern. In this regard, NIV finds a significant role when used as the initial mode of respiratory support in appropriate patients by potentially averting the need for IPPV. One of the seemingly earliest case series of NIV use in MG reports a significant reduction in need for intubation as well as hospital stay.[8] Subsequent literature has gone on to suggest reductions in ICU length of stay (LOS), mean days requiring respiratory assistance, and also the incidence of pulmonary complications.[9,10] These are largely case series and retrospective cohorts that are rather considered hypothesis generating. It will be highly ambitious to design a large-scale randomized trial in this group of relatively uncommon disease.

Patients with MG who could potentially benefit from NIV support include:
- Myasthenic crisis (MC), defined as MG with life-threatening respiratory insufficiency
- MG on IPPV as a weaning mode and prophylactic NIV
- Generalized MG with unsatisfactory pharmacological control
- MG with other respiratory comorbidities
- MG with respiratory stress which happens during sleep (physiologic)

Bilevel positive airway pressure is the mode of NIV that has been largely used and reported. This combines the benefit of EPAP which helps to maintain upper airway patency and prevents alveolar atelectasis, and IPAP which reduces the work of breathing by supporting the fatiguing respiratory muscles. These positive pressure levels require careful bedside titration guided by respiratory dynamics and therefore clinical improvement. In general, the pressure requirements so far reported were from 4 to 6 cm H_2O EPAP and 10 to 16 cm H_2O IPAP.[8-10] Needless to say, the pressure requirement closely correlates with the severity of respiratory insufficiency. A face mask was used in most patients reported in available literature and some patients were transitioned over to nasal mask upon improvement. Supplemental oxygen was used to maintain an SpO_2 ≥90%. All principles and contraindications pertaining to the general use of NIV shall apply in these patients with MG as well. In particular, one has to be wary of poor cough effort and secretion handling as this could be a significant limitation amounting to NIV failure.

While treating patients with MC, one has to carefully adhere to the principles of NIV trial (described elsewhere). NIV shall not be used to inappropriately delay intubation in the event of failure of NIV trial as this has in general shown to worsen outcomes. Similarly, judicious choice of patients for using NIV as a weaning mode is paramount to success of therapy. Weaning shall clearly not be attempted using NIV in those with copious respiratory secretions and impaired cough (bulbar weakness). Prophylactic NIV following extubation in those at high risk of extubation failure also seems to be another potential option. These patients can further be weaned off respiratory assistance using intermittent NIV.[11] It needs to be stressed that there is neither enough experience nor evidence to substantiate the practice of prophylactic NIV considering the fact that extubation failure can amount to serious in-hospital morbidity in patients with MG.[11]

With better avenues for therapy and improved healthcare, greater numbers of patients with MG can be expected to live on to advanced ages with increasing comorbidities, notably respiratory disorders including CSA and OSA, chronic obstructive pulmonary disease (COPD), and recurrent respiratory infections or cardiac diseases such as heart failure from various causes. Each one of these comorbidities could be a potential indication for NIV over and above MG. Further to this, the disorders by themselves or by way of medication can also have an adverse impact on MG, thereby increasing the dependence on NIV.

Another interesting phenomenon and possible avenue for use of NIV in MG constitutes the physiological stress of sleep in these patients especially following recovery from a MC. Diminished output from the respiratory center during rapid eye movement (REM) sleep can compromise upper airway patency as well as intercostal and accessory muscle power thereby affecting ventilation. While there seems to be enough reasoning for the application of NIV, evidence is bleak.

Despite the growing popularity of NIV in general and in patients with neuromuscular diseases, it appears to be offered much less often than can be expected.[12]

Predictors of NIV Outcome

Hypercapnia (pCO_2 >45 mm Hg) at the time of NIV initiation was shown to be a predictor of NIV failure.[9] A lower severity of illness (APACHE II score <6) and serum bicarbonate level <30 mmol/L have been shown to be associated with NIV success.[11] In addition to the above findings, it is reasonable to consider that careful patient selection, expertise in NIV therapy, and prompt intubation in the event of failure of NIV trial can all have a favorable impact on outcomes.

TETRAPLEGIA/QUADRIPLEGIA

The term tetraplegia or quadriplegia rather includes myriad disorders arising from diverse etiopathologies. These can be broadly classified into the upper motor neuron (UMN) type, lower motor neuron (LMN) type, and from miscellaneous causes. Some of the commonly encountered problems are listed in **Table 2** which is not exhaustive. DMD and MG, described earlier in this chapter are prototypes for LMN disorders affecting muscle and the NM junction, respectively.

Chapter 17: Noninvasive Ventilation in Neuromuscular Disease

Table 2: Causes of tetraplegia/tetraparesis.

Level of lesion		Example
UMN	Cortex	Bilateral MCA stroke
	Cervical spinal cord	Trauma, tumors, multiple sclerosis
	Motor neuron	Motor neuron disease (MND), poliomyelitis
LMN	Peripheral nerve	Guillain–Barré syndrome (GBS), critical illness neuropathy
	NMJ	Myasthenia gravis (MG), organophosphorus poisoning
	Muscle	Critical illness myopathy, muscle dystrophy, storage disorders
Misc.		Hypokalemic periodic paralysis, alcoholic myopathy, endocrine muscle weakness

UMN: upper motor neuron; LMN: lower motor neuron; NMJ: neuromuscular junction

This section will elaborate on pathophysiology of UMN type of lesions and role of NIV in the management. The most common cause for UMN type tetraplegia is spinal cord injuries (SCI).

Pathophysiology

Spinal cord injuries are not uncommon. The level of injury is denoted by the lowest level of spinal cord segment with normal motor functions.[13] Respiratory complications are due to acute respiratory muscle paralysis **(Table 3)**. The higher the level of injury, the higher incidence of complications and higher morbidity/mortality occurs. The disability from spinal cord injuries occurs as two phases—an acute phase and a chronic phase. The acute phase of spinal injury is the immediate post-injury period, in which patient is in a state of spinal shock with autonomic imbalance, poor circulation, and perfusion to the muscles. The chronic phase of spinal injury happens once they recover with residual deficits.

Table 3: Level of spinal cord injury and disability.

Level of injury	Muscles affected	Process affected	Remarks
C3, 4, 5	Diaphragm	Inspiration: Low vital capacity	Needs initial invasive ventilation, difficult to wean off ventilation
C4–C8	Accessory muscles Scalene	Inspiration	May breathe independent after initial ventilation, passive expiration
T1–T11	Intercostal muscles	Inspiration at low volumes, Expiration at high volumes	Poor cough effort
T6–L1	Abdominal muscles	Exhalation	Poor cough effort

In the acute phase,[14] most patients are on invasive ventilation within a week, when the glycogen stores of the diaphragm get exhausted. The sole triggers are inability to clear secretions and gradual diaphragmatic weakness. After an initial lag of about a month of optimized ventilation with optimal physiotherapy and nutrition, the respiratory mechanics and lung volumes improve to a certain extent **(Table 4)**. This is when they are assessed for weaning and extubation. The readiness to wean is assessed with peak expiratory flow rate. A cough flow of 220 L/min is a good marker of readiness to decannulate/extubate. Other factors are decreased secretion load, cooperation of the patient, and vital capacity of about 15 mL/kg. Poor markers are high level of cord injury, age >50 years and vital capacity <1 L. In patients with diaphragmatic palsy and abdominal muscles weakness, supine position is preferred during extubation,[15] as the abdominal contents push the diaphragm up to aid breathing attempts.

The chronic phase is more challenging for the caregivers, the objective being to wean the patients off invasive ventilation to NIV, thus avoiding tracheostomy, poor quality of life, and lifetime institutionalization.

Table 4: Changes in respiratory physiology in tetraplegia.

Parameters	Acute phase	Chronic phase	Trend
Vital capacity	Decrease by 30%	Improve after about 3 weeks	Improves
Inspiratory capacity	Decrease by 25%	Decrease by 25%	Improves
Expiratory reserve volume	Almost nil	Decrease to 75%	Improves
Peak inspiratory pressure	Up to –30 cm H_2O	Up to –60 cm H_2O	Improves
Peak expiratory pressure	Less than +30 cm H_2O	Around +30 cm H_2O	Almost the same

Role of NIV

The role of NIV is not much different from that in patients with Duchenne's. The issues those need to be addressed are:
- Atelectasis/hypoventilation secondary to poor inhalation due to paralysis of the diaphragm.
- Clearance of secretions due to poor cough effort.

Noninvasive ventilation helps in treating the OSA[16,17] components, which is more prevalent in patients with SCI. NIV, hence, prevents hypoventilation and atelectasis. Clearance of secretion can be facilitated by using mechanically assisted cough devices, a device which synchronizes with patient's breath cycle with vibrations causing loosening up of secretions. This along with the mechanical insufflation and exsufflation,[18] helps in clearance of the secretions.

Predictors of NIV Outcome

Noninvasive ventilation is successful when there is adequate clearance of carbon dioxide to a $PCO_2 < 50$ mm Hg and SPO_2 about 95% during the day. If less than this or in case of sudden deterioration, pneumonia or thromboembolism should be strongly suspected and intubation needs to be considered.

Novel Techniques

The newer techniques which are seen to be effective in patients with tetraplegia are GPB and breathe stacking. GPB takes care of brief needs during ventilator failure. Breath stacking is a method of using a resuscitation bag connected to the mouth piece and giving 2–3 breaths just before exhalation restoring adequate lung volumes and clearance of secretions. Electrical diaphragmatic pacing[19,20] is a method of implanting pacers adjacent to the paralyzed diaphragm, which can be stimulated by external signals. This helps in better wheel chair mobility, improved speech, and clearance of secretions. Disadvantages are need for surgical procedure (thoracotomy) and extensive postoperative training.

CONCLUSION

With improvement in our understanding and experience in the use of NIV, its scope of application has been ever expanding. It should be noted that many of these indications are not backed by sound evidence. At this time point, we cannot stress enough the importance of adhering to the general principles of NIV use which emphasizes on preventing delay in intubation for assisted invasive ventilation in the event of failure of a NIV trial. Careful patient selection, a detailed knowledge regarding contraindications, and promptness in identifying NIV failure are paramount not only to the success of therapy but also to patient safety. In the absence of clear-cut indications and expertise in handling NIV, elective invasive ventilation is a far safer option.

REFERENCES

1. Begin R, Bureau MA, Lupien L, Lemieux B. Control of breathing in Duchenne's muscular dystrophy. Am J Med. 1980;69(2):227-34.
2. Toussaint M, Steens M, Soudon P. Lung function accurately predicts hypercapnia in patients with Duchenne muscular dystrophy. Chest. 2007;131(2):368-75.
3. Gomez-Merino E, Bach JR. Duchenne muscular dystrophy: prolongation of life by noninvasive ventilation and mechanically assisted coughing. Am J Phys Med Rehabil. 2002;81(6):411-5.
4. Rideau Y, Delaubier A, Guillou C, Renardel-Irani A. Treatment of respiratory insufficiency in Duchenne's muscular dystrophy: nasal ventilation in the initial stages. Monaldi Arch Chest Dis. 1995;50(3):235-8.
5. Guilleminault C, Philip P, Robinson A. Sleep and neuromuscular disease: bilevel positive airway pressure by nasal mask as a treatment for sleep disordered breathing in patients with neuromuscular disease. J Neurol Neurosurg Psychiatr. 1998;65(2):225-32.
6. McKim DA, Griller N, LeBlanc C, Woolnough A, King J. Twenty four hour noninvasive ventilation in Duchenne muscular dystrophy: A safe alternative to tracheostomy. Can Respir J. 2013;20(1):e5-e9.
7. Baydur A, Layne E, Aral H, Krishna Reddy N, Topacio R, Frederick G, et al. Long term non-invasive ventilation in the community for patients with musculoskeletal disorders: 46 year experience and review. Thorax. 2000;55(1):4-11.
8. Rabinstein A, Wijdicks EF. BiPAP in acute respiratory failure due to myasthenic crisis may prevent intubation. Neurology. 2002;59(10):1647-9.
9. Seneviratne J, Mandrekar J, Wijdicks EFM, Rabinstein AA. Noninvasive ventilation in myasthenic crisis. Arch Neurol. 2008;65(1):54-8.
10. Agarwal R, Reddy C, Gupta D. Noninvasive ventilation in acute neuromuscular respiratory failure due to myasthenic crisis: case report and review of literature. Emerg Med J. 2006;23(1):e6.
11. Wu JY, Kuo PH, Fan PC, Wu HD, Shih FY, Yang PC. The role of non-invasive ventilation and factors predicting extubation outcome in myasthenic crisis. Neurocrit Care. 2009;10(1):35-42.
12. Alshekhlee A, Miles JD, Katirji B, Preston DC, Kaminski HJ. Incidence and mortality rates of myasthenia gravis and myasthenic crisis in US hospitals. Neurology. 2009;72(18):1548-54.
13. Wyndaele M, Wyndaele JJ. Incidence, prevalence and epidemiology of spinal cord injury: what learns a worldwide literature survey? Spinal Cord. 2006;44(9):523-9.
14. Berlly M, Shem K. Respiratory management during the first five days after spinal cord injury. J Spinal Cord Med. 2007;30(4):309-18.
15. Frisbie JH, Brown R. Waist and neck enlargement after quadriplegia. J Am Paraplegia Soc. 1994;17(4):177-8.
16. Olson EJ, Simon PM. Sleep-wake cycles and the management of respiratory failure Curr Opin Pulm Med. 1996;2(6):500-6.
17. Bascom AT, Sankari A, Goshgarian HG, Badr MS. Sleep onset hypoventilation in chronic spinal cord injury. Physiol Rep. 2015;3(8):e12490.
18. Bach JR. Mechanical insufflation-exsufflation: comparison of peak expiratory flows with manually assisted and unassisted coughing techniques. Chest. 1993;104(5):1553-62.
19. Onders RP, Khansarinia S, Weiser T, Chin C, Hungness E, Soper N. Multicenter analysis of diaphragm pacing in tetraplegics with cardiac pacemakers: positive implications for ventilator weaning in intensive care units. Surgery. 2010;148(4):893-8.
20. DiMarco AF. Diaphragm pacing in patients with spinal cord injury. Top Spinal Cord Inj Rehabil. 1999;5:6-20.

Chapter 18

Noninvasive Ventilation in Chest Wall Deformities and Chest Trauma

Suneel Kumar Garg, Prashant Singh, Gunjan Chanchalani, Amit Goel

■ INTRODUCTION

Patients with chest wall deformities have poor chest wall compliance, which is the main cause of morbidity and mortality in these patients. Low compliance coupled with mechanical disadvantage to the respiratory muscles can lead to both acute and chronic respiratory failure.

Neuromuscular and chest wall disorders often exist together and they make an important group of conditions that can cause acute respiratory failure. This is best recognized in scoliosis, kyphosis, following a thoracoplasty, and in various muscular dystrophies.[1]

This chapter reviews the pathophysiological mechanisms responsible for respiratory failure in patients with chest wall deformities and the place of noninvasive ventilation (NIV) in acute respiratory failure (ARF) and for prolonged domiciliary support.

■ MECHANISM UNDERLYING RESPIRATORY FAILURE IN CHEST WALL DEFORMITY

The pathophysiology involving chest wall deformity is related mainly to the restrictive nature of deformity along with imposition of excess elastic loads placed on the respiratory muscles. In conditions like kyphoscoliosis, the load on the muscles is chronic and progressive, but the load is acute in conditions like flail chest. If the respiratory muscles have limited time to adapt to the increased work of breathing, it may lead to acute respiratory failure.[2]

The primary mechanisms involved are:
- Reduced chest wall compliance
- Decreased functional residual capacity (FRC)
- Increased elastic load on the respiratory muscles
- Mild to moderate reductions in maximal static inspiratory (PI_{max}) and expiratory pressures (PE_{max}), with consequent reduction in vital capacity
- Increased work of breathing.

These factors lead to shallow tidal volumes, and thus predispose to development of atelectasis and subsequently worsening of lung compliance, in the absence of intrinsic lung disease.

As age advances, chest wall compliance decreases further, causing worsening of the respiratory mechanics, even though the chest wall deformity may remain constant. The work of breathing increases with increased oxygen cost of breathing with decreased ventilatory reserve, predisposes to fatigue and contributes to respiratory failure.

Chapter 18: Noninvasive Ventilation in Chest Wall Deformities and Chest Trauma

Normocapnic hypoxemia is the most common gas exchange abnormality found in patients with chest wall deformities. Patient can desaturate with even minimal activity. Hypoxemia is usually secondary to the ventilation perfusion mismatch, and less commonly due to shunt associated with atelectasis.[3] In severe cases, hypoventilation leads to chronic hypercapnia, initially detected only during sleep or with exercise. With aging as the disease progresses, hypercapnia is seen at rest as well as when awake.

PLACE OF NIV IN CHEST WALL DEFORMITIES

In Acute Respiratory Failure

Indications of use of NIV in acute respiratory failure in patients with chest wall deformity include acute onset dyspnea, acute respiratory acidosis and lethargy. NIV is indicated in acute cases, when $PaCO_2$ >45 mm Hg, even though the patient is not acidotic. It should also be considered in patients with normal $PaCO_2$ with reduced vital capacity and tachypnea. Delay in application of NIV in such cases can lead to respiratory muscle fatigue and acute respiratory failure.[4]

The usual contraindications of NIV should be excluded like severe inability to swallow; uncontrollable airway secretions; life-threatening hypoxemia; severely impaired mental status; hemodynamic instability; recent facial, upper airway, or upper gastrointestinal tract surgery; or bowel obstruction. A close monitored trial should be given before switching to invasive ventilation, if the trial fails. Once the acute illness is treated, patients should be extubated to NIV promptly.

In a randomized cohort trial in ICU, the success rate of NIV in kyphoscoliosis patients with ARF was found to be 76.4%.[5] Patients with NIV failure had a higher frequency of sepsis and septic shock. Higher APACHE-II score, high respiratory rate, low Glasgow Coma Scale, and lower pH values were the predictors of NIV failure. However, mortality was much higher in NIV failure, compared to patients who were invasively ventilated initially. This shows that choosing the right patient is very important for NIV success and for improved outcomes.

In Chronic Respiratory Failure

Long-term domiciliary NIV is almost always indicated following an episode of hypercapnic respiratory failure. Benefits of long-term NIV include; improvements in gas exchange, sleep efficiency, quality of life, and survival.[2] **(Table 1)**.

Initial studies of the use of NIV in chest wall deformities were mainly retrospective in nature and showed a longer survival with the use of NIV over oxygen therapy alone.[6,7] However, a Cochrane review published in 2007, concluded that the benefit of NIV in chest wall deformities is weak but consistent, with short-term alleviation of symptoms of chronic hypoventilation.[8]

In comparison to use of long-term oxygen therapy in these patients, NIV scored better in terms of gas exchange indices and pulmonary function tests. Buyse et al.[9] found a 54% increase in PaO_2, 21% fall in $PaCO_2$, 47% rise in vital capacity, and 33% rise in maximal static inspiratory mouth pressure, with the use of NIV as compared to long-term oxygen therapy (LTOT) in kyphoscoliosis. Also, the 1-year survival was much higher in the LTOT group compared to NIV group (100% vs 66%).

Table 1: Therapeutic benefits of NIV in patients with chest wall deformities.[2]

Gas exchange indices	
PaO_2	Increase
$PaCO_2$	Decrease
Bicarbonate	Decrease
Pulmonary function tests	
FVC	No change
FEV1	No change
TLC	No change
FRC	No change
Respiratory mechanics	
PIm_{ax}, PE_{max}	No change or slight increase
Twitch P_{di}	No change
Chest wall compliance	No change
Lung compliance	No change
Hemodynamic parameters	
PAP	Decrease
Ventilatory control	
Hypercapnic ventilatory	Improved response
Sleep	
Epworth sleepiness scale	Decrease
Quality of life	Improvement
Survival	Increase

(FEV1: forced expiratory volume in one second; FRC: functional residual capacity; FVC: forced vital capacity; P_{di}: transdiaphragmatic pressure; PAP: pulmonary artery pressure; PE_{max}: maximum expiratory pressure; PI_{max}: maximum inspiratory pressure; TLC: total lung capacity)

Similar results were reflected in patient experiences of symptoms and quality of life. Use of domiciliary NIV in restrictive thoracic disorders has shown to significantly improved the quality of life and emotional status of patients, and ameliorated symptoms of dyspnea, and fatigue.[10] Marti and coworkers[11] concluded that $PaCO_2 \geq 50$ mm Hg at 1 month of home ventilation and comorbidity (Charlson comorbidity index ≥ 3) were independent predictors of mortality in chest wall disease treated with home NIV ventilation.

These advantages however have been shown to rapidly reverse on discontinuation of NIV. Patients having total lung capacity ≤ 65% of predicted and who have been initially stabilized with NIV, have shown to rapidly progress to nocturnal followed by diurnal respiratory failure within days, upon discontinuation of NIV.[12] Thus, it is not advisable to withhold NIV for >24–48 hours in such patients.

Noninvasive Ventilation Settings

Higher levels of IPAP are needed in this group of patients, usually up to 20-30 cm H_2O.

Delivery of inadequate TV is common. Since these patients have low lung compliance (high elastance), which can lead to inspiration ending too early, on a spontaneously cycled ventilator. Using longer inspiratory times helps to deliver better volumes.

Budweiser et al.[10] found that use of pressure support >15 cm H_2O, accentuated the fall in $PaCO_2$. They showed that the inspiratory positive airway pressure (IPAP)–expiratory positive airway pressure (EPAP)/weight ratio correlated with the fall in $PaCO_2$ at the first visit after hospital discharge with long-term NIV.

Marti et al.[11] found an improvement in lung functions and 6 min walk distance with pressure support of 15 cm H_2O, with pressure cycled NIV devices during long-term treatment.

Use of newer modes like average volume assured pressure support (AVAPS) in kyphoscoliotic patients, have shown to improve daytime and nocturnal gas exchange, both immediate as well as in long-term. This mode has shown a significant improvement of diurnal PaO_2 and $PaCO_2$, mean blood oxygen saturation during sleep on the 5th day of NIV and after 1 year of NIV, along with increase in forced vital capacity after 1 year.[13]

KEY POINTS

- The primary mechanisms of respiratory failure in patients with chest wall deformities involve reduced chest wall compliance, decreased FRC, increased elastic load on the respiratory muscles etc.
- Poor chest wall compliance is the main cause of morbidity and mortality in these patients.
- Normocapnic hypoxemia is the most common gas exchange abnormality found in patients with chest wall deformities.
- Indications of use of NIV for acute respiratory failure in these group of patients include acute onset dyspnoea, acute respiratory acidosis and lethargy.

NONINVASIVE VENTILATION IN TRAUMA

Nearly 16.6% of all deaths are caused by trauma, making trauma as 6th leading cause of death in India.[14] These are a heterogeneous patient population with diverse respiratory needs. Chest trauma and pulmonary contusions remains the most common cause of death in up to 25% of patients with multiple system trauma.[15,16]

Pathophysiology of Acute Respiratory Failure in Trauma

Two major mechanisms responsible for ARF following trauma are:
1. The direct involvement of the thoracic cage or lung parenchyma, such as in the case of multiple rib fractures, flail chest, pulmonary contusions, pneumothorax and injury to airway structures, major vessels, heart and pericardium, diaphragm and other structures of the mediastinum.
2. The leakage of edema fluid into the lung and inflammatory cellular infiltrates associated with altered surfactant composition and diffusion abnormalities. This is typically seen in lung involvement from nonthoracic trauma associated with shock, disseminated intravascular coagulation, sepsis, large transfusion of blood products, and acute pancreatitis.

Both pathogenic events may converge on a common pathophysiological pathway and cause differing degrees of respiratory dysfunction.

In spontaneously breathing patients, the trauma-induced alteration of the chest wall mechanics decreases the tidal volume interfering with the cough reflex, predisposing to the retention of secretions, atelectasis and pneumonia. An associated pulmonary contusion can dramatically contribute to intrapulmonary shunt, worsening of gas exchange, causing a variable degree of disarrangement in ventilation and gas exchange.[17] This is particularly evident in patients with flail chest who present with hypoxemic ARF and are at high risk for respiratory impairment.[18]

Flail chest occurs when 3 or more consecutive ribs are fractured at two separate sites, causing that segment of the chest wall to become disconnected from the rest of the thoracic cage. This results in paradoxical movement of the flail segment from rest of the rib cage. The negative inspiratory pressure during spontaneous breathing results in the inward pulling of the flail segment and the positive pressure during expiration results in its pushing outwards. This leads to atelectasis, V/Q mismatch, shunt (due to lung contusion), and hemothorax,[17] ultimately resulting in hypoxemic respiratory failure.[18]

Management

Trauma management has been guided according to the mechanism of injury, its anatomic involvement, and the staging of the injury. Management include pulmonary toilet, control of chest wall pain, surgical stabilization and fluid therapy. The intensity and modality of respiratory and ventilatory supports mainly depend on the severity of respiratory dysfunction, extent of pulmonary contusions, the degree of gas exchange impairment, associated injuries and the feasibility of NIV as the first line approach.

The goal should be to avoid endotracheal intubation (ETI) and complications associated with it.[19,20] The application of positive pressure to the airways, either by NIV or Continuous Positive Airway Pressure (CPAP), may reduce the need for ETI in such patients.

A study done by Hernandez et al. showed that, when NIV is applied early, the beneficial results can be ascribed to the ease of the recruitment of contused lung regions.[21] By increasing the intrathoracic pressure, NIV increases the functional residual capacity, improves oxygenation, reduces the work of breathing and does not significantly alter the hemodynamics.

High-flow CPAP has been shown to provide a true "internal pneumatic stabilization" and less chest wall distortion when compared with intermittent mandatory ventilation.[22]

Numerous studies have also shown that the use of NIV in patients with hypoxemic ARF is associated with fewer complications, reduced mechanical ventilation, and length of ICU stay.[23]

Patients with blunt chest trauma should be stabilized in first 48 to 72 hours of presentation before giving trial of NIV, as failure of NIV has been reported mostly following this period.[21] Thus, for patients who are unresponsive to NIV, it should be discontinued as soon as possible within the first 24 hours and ETI should be considered early to mitigate the potential for harm.

Early research studied the role of CPAP in the "internal pneumatic stabilization" of the flail segment and found that use of CPAP caused less chest wall distortion and less pulmonary complications like atelectasis and pneumonia.[22] The positive pressure provided thus helps to improve gas exchange and reduce respiratory insufficiency. Compared to invasive ventilation, use of CPAP has shown to decrease the length of ICU stay, lesser infections and lower rates of complications.[24,25] As compared to high-flow nasal oxygen, patients on NIV require to be intubated less often due to hypoxemia.[21] However, there is no mortality benefit proven.

The main principles of use of NIV in flail chest are:
- Adequate pain relief
- To rule out contraindications to NIV like apnea, hemodynamic instability, faciomaxillary injury, esophageal injury, vomiting, low sensorium, excessive airway secretions and poor cough
- Close monitoring
- Repeated bedside evaluation to recognize failure of NIV and respiratory insufficiency.

There has been a scarcity of randomized controlled trials on ventilatory management of patients with posttraumatic hypoxemic respiratory failure. This is reflected by a low-grade recommendation for the use of NIV in trauma patients by the British Thoracic Society guidelines[26] and "no recommendation" by Canadian Critical Care Trials Group/Canadian Critical Care Society Noninvasive Ventilation Guidelines Group[19] due to a lack of sufficient evidence.

KEY POINTS

- In the absence of contraindications, patients with moderate trauma-related ARF should be put on NIV as the first-choice treatment; however close monitoring and promptly available ETI is warranted.
- Optimum pain control is the key to success for faster recovery.
- Risks associated with ETI can be avoided when NIV is applied judiciously and by avoiding prophylactic intubation.
- Primary aim of ventilation is to improve oxygenation, unload respiratory muscles and relieve dyspnea.
- Not clearly evident about the modality of NIV, but NPPV has been shown to be more effective than CPAP alone in optimizing lung functions.

REFERENCES

1. American Thoracic Society. Springer book, 2nd edition, page 3233-35.
2. Fishman's Pulmonary Diseases and Disorders. 5th edition.
3. Kafer ER. Idiopathic scoliosis: Gas exchange and the age dependence of arterial blood gases. J Clin Invest. 1976;58:825-33.
4. Ghosh D, Elliott MW. Acute non-invasive ventilation—getting it right on the acute medical take. Clinical Medicine. 2019;19(3):237-42.
5. Adiguzel N, Karakurt Z, Gungor G, et al. Management of kyphoscoliosis with respiratory failure in the intensive care unit and during long term follow up. Multidiscip Respir Med. 2012;7(1):30.
6. Jager L, Franklin KA, Midgren B, Lofdahl K, Strom K. Increased survival with mechanical ventilation in post-tuberculosis patients with the combination of respiratory failure and chest wall deformity. Chest. 2008;133(1):156-60.
7. Marti S, Pallero M, Ferrer J, Rios J, Rodriguez E, Morell F, et al. Predictors of mortality in chest wall disease treated with non-invasive home mechanical ventilation. Respir Med. 2010;104(12):1843-49.
8. Annane D, Orlikowski D, Chevret S, Chevrolet JC, Raphael JC. Nocturnal mechanical ventilation for chronic hypoventilation in patients with neuromuscular and chest wall disorders. Cochrane Database Syst Rev. 2007(4):CD001941.

9. Buyse B, Meersseman W, Demedts MM. Treatment of chronic respiratory failure in kyphoscoliosis: oxygen or ventilation? The European respiratory journal. 2003;22(3): 525-8.
10. Budweiser S, Heinemann F, Fischer W, Dobroschke J, Wild PJ, Pfeifer M. Impact of ventilation parameters and duration of ventilator use on non-invasive home ventilation in restrictive thoracic disorders. Respiration. 2006;73:488-94.
11. Martí S, Pallero M, Ferrer J, et al. Predictors of mortality in chest wall disease treated with non-invasive home mechanical ventilation. Respir Med. 2010;104(12):1843-9.
12. Petitjean T, Philit F, Germain-Pastenne M, et al. Sleep and respiratory function after withdrawal of non-invasive ventilation in patients with chronic respiratory failure. Respir Care. 2008;53(10):1316-23.
13. Piesiak P, Brzecka A, Kosacka M, et al. Efficacy of non-invasive volume targeted ventilation in patients with chronic respiratory failure due to kyphoscoliosis. Adv Exp Med Biol. 2015;838:53-8.
14. Road Traffic Accidents and Injuries in India. Economic & Political weekly. 2018;53:14.
15. Szucs-Farkas Z, Kaelin I, Flach PM, Rosskopf A, Ruder TD, Triantafyllou M, et al. Detection of chest trauma with wholebody low dose linear slit digital radiography: a multi-reader study. Am J Roentgenol. 2010;194:W388-W395.
16. Wanek S, Mayberry JC. Blunt thoracic trauma: flail chest, pulmonary contusion, and blast injury. Crit Care Clin. 2004;20:71-81.
17. Davignon K, Kwo J, Bigatello LM. Pathophysiology and management of the flail chest. Minerva Anestesiol. 2004;70:193-9.
18. Keenan SP, Mehta S. Non-invasive ventilation for patients presenting with acute respiratory failure: the randomized controlled trials. Respir Care. 2009;54:116-26.
19. Keenan SP, Sinuff T, Burns KE, Muscedere J, Kutsogiannis J, Mehta S, et al. Clinical practice guidelines for the use of non-invasive positive-pressure ventilation and non-invasive continuous positive airway pressure in the acute care setting. CMAJ. 2011;183:E195-214.
20. Papadakos PJ, Karcz M, Lachmann B. Mechanical ventilation in trauma. Curr Opin Anaesthesiol. 2010;23:228-32.
21. Hernandez G, Fernandez R, Lopez-Reina P, Cuena R, Pedrosa A, Ortiz R, et al. Non-invasive ventilation reduces intubation in chest trauma-related hypoxemia: a randomized clinical trial. Chest. 2010; 137:74-80.
22. Tanaka H, Tajimi K, Endoh Y, Kobayash K. Pneumatic stabilization for flail chest injury: an 11-year study. Surg Today. 2001;31:12-7.
23. Brochard L. Non-invasive ventilation for acute respiratory failure. JAMA. 2002;288:932-35.
24. Bolliger CT, Van Eeden SF. Treatment of multiple rib fractures. Randomized controlled trial comparing ventilatory with nonventilatory management. Chest. 1990;97:943-8.
25. Gunduz M. A comparative study of continuous positive airway pressure (CPAP) and intermittent positive pressure ventilation (IPPV) in patients with flail chest. Emerg Med J. 2005;22:325-9.
26. British Thoracic Society Standards of Care Committee. Noninvasive ventilation in acute respiratory failure. Thorax. 2002;57:192-211.

Chapter 19

Noninvasive Ventilation in Immunocompromised Patients and Patients on Palliative Care

Supradip Ghosh, Ripenmeet Salhotra, Sonali Ghosh

■ INTRODUCTION

Noninvasive ventilation (NIV) has now established itself as the first line respiratory support for a number of clinical conditions. In patients with acute de novo hypoxemic respiratory failure, NIV at least in theory, has an advantage over conventional low flow oxygen therapy, as it can potentially recruit lung with application of positive pressure and keep the lung recruited with appropriate use of positive end expiratory pressure (PEEP), can improve hypoxia and thus sense of dyspnea and provide relief to respiratory muscle fatigue. In immunocompromised patients with hypoxemic respiratory failure, application of NIV can potentially avoid intubation and thus avoid risks associated with invasive mechanical ventilation including airway injury, excess sedation, ventilator associated pneumonia and neuromuscular weakness. NIV also have the advantage of keeping a patient awake and allowing him or her oral feeding and ability to communicate. On the other hand, over-reliance on NIV has the potential of delaying intubation unnecessarily. Application of NIV in a patient with high respiratory drive can also increase the risk of barotrauma.[1] NIV may also have an important role in palliative care by decreasing the sense of dyspnea without intubating a terminally ill patient. In this chapter, we shall briefly review current evidence on the use of NIV in immunocompromised patients and in the setting of palliative care.

■ NONINVASIVE VENTILATION IN IMMUNOCOMPROMISED PATIENTS

Immunocompromised states include a heterogenous group of conditions where the immunity of the subject is inadequate to defend against various infections. Various examples are subjects with hematological malignancies, those receiving hematopoietic stem cell transplant (HSCT) or solid organ transplant (SOT), or receiving chemotherapy or other immunosuppressive agents like corticosteroids, suffering from acquired immunodeficiency syndrome (AIDS) or patients with asplenia or primary immunodeficiencies. Acute respiratory failure (ARF) is the leading cause of intensive care unit (ICU) admission in these patients. While early initiation of ICU care in this group of patients improves mortality, selection of appropriate initial oxygenation and ventilation strategy remains a challenge. Traditionally NIV is considered as the first line respiratory support in this group of patients as it can avoid complications of invasive mechanical ventilation (IMV). However, emerging evidences have started challenging this traditional view. Moreover, role of newer technologies like delivery of high flow humidified oxygen by nasal cannula is evolving.

Evidence for Noninvasive Ventilation in Immunocompromised Patients (Table 1)

Acute respiratory failure leading to ICU admission is associated with high mortality in the immunocompromised subjects. It is even worse in the subset which requires intubation and IMV. Researchers have tried to find out the optimal respiratory support for these vulnerable group of patients and whether NIV could improve the outcomes by avoiding IMV and its complications.

Two small single-center randomized controlled trials (RCTs) published in early 2000s demonstrated positive patient outcomes with early use of NIV in immunocompromised patients with hypoxemic respiratory failure in protective ICU setting. Hilbert and colleagues compared NIV with standard oxygen therapy via face mask in immunosuppressed patients with respiratory failure.[2] Etiology of immunosuppression was hematological malignancy in most cases but also included HIV, SOT and patients on corticosteroids. Need for intubation, the primary outcome of the study, was significantly lower in NIV group compared to oxygen therapy group (12 vs 20 of 26 patients in each group, P = 0.03). Use of NIV could also reduce major complications, ICU and inhospital mortality. In another small study of 40 SOT patients with acute respiratory failure, Antonelli and colleagues evaluated the effect of NIV on need for intubation.[3] Etiology of ARF was acute respiratory distress syndrome (ARDS) in about 40% and atelectasis in another 25%. Application of NIV significantly reduced the need for endotracheal intubation (20% vs 70%, P = 0.02). Application of NIV also reduced ICU mortality and length of stay in ICU.

In a small study of 40 patients of hematological malignancy with ARF admitted in the wards, Squadrone and colleagues investigated the role of continuous positive airway

Table 1: Summary of trials of NIV use in immunocompromised patients.

Study	Setting/ Number of patients	Patients	Severity of ARF PaO_2/FiO_2	Results	Comments
Hilbert et al.[2]	Single center/ICU/52	Mixed (mostly hematological)	<200	Lesser rate of intubation and mortality in NIV	Small study, very high mortality in control group
Antonelli et al.[3]	Single center/ICU/40	SOT recipients	<200	Lesser rate of intubation and mortality in NIV	All post-SOT patients, atelectasis present in 25%, small study
Squadrone et al.[4]	Single center/ward/40	Hematologic	282, 256	Lesser ICU admission, mechanical ventilation in CPAP	"Prophylactic" CPAP in less sick patients in wards
Wermke et al.[6]	Single center/ward/86	HSCT recipients	<300	No difference	"Prophylactic" NIV in less sick patients in wards
Lemiale et al.[7]	Multicenter/ICU/374	Mixed	136, 156	No difference	Largest trial HFNC used more often in control group

(ARF: acute respiratory failure; CPAP: continuous positive airway pressure; HFNC: high flow humidified oxygen by nasal cannula; HSCT: hematopoietic stem cell transplant; NIV: noninvasive ventilation; SOT: solid organ transplant)

pressure (CPAP) (compared to oxygen therapy alone) in reducing need for ICU admission and mechanical ventilation.[4] Application of CPAP was found to reduce need for ICU admission. Amongst patients who needed ICU admission, CPAP could reduce the need for intubation and IMV.

Based on these trials, NIV was considered as a treatment of choice for patients with significant immunosuppression and respiratory failure in many centers across the world. But these older data, needs to be relooked in more modern setting, with significant improvement in overall care of immunocompromised patients both in wards and ICU and a large improvement in care of patients on invasive mechanical ventilation.[5] In fact, results of these earlier trials were not replicated in some more recent studies. Wermke and colleagues compared early NIV with oxygen in patients of HSCT with respiratory failure.[6] Despite improvement in oxygenation earlier on, application of NIV was not associated with need for ICU admission, rate of intubation or any survival parameters. In the most recent and the largest multicenter study evaluating role of NIV in immucompromised patients with ARF, Lemiale and colleagues randomized 376 patients to receive either NIV or oxygen therapy. Majority (60%) of these patients were suffering from hematological malignancy.[7] Mean $PaO_2 : FiO_2$ ratios at randomization were 130 and 156 respectively in oxygen and NIV groups. The 28-day mortality was not different between the two groups (24.1% in NIV and 27.3% in oxygen group). Secondary outcomes including rate of intubation (38.2% in NIV vs. 44.8% in oxygen group) were again not significantly different in two groups. It was a well conducted RCT with high protocol adherence among institutions with expertise in delivering NIV and caring for immunocompromised patients. However, the authors acknowledged a few shortcomings like the lower than expected mortality rate might have reduced the power of the study resulting in no significant difference in the primary outcome. Another issue was the use of HFNC more often in the oxygen than NIV arm (44.3% vs 31.4%, P = 0.01), which might have influenced the results. The study was also criticized for improper use of NIV (<12 hours a day).

A recent meta-analysis pooled the data from these five RCTs and found that NIV was associated with a significant reduction in short-term mortality and intubation rates but not long-term mortality.[8] The joint European/American guidelines recommend early NIV for immunocompromised patients with ARF (conditional recommendation, moderate certainty of evidence).[9] However, as seen above only, older data showed benefit of NIV in immunocompromised subjects.[2-4] The two most recent RCTs suggest no difference in outcomes from use of NIV.[6,7] Several recent observational trials too found no benefit of NIV in this setting. Besides NIV failure leading to invasive mechanical ventilation was associated with worse outcomes in this subset of patients.[10]

Patients at Higher Risk of Noninvasive Ventilation Failure

Several studies have identified factors associated with success or failure of NIV in immunosuppressed. In a retrospective study of 99 patients of hematological malignancy who received NIV for ARF, Adda and colleagues evaluated the risks of NIV failure.[11] Multivariate analysis identified higher respiratory rate on NIV, delay in application of NIV, presence of ARDS, need for vasopressor or renal replacement therapy as independent predictors of NIV failure. In another prospective multicenter study, ARF of unknown etiology was associated with failure of NIV and

> **Box 1:** Factors associated with NIV failure in immunosuppressed in various studies.
> - Moderate to severe ARDS
> - Use of vasopressors
> - Renal failure requiring dialysis
> - High SAPS 2 score
> - ARF of unknown etiology
> - High respiratory rates

high mortality whereas bacteremia on admission (allowing directed antibiotic therapy) was associated with successful NIV.[12] Factors associated with NIV failure in immunocompromised patients are enumerated in **Box 1**.

Role of High-flow Nasal Cannula in Immunocompromised Patients

Recent years have seen an increase in use of high-flow nasal cannula (HFNC) as a mode of respiratory support in patients in acute hypoxic (nonhypercapnic) respiratory failure. This new type of respiratory support provides heated and humidified oxygen at various concentrations and high flows through nasal cannulae. Beneficial effects on gas exchange and respiratory function results from provision of stable fraction of inspired oxygen, generation of some positive end expiratory pressure (PEEP) and elimination of dead space among others. Besides it is more comfortable to patients as compared to NIV.

In the landmark "FLORALI" (High Flow Nasal Oxygen Therapy in Resuscitation of Patients with Acute Lung Injury) study, 310 patients with hypoxemic respiratory failure from 23 ICUs in France and Belgium, were randomly assigned to three groups–HFNC group, NIV group and conventional low flow oxygen therapy group.[13] Intubation rate were significantly lower in HFNC group. Interestingly patients in the NIV group had higher risk of mortality at 90-days compared to both oxygen therapy groups.[13] In a post hoc analysis of subset of immunocompromised patients from FLORALI, incidence of intubation was higher in NIV group, though there was no significant difference in HFNC and oxygen groups.[14] Similarly, Coudroy and colleagues reported fewer intubations with HFNC than NIV in an observational cohort of immunosuppressed patients with ARF.[15] However, in the recently published multicenter "HIGH" study in which 778 immunocompromised patients with ARF were randomized to receive either HFNC or conventional low-flow oxygen therapy, HFNC failed to show reduction in 28-day mortality or rate of intubation.[16]

Recommendation

- Current evidence does not support the use of NIV as the first-line respiratory support in immunocompromised patients with acute hypoxemic respiratory failure.
- HFNC is perhaps a better initial modality of choice in these patients.
- If considered as the initial modality, NIV should be used only in subgroup of patients with no risk of NIV failure **(Table 1)** under careful monitoring. Efforts should be made to recognize early NIV (and HFNC) failure and avoid delaying intubation.

NONINVASIVE VENTILATION IN PALLIATIVE CARE

Noninvasive ventilation is now increasingly being used in palliative care settings when endotracheal intubation is considered inappropriate. A taskforce of Society of Critical Care Medicine looking into role of NIV in palliative care settings, had identified three distinct subgroup of patients.[17] Type 1 patients where NIV is used as a lifesaving therapy to manage potentially modifiable conditions. Type 2 patients where there is a clear "Do not intubate" order but there is no other limitation of therapy, NIV can be used as a salvage therapy for potentially surviving hospitalization. In this subgroup of patients, NIV can be used as part of home care therapy in order to optimize the quality of life. Type 3 patients where palliative NIV is to attenuate symptoms of respiratory distress in patients who are expected to die. However, application of NIV is not without risk in this category of patients. NIV interface can cause pressure injury of skin resulting in skin peeling, claustrophobia and difficulty in feeding. Ultimate goal of NIV in this setting should be to decrease respiratory distress. An optimized NIV setting has the potential to reduce need for sedative and opioids potentially minimizing their side effects.

Evidence for NIV in Palliative Care Setting

In the first prospective study, NIV was investigated in 23 patients with solid organ malignancy receiving palliative care and were affected by severe hypoxic or hypercapnic respiratory failure.[18] Most of these patients received NIV in protective environments like ICU; only 4 received treatment in palliative care unit. After one hour, NIV significantly improved PaO_2/FiO_2 ratio and the Borg dyspnea score. In 13 of 23 patients, NIV was successful and all of them were discharged home alive. In rest of the 10 patients, NIV was discontinued due to intolerance, progressive worsening of ABG, sudden death, irreversible vomiting and need for deep sedation due to severe metastatic pain. Two of these patients gave consent for intubation. Overall mortality in NIV failure group was 90%.

In a randomised feasibility study, Nava and colleagues recruited 200 patients from 7 centers in Italy, Spain, and Taiwan, who had solid tumors and acute respiratory failure and had a life expectancy of <6 months and randomly allocate them to receive either NIV or oxygen therapy (using a Venturi or a reservoir mask).[19] Primary end points of the study were to assess the acceptability of NIV used solely as a palliative measure, to assess its effectiveness in reducing dyspnea and the amount of opiates needed compared with oxygen therapy. The study showed a clear decrease in Borg dyspnea score (mostly in the first hour after randomization and in hypercapnic subgroup) in the NIV group. Total dose of morphine in first 48 h was lower in the NIV group than in the oxygen group. Adverse events leading to NIV discontinuation were mainly related to mask intolerance and anxiety. In another feasibility study, Hui and colleagues, randomized 30 patients with advanced cancer and persistent dyspnea to either HFNC or NIV for two hours.[20] Primary outcome was reduction of dyspnea, assessed dyspnea with a numeric rating scale (NRS) and modified Borg scale (MBS) before and after the intervention. Both interventions were shown to be associated with improvements in both NRS and MBS, but reductions of dyspnea NRS and MBS were no significant different between two groups.

The joint European/American guidelines suggests offering NIV in dyspneic patients for palliation in the setting of terminal cancer or other terminal illnesses (conditional recommendation, moderate certainty of evidence).[9]

Role of HFNC in Palliative Care Settings

A few small-scale observational studies have shown role of HFNC in this set up. Spectrum of patients in these studies range from patients who are very sick with underlying pulmonary fibrosis, cardiopulmonary disease to advanced malignancy. In one study, Peters and colleagues, applied HFNC to 50 patients with "Do not intubate" order.[21] HFNC was shown to reduce respiratory rate and improve oxygen saturation. 18% of these patients were finally switched over to NIV, whereas in 82% HFNC were continued. Epstein and colleagues studied use of HFNC in 183 cancer patients (50% of them with DNR orders). Use of HFNC showed improvement in hypoxia but results were not statistically significant.[22]

In the RCT done by Hui and colleagues, in addition to reduction in dyspnea NRS and MBS, HFNC was also associated with improvement in oxygen saturation and reduction of respiratory rate but both were not statistically significant when compared with NIV.[20]

REFERENCES

1. Ghosh S. NIV induced Acute Lung Injury. In: Todi S, Mehta Y, Zirpe K, Dixit S (Eds). Critical Care Update 2019. Jaypee Brothers Medical Publishers (P) Ltd, New Delhi. 2019.
2. Hilbert G, Gruson D, Vargas F, Valentino R, Gbikpi-Bennisan G, Dupon M, et al. Noninvasive ventilation in immunosuppressed patients with pulmonary infiltrates, fever, and acute respiratory failure. N Engl J Med. 2001; 344(7):481-7.
3. Antonelli M, Conti G, Bufi M, Costa MG, Lappa A, Rocco M, et al. Noninvasive ventilation for treatment of acute respiratory failure in patients undergoing solid organ transplantation: a randomized trial. JAMA. 2000;283:235-41.
4. Squadrone V, Massaia M, Bruno B, Marmont F, Falda M, Bagna C, et al. Early CPAP prevents evolution of acute lung injury in patients with hematologic malignancy. Intensive Care Med. 2010;36(10):1666-74.
5. De Jong A, Hernandez G, Chiumello D. Is there still a place for noninvasive ventilation in acute hypoxemic respiratory failure? Intensive Care Med. 2018;44(12):2248-50.
6. Wermke M, Schiemanck S, Höffken G, Ehninger G, Bornhäuser M, Illmer T. Respiratory failure in patients undergoing allogeneic hematopoietic SCT—a randomized trial on early non-invasive ventilation based on standard care hematology wards. Bone Marrow Transplant. 2011;47(4):574-80.
7. Lemiale V, Mokart D, Resche-Rigon M, Pène F, Mayaux J, Faucher E, et al. Effect of noninvasive ventilation vs oxygen therapy on mortality among immunocompromised patients with acute respiratory failure. JAMA. 2015;314(16):1711-9.
8. Huang HB, Xu B, Liu GY, Lin JD, Du B. Use of noninvasive ventilation in immunocompromised patients with acute respiratory failure: a systematic review and meta-analysis. Critical Care. 2017;21:4.
9. Rochwerg B, Brochard L, Elliott MW, Hess D, Hill NS, Nava S, et al. Official ERS/ATS clinical practice guidelines: noninvasive ventilation for acute respiratory failure. Eur Respir J. 2017; 50:1602426.
10. Azoulay E, Pickkers P, Soares M, Perner A, Rello J, Bauer PR, et al. Acute hypoxemic respiratory failure in immunocompromised patients: the Efraim multinational prospective cohort study. Intensive Care Med. 2017;43(12):1808-19.
11. Adda M, Coquet I, Darmon M, Thiery G, Schlemmer B, Azoulay E. Predictors of noninvasive ventilation failure in patients with hematologic malignancy and acute respiratory failure. Crit Care Med. 2008;36(10):2766-72.
12. Molina R, Bernal T, Borges M, Zaragoza R, Bonastre J, Granada RM, et al. Ventilatory support in critically ill hematology patients with respiratory failure. Crit Care. 2012;16(4):1-7.
13. Frat JP, Thille AW, Mercat A, Girault C, Ragot S, Perbert S, et al. High-flow oxygen through nasal cannula in acute hypoxemic respiratory failure. N Engl J Med. 2015;372:2185-96.

14. Frat JP, Ragot S, Girault C, Perbet S, Prat G, Boulain T, et al. Effect of non-invasive oxygenation strategies in immunocompromised patients with severe acute respiratory failure: a post-hoc analysis of a randomized trial. Lancet Respir Med. 2016;4(8):646-52.
15. Coudroy R, Jamet A, Petua P, Robert R, Frat JP, Thille AW. High-flow nasal cannula oxygen therapy versus noninvasive ventilation in immunocompromised patients with acute respiratory failure: an observational cohort study. Ann Intensive Care. 2016;6(1):45.
16. Azoulay E, Lemiale V, Mokart D, Nseir S, Argaud L, Pene F, et al. Effect of High-Flow Nasal Oxygen vs Standard Oxygen on 28-Day Mortality in Immunocompromised Patients with Acute Respiratory Failure: The HIGH Randomized Clinical Trial. JAMA. 2018;320(20):2099-2107.
17. Curtis JR, Cook DJ, Sinuff T, White DB, Hill N, Keenan SP, et al. Non-invasive positive pressure ventilation in critical and palliative care settings: understanding the goals of therapy. Crit Care Med. 2007;35(3):932-9.
18. Cuomo A, Delmastro M, Ceriana P, Nava S, Conti G, Antonelli M, et al. Non-invasive mechanical ventilation as a palliative treatment of acute respiratory failure in patients with end-stage solid cancer. Palliat Med. 2004;18(7):602-10.
19. Nava S, Ferrer M, Esquinas A, Scala R, Groff P, Cosentini R, et al. Palliative use of non-invasive ventilation in end-of-life patients with solid tumours: a randomised feasibility trial. Lancet Oncol. 2013;14(3):219-27.
20. Hui D, Morgado M, Chisholm G, Withers L, Nguyen Q, Finch C, et al. High-flow oxygen and bilevel positive airway pressure for persistent dyspnea in patients with advanced cancer: a phase II randomized trial. J Pain Symptom Manage. 2013;46(4):463-73.
21. Peters SG, Holets SR, Gay PC. High-flow nasal cannula therapy in do-not-intubate patients with hypoxemic respiratory distress. Respir Care. 2013;58(4):597-600.
22. Epstein AS, Hartridge-Lambert SK, Ramaker JS, Voigt LP, Portlock CS. Humidified high-flow nasal oxygen utilization in patients with cancer at Memorial Sloan-Kettering Cancer Center. J Palliat Med. 2011;14(7):835-9.

Chapter 20

Noninvasive Ventilation in Pneumonia

Vikas Marwah, Priyanka Singh, Amit Singh Vasan

■ INTRODUCTION

Community acquired pneumonia (CAP) is a common, acute, and severe infection of lung parenchyma. The incidence of pneumonia is estimated to be 1.5–14 cases per 1,000 person years. Studies indicate that India accounts for 23% of global pneumonia burden and 36% of World Health Organization health burden.[1] Despite availability of guidelines directed antimicrobial therapy, it is an important cause of mortality and morbidity.[2] Severe CAP (sCAP) is essentially pneumonia which requires admission to the intensive care unit (ICU) or carries high mortality risk.[2] The mainstay of management of pneumonia is antibiotic therapy. Ventilatory support is required for patients who develop acute respiratory failure (ARF).[2] Mortality in CAP is determined by development of sepsis and onset of ARF.[3] Incidence of ARF has been reported in 58-87% of patients with severe CAP.[4] ARF, is characterized by an impaired gas exchange between the lungs and the blood. It can be managed by providing oxygen via a nasal cannula or face mask, followed by application of positive pressure throughout the respiratory cycle in occurrence of failure. Positive end expiratory pressure (PEEP) can be delivered either via endotracheal intubation (mechanical ventilation) or a noninvasive interface by noninvasive ventilation (NIV). Since mechanical ventilation is associated with an increased risk of complications, viz. ventilator-associated pneumonia (VAP), ventilator-induced lung injury, and increased need of sedation, NIV could have a role in avoiding intubation and its complications.[3]

■ EVIDENCE FOR USE OF NONINVASIVE VENTILATION IN PNEUMONIA

Though use of NIV in pneumonia may be a common practice in many ICUs. Available evidence for use of NIV in pneumonia are conflicting, thereby authors do not explicitly support or overtly oppose use of NIV in severe CAP. A cautious NIV attempt may be justified in CAP with the key point being patient selection.[5]

The rate of NIV failure in patients with pneumonia in various studies is widely variable, being lower in controlled clinical trials (21–26%) than observational studies (33–66%).[2] Vanoni et al. performed a systematic review of available literature focused on ARF in CAP between 1 Jan 1997 to 31 Aug 2017. When the data was analyzed, NIV success rates showed heterogenous results ranging from 20% to 76%. NIV failure was associated with higher mortality, prolonged ICU and hospital stay, and a higher rate of complications, (e.g. sepsis). The majority of the studies included in the review chose NIV failure as the primary endpoint,

(i. e. need for endotracheal intubation and mechanical ventilation).[3] A retrospective study was performed by Murad et al. on 209 patients using inhospital mortality as the primary outcome and reported the highest NIV failure rate of 76%.[6] A prospective study by Nicolini et al. in 2014 in 127 patients with sCAP and severe acute respiratory failure [oxygen arterial pressure/oxygen inspiratory fraction ratio (PaO_2/FiO_2) <250] reported lowest NIV failure rate (25%).[7] In a study by Carrillo et al. 184 consecutive patients were assessed where in 102 had "de novo" ARF, and 82 patients had previous cardiac or respiratory disease. Patients with "de novo" ARF failed NIV more frequently than patients with previous cardiac or respiratory disease (47, 46% vs 21, 26%, $p = 0.007$).[2] De novo ARF is defined as hypoxemic respiratory failure occurring in patients without chronic cardiopulmonary disease.[8] An RCT by Confalonieri et al. showed that in selected patients with ARF caused by severe CAP, NIV was associated with a significant reduction in the rate of intubation (21% vs 50%; $p = 0.03$) and duration of ICU stay (1.8 vs 6.6 days, $p = 0.04$).[4] This benefit, however, was almost entirely explained by the subgroup of patients with COPD or hypercapnic ARF.[9] Subgroup of patients with COPD showed a survival advantage at 2 months (88.9% vs 37.5%; $p = 0.05$).[4] The efficacy of NIV in ARF due to CAP when compared with other proven indications such as COPD and cardiogenic pulmonary edema showed the highest intubation rate occurred in patients with pneumonia.[10,11]

Hangyong et al. conducted a prospective, multicenter, randomized controlled trial (RCT) of NIV compared with conventional administration of oxygen through a Venturi mask for pneumonia induced mild early ARDS. Two hundred subjects were randomized to NIV (n = 102) or control (n = 98) groups from 21 centers. NIV did not decrease the proportion of patients requiring intubation than in the control group (11/102 vs 9/98, 10.8% vs 9.2%, $p = 0.706$).[12] Similarly, an RCT by Honrubia et al.[13] testing NIV as an alternative to invasive ventilation in patients with various types of ARF found that the subgroup with pneumonia did very poorly, with all 8 patients randomized to NIV requiring intubation. In contrast Ferrer et al.[14] showed that, NIV can be successful in community acquired pneumonia provided a very careful selection of the patient is performed (exclusion of hemodynamic instability, several organ failures, lack of cooperation, abundant secretions etc.).

Given the uncertainty of evidence, no recommendation on the use of NIV for de novo ARF were offered by European Respiratory Society/American Thoracic Society (ERS/ATS) guidelines. Pooled analysis demonstrated that NIV use led to a decrease in mortality (RR 0.83, 95% CI 0.65–1.05) and the need for intubation (RR 0.75, 95% CI 0.63–0.89), although these were both based on a low certainty of evidence.[15]

The wide variation in NIV outcomes is possibly due to variation in selection criteria of patients and conduct of studies in center with major experience in the use of NIV. Therefore, these results cannot be extrapolated to less trained and equipped hospitals and offer low certainty of evidence.[2]

REASONS FOR NIV FAILURE IN ARF DUE TO PNEUMONIA

The rationale of applying NIV is to improve oxygenation, to decrease dyspnea and the work of breathing and to avoid intubation.[8] Several mechanisms have been implicated for failure of NIV in de novo ARF:
- Positive effects achieved in terms of alveolar recruitment and reduction of work of breathing disappear immediately with the interruption of NIV.

- The end inspiratory transpulmonary pressure during NIV cannot be known and also the measurement of its surrogate, i.e. dynamic transpulmonary pressure using esophageal balloon is not clinically feasible. Tidal volume in spontaneously breathing patient in such a setting is dependent upon both airway pressure delivered by ventilator and respiratory muscle pressure generated by patient's respiratory drive. Thus, it is difficult to attain ideal low tidal volume. Concept of patient self-inflicted lung injury is a novel entity implicated in such a scenario as high respiratory drive may contribute to higher tidal volumes.
- Noninvasive ventilation by improving gas exchange and dyspnea may offer false optimism and delay clinical decision and timing of intubation.[8]

Recommendations

- Authors recommend use of NIV in the ICU with caution in selected patients with community-acquired pneumonia particularly in those with associated COPD (Level 2A).[9]
- Noninvasive ventilation in recipients of solid organ transplantation with acute hypoxemic respiratory failure (AHRF) is also associated with a significant reduction in intubation rate (20% vs 70%; $p = 0.002$), fatal complications (20% vs 50%; $p = 0.05$), length of ICU stay (5.5 vs 9; $p = 0.03$), and ICU mortality (20% vs 50%; $p = 0.05$).[16]
- Noninvasive ventilation requires the ability of clinicians to choose patients case-by-case. A trial of NIV may be offered to a patient with community-acquired pneumonia if they are being managed by an experienced clinical team, patients are carefully selected, cooperative (no contraindications such as abnormal mental status, shock or multiorgan system failure, associated major organ dysfunction, cardiac ischemia or arrhythmias, and with no limitations in clearing secretions). They should be closely monitored in the ICU, reassessed early after starting NIV and intubated promptly if they are not improving. The main risk of NIV for the indication of de novo ARF is to delay a needed intubation.
- Noninvasive ventilation has also been used in patients with ARF due to influenza A H1N1 infection, with failure rates ranging between 13% and 77%. Given the uncertainty of evidence for use of NIV in ARF due to pandemic viral illness no recommendations are offered.[15]

Predictors of Noninvasive Ventilation Failure (Flowchart 1)

Various studies have seen the failure trends and authors recommend that these be monitored carefully as predictors of NIV failure.[2] If predictors for NIV failure are present, avoiding delayed intubation of patients with "*de novo*" ARF would potentially minimize mortality.[16]
- Higher APACHE II scores and vasopressor use at 2 h after initiation of NIV.[6]
- More severe scores at admission (SAPS II and CURB 65), more extensive radiologic findings (Opravil score) ($p < 0.003$) and a higher lactate dehydrogenase (LDH), Greater respiratory impairment at admission (lower PaO_2/FiO_2 ratio, higher A-aDO2), and after 1 h of NIV ($p < 0.001$).[7] Opravil score grades the severity of pulmonary infiltrate on chest radiograph. Each lung is divided into four equal quadrants. Each quadrant is scored on a scale of 0–3, maximum score being 24 for both lungs. 0: normal, 1: subtle increase in interstitial markings, 2: prominent interstitial markings, 3: confluent interstitial and acinar opacities.[17]
- Worsening radiologic infiltrate 24 h after admission, maximum Sepsis-Related Organ Failure Assessment (SOFA) score and; after 1 h of NIV, higher heart rate and lower PaO_2/FiO_2 and bicarbonate independently predicted NIV failure.[2]

- Higher severity score, older age, or a failure to improve after 1 h of treatment.[15]
- Oxygenation index (OI; FiO_2 × mean airway pressure × $100/PaO_2$) is an early predictor of NIV failure. In patients who worsen or do not improve OI after 1 h NIV, in fact, intubation should be an early alternative. Higher SAPS II at admission and lower pH values before NIV have poor outcomes.[5]
- The severity of hypoxemia and the coexistence of other acute organ failure.[16]
- Higher tidal volumes before intubation.[15]
- Minute ventilation greater than 11 L/min at 48 h was the independent risk factor for NIV failure.[12]

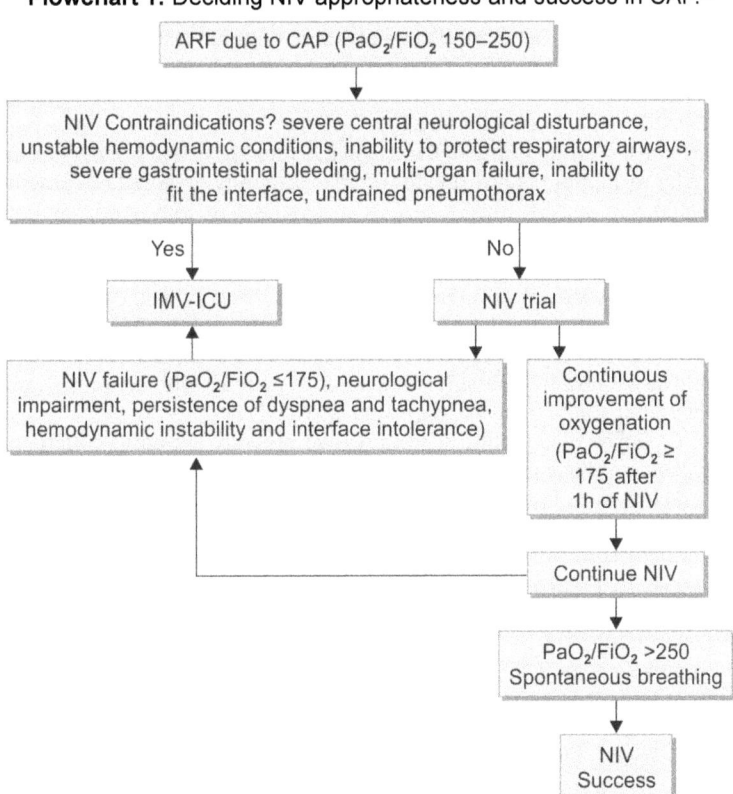

Flowchart 1: Deciding NIV appropriateness and success in CAP.[18]

(ARF: acute respiratory failure; CAP: community acquired pneumonia; ICU: intensive care unit; IMV: invasive mechanical ventilation; NIV: noninvasive ventilation)

KEY POINTS

Specific risks have been described with NIV and there is not enough evidence to recommend its use for all patients of pneumonia. An experienced clinical team may offer a trial of NIV in selected, closely monitored ICU patients so that they can be intubated promptly in case of lack of improvement. Predictors of NIV failure should be monitored judiciously to prevent delay in intubation. In conclusion, further research and larger RCT are needed to better evaluate the use of NIV in patients with CAP.

REFERENCES

1. Nayar S, Hasan A, Waghray P, Ramananthan S, Ahdal J, Jain R. Management of community-acquired bacterial pneumonia in adults: Limitations of current antibiotics and future therapies. Lung India. 2019;36(6):525-33.
2. Carrillo A, Gonzalez-Diaz G, Ferrer M, Martinez-Quintana ME, Lopez-Martinez A, Llamas N, et al. Non-invasive ventilation in community-acquired pneumonia and severe acute respiratory failure. Intensive Care Med. 2012;38(3):458-66.
3. Vanoni NM, Carugati M, Borsa N, Sotgiu G, Saderi L, Gori A, et al. Management of Acute Respiratory Failure Due to Community-Acquired Pneumonia: A Systematic Review. Med Sci. 2019;7(1):10.
4. Confalonieri M, Potena A, Carbone G, Porta RD, Tolley EA, Umberto Meduri G. Acute respiratory failure in patients with severe community-acquired pneumonia: a prospective randomized evaluation of noninvasive ventilation. Am J Respir Crit Care Med. 1999;160(5):1585-91.
5. Carron M, Freo U, Zorzi M, Ori C. Predictors of failure of noninvasive ventilation in patients with severe community-acquired pneumonia. J Crit Care. 2010;25(3):540-e9.
6. Murad A, Li PZ, Dial S, Shahin J. The role of noninvasive positive pressure ventilation in community-acquired pneumonia. J Crit Care. 2015;30(1):49-54.
7. Nicolini A, Ferraioli G, Ferrari-Bravo M, Barlascini C, Santo M, Ferrera L. Early non-invasive ventilation treatment for respiratory failure due to severe community-acquired pneumonia. Clin Respir J. 2016;10(1):98-103.
8. Scala R, Pisani L. Noninvasive ventilation in acute respiratory failure: which recipe for success? Eur Respir Rev. 2018;27(149):180029.
9. Chawla R, Chaudhry D, Kansal S, Khilnani GC, Mani RK, Nasa P, et al. Guidelines for noninvasive ventilation in acute respiratory failure. Indian J Crit Care Med. 2013;17(5):42-70.
10. Antonelli M, Conti G, Moro ML, Esquinas A, Gonzalez-Diaz G, Confalonieri M, et al. Predictors of failure of noninvasive positive pressure ventilation in patients with acute hypoxemic respiratory failure: a multi-center study. Intensive Care Med. 2001;27(11):1718-28.
11. Domenighetti G, Gayer R, Gentilini R. Noninvasive pressure support ventilation in non-COPD patients with acute cardiogenic pulmonary edema and severe community-acquired pneumonia: acute effects and outcome. Intensive Care Med. 2002;28(9):1226-32.
12. He H, Sun B, Liang L, Li Y, Wang H, Wei L, et al. A multicenter RCT of noninvasive ventilation in pneumonia-induced early mild acute respiratory distress syndrome. Crit Care. 2019;23(1):300.
13. Honrubia T, López FJ, Franco N, Mas M, Guevara M, Daguerre M, et al. Noninvasive vs conventional mechanical ventilation in acute respiratory failure: a multicenter, randomized controlled trial. Chest. 2005;128(6):3916-24.
14. Ferrer M, Esquinas A, Leon M, Gonzalez G, Alarcon A, Torres A. Noninvasive ventilation in severe hypoxemic respiratory failure: a randomized clinical trial. Am J Respir Crit Care Med. 2003;168(12):1438-44.
15. Rochwerg B, Brochard L, Elliott MW, Hess D, Hill NS, Nava S, et al. Official ERS/ATS clinical practice guidelines: noninvasive ventilation for acute respiratory failure. Eur Respir J. 2017;50(2):1602426.
16. Dhar R, Ghosh D, Krishnan S. Noninvasive ventilation in hypoxemic respiratory failure. J Assoc Chest Physicians. 2016;4(2):50.
17. Trivedi TH. Relying on Radiological Findings in Critically Ill H1N1Infected Patients-how Logical. J Assoc Physicians India. 2013;61:9-10.
18. Nicolini A, Cilloniz C, Piroddi IM, Faverio P. Noninvasive ventilation for acute respiratory failure due to community-acquired pneumonia: A concise review and update. Community Acquired Infection. 2015;2(2):46-50.

Section 3

Noninvasive Ventilation in Specific Situations

21. Noninvasive Ventilation during Transport
22. Noninvasive Ventilation during Intensive Care Unit Procedures
23. Ambulation on Noninvasive Ventilation in Critically Ill Patients
24. Sedation during Noninvasive Ventilation
25. Humidification and Aerosol Therapy in Noninvasive Ventilation

Chapter 21

Noninvasive Ventilation during Transport

Suresh Ramasubban

▮ INTRODUCTION

Critically ill patients require intrahospital as well as interhospital transport. Intrahospital transport primarily involves movement out of the intensive care units (ICU) for diagnostic and therapeutic procedures, predominantly to radiology and operating room (OR). Interhospital transport is generally for upgraded treatment facilities of a critically ill patient. Transport also involves emergency retrievals from home and other sites. Transport of critically ill patients is a challenge as these patients have deranged physiology and this gets worse during transport. Transport requires expertise and meticulous planning to ensure safety of the patients. Simple audits done in the United Kingdom have revealed that almost 15% of patients are received with hypotension and hypoxia, which were avoidable if safe transport principles had been followed.[1] A majority of the critically ill patient have respiratory failure as their primary deranged physiological organ system. This subset of critically ill patients requires special considerations during transport.

Noninvasive ventilation (NIV) has been one of the most important innovation in medicine that has revolutionized the management of respiratory failure. Indicated in a number of conditions leading to acute respiratory failure (ARF), use of NIV has become the gold standard in management of an acute exacerbation of chronic obstructive pulmonary disease (AECOPD) and acute decompensated heart failure (ADHF), which form the majority of admissions to the intensive care units (ICU).[2] Also, there is a spurt in the indications for NIV for varying conditions ranging from chest trauma to immunocompromised patients to facilitate end of life care. As the indications for NIV in ARF are increasing, consequently the need for transport of these patients on NIV also seems to be increasing. NIV use in the prehospital situation also has beneficial effect in preventing intubations and improves vital signs.[3]

▮ INTERHOSPITAL TRANSFER

Interhospital transfers and emergency retrievals are the domain of emergency medicine physicians and intensivists are not generally involved, however occasionally intensivists are requested to provide care during transport to another facility for upgraded treatment. Interhospital transport should be undertaken only after full assessment and discussion with all the stakeholders. Guidelines exist regarding timing of transfer for certain conditions like head injury, acute coronary syndromes and others, however for most other conditions safety of transport should follow the general guidelines for safe transfer. The general guidelines for safe transfer include the presence of staff well versed with transfers, appropriate equipment and vehicle, stabilization of the patient before transfer, continuous and extensive monitoring during transfer, continuing care during transfer (which includes continuing NIV, if patient was on NIV prior to transfer) and a good handover at the receiving hospital (**Table 1**). The details of a safe transfer are beyond the scope of this review; however, it is prudent to mention regarding stabilization before transfer with reference to respiratory failure and NIV.

Table 1: Guidelines for safe transfer of critically ill patient.
- Well trained and experienced staff in transportation of critically ill
- Appropriate equipment
- Stabilization of patient before transfer
- Monitoring during transfer
- Continuing care during transfer
- Handover
- Documentation.

Intubating a patient while in transit in a moving vehicle, aircraft etc. is very difficult, so while transporting a patient with ARF over a long distance without an unprotected airway, requires sound decision making. If the patient is very likely to lose his airway or develop respiratory failure in transit, then it is better to obtain an airway by intubation, prior to departure. Safety of transporting patients with ARF who are being managed by NIV had conflicting data. Recent reports from the Australian Helicopter Medical services,[4] involving 3018 missions, in which there were 106 cases of NIV therapy during the retrieval revealed that none of these patients died or were intubated enroute. These results demonstrate the growing safety of NIV in interhospital transport using NIV in patients with ARF, key however being proper patient selection.

■ INTRAHOSPITAL TRANSFER

Intrahospital transfer of patients on NIV usually are made from the Emergency department to ICU, from one unit to another or from ICU to radiology or endoscopy. Transport to and back from these locations to the ICU requires knowledge of the hospital layout as the time spent outside the controlled environment of the ICU depends on this. The time taken outside of the ICU generally is 10–15 min for transport from one unit to another, however, during transfer to radiology for diagnostics can involve 30–90 min outside the ICU. Even though intrahospital transfers offer more resources, space and equipment as compared to interhospital transports, principles of transfer remain the same. Before transferring a patient on NIV, it is important to go through some key elements and equipment.[5]

- *Patient selection prior to transport*: The indications of NIV for ARF should be reviewed prior to undertaking intrahospital transport of patients on NIV. Patients who are hemodynamically unstable, have impaired consciousness and are unable to protect their airways should preferably be not transported while on NIV. Patients who are not responding or those who are partial responders to NIV are poor candidates for transfer on NIV. Patients who do not have a class I indication for NIV and have ARF managed with NIV should also be closely evaluated prior to decision for transport, preferably these patients should avoid transfer while on NIV. Similarly, patients intolerant to NIV due to asynchrony or patients with persistent dyspnea on NIV should be stabilized further before transfer. In other words, the indications and contraindications of NIV should be carefully investigated, before initiating transfer on NIV (**Table 2**).

Table 2: Contraindications for transfer of patient on noninvasive ventilation.

- Unable to maintain adequate oxygenation and ventilation on noninvasive ventilation during transport
- Hemodynamic instability
- Unable to monitor patient's cardiorespiratory status during transport
- Unable to maintain control of airway during transport (e.g.,-Upper GI bleed, severe encephalopathy, excessive secretions)
- Inadequate staff available for transfer
- Lack of trained staff
- Lack of communication and coordination amongst various departments.

- *Preparation for transport*: Once the indications of NIV are confirmed and in the absence of any contraindications for NIV, pretransfer preparation and planning is commenced. Necessary staff for transport needs to be assembled. Transfer should be accompanied by one physician and a nurse or a respiratory therapist, who is trained in airway management and CPR. The transport team should be comfortable with NIV equipment and interfaces. Communication with the receiving unit is of the essence, to ensure an available bed on reaching the transfer destination.
- *Equipment for transfer*: The accompanying equipment should be portable, lightweight, compact and easily transportable through corridors and lifts. Positioning the equipment properly and securing it is vital, to prevent it from falling off the patient's bed during transport. The equipment includes an airway kit, resuscitation kit, oxygen source, monitor and of course NIV device and interface. The practical checking of equipment prior to transport should include:
    - Verify the availability and functioning of equipment needed for intubation, like laryngoscopes, ventilation bag, and medications required for intubation.
    - Ensure adequate oxygen supply. A general rule for oxygen requirements should consider the formula: 2 × transport time (min) × (minute ventilation × FiO_2) + ventilator driving gas + leak compensation.[6]
    - Ensure the presence of a monitor that provides heart rate and ECG monitoring and allows to continue invasive monitoring devices like arterial blood pressure (ABP).
    - Continuous pulse oximetry.
    - If using a Boussignac CPAP, i.e. CPAP high flow device, ensure proper functioning of the manometer and a suitable flow meter and correct connection of the hose, filter, and oxygen source (**Figs. 1 and 2**).
    - If using a mechanical device CPAP, check the battery charge status, monitor the set parameters and alarms, ensure correct interface fitting and finally ensure the proper connection between different parts.
    - Verify the availability of appropriate medications for resuscitation, sedation and rapid sequence intubation.
- *Noninvasive ventilators*: Three major categories of ventilators are available for delivery of NIV: bilevel ventilators, critical care ventilators, and intermediate ventilators. Bilevel ventilators work with a single limb circuit with a passive exhalation valve. Critical care

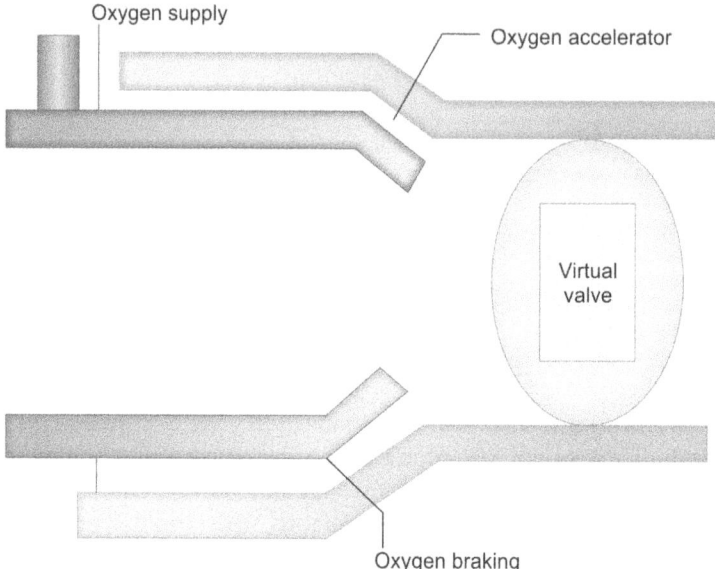

Fig. 1: Boussignac CPAP: Working principle (Jet turbine principle).
(*Courtesy*: Vygon catalogue: Vygon.com)

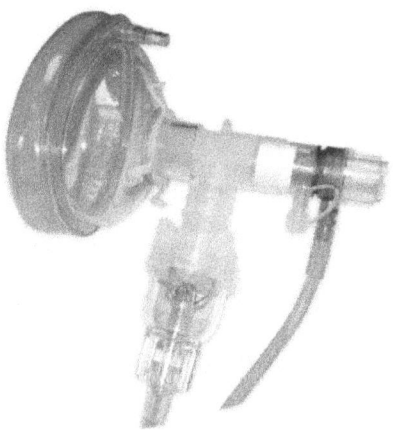

Fig. 2: Boussignac CPAP mask.
(*Courtesy*: richardsmedical.com)

ventilators have a dual limb circuit and have an active exhalation valve. Intermediate ventilators are usually used for transport and they may have a passive exhalation port or an active exhalation valve. It is therefore crucial to understand the potential danger of working with various ventilators, interfaces and tubing and the catastrophe of failing to match the appropriate ventilator with tubing. Therefore, it is mandatory to label circuits as "use with vented masks" or "use only with nonvented masks". Also, it is important to know the battery life of different equipment and take appropriate care to ensure no equipment failure during transport. Back up with a manual resuscitator is mandatory for transport.

- *Interface*: There are various interfaces available for the delivery of NIV. These include; nasal masks, oronasal masks, full face masks, helmets, and nasal pillows. However, for delivery of NIV in ARF, an oronasal mask is the preferred interface. However, if a patient is well suited to another device prior to transport, it is prudent to continue the same device for transport. Interface also includes the circuit; the circuit can be single limb or dual limb. A single limb circuit needs passive exhalation ports, so it is used with a vented mask while a dual limb circuit is generally used with devices which have an active exhalation valve, therefore a nonvented mask is used. Leak compensation is built-in into the bilevel ventilators and sometimes the algorithm uses only a manufacturer suggested interface with a bilevel machine. One needs to be aware of this before mixing and matching bilevel ventilators and interfaces of different manufacturers. It is generally preferred to use the manufacturer recommended interface for a bilevel ventilator.
- *Mode*: Most NIV work on a pressure targeted mode, either a pressure support (PS) or a pressure control (PC) mode. During transport, there is no specific recommendation for a mode, so it is prudent to continue with the same mode that the patient was on before transport. If ventilation change is necessary for transport, due to change of ventilator or interface, then monitoring on the transport NIV mode for 5–10 min prior to start of transport is necessary. Once stability is noted on the transport mode, then only should one proceed for transport.
- *Monitoring*: The purpose of monitoring during transport is to prevent the potential complications as listed in **Table 3**. The complications include circuit disconnect and loss of PEEP and a consequent hypoxemia/hypoventilation, positional changes leading to aspiration, hypoxemia and hypotension, arrhythmias due to acidosis or hypoxia and the other attendant complications of transport like accidental removal of catheters and intravenous medications. Blood gas monitoring during transport is not feasible, thus an arterial blood gas sample should be analyzed before transport, provided the patients clinical condition demands it. During transport, monitoring of the respiratory status is paramount and includes respiratory rate, oxygen saturation, asynchrony, dyspnea, and patient comfort.

Table 3: Complications of transporting patients on noninvasive ventilation (NIV)
- Hypoxemia due to loss of PEEP/CPAP
- Hypotension/Hypoxemia/Aspiration due to change of position
- Arrhythmias
- Disconnection of ventilatory support due to transport
- Disconnection of monitoring equipment due to transport

CONCLUSION

Noninvasive ventilation is increasingly used in patients with ARF and there is naturally an increasing requirement for transport of these patients. Transport on NIV is a challenge and can have significant potential complications which can be catastrophic and hence knowing the indications and contraindications for transfer on NIV is important. Interhospital as well as intrahospital transfer on NIV includes meticulous planning and communication and the general principles of safe transfer are well applicable in this regard. Equipment checks and having backup is mandatory for a safe transfer. A thorough knowledge of ventilators, interfaces and the circuits are necessary for safe transport on NIV. Intensivists who are responsible for transport need to be aware of the issues that have been highlighted in this review.

REFERENCES

1. Wallace PGM, Ridley SA. Transport of critically ill patients. BMJ. 1999;319(7206):368-71.
2. Ram FS, Picot J, Lightowler J. Non-invasive ventilation for treatment of respiratory failure due to acute exacerbation of chronic obstructive pulmonary disease. Cochrane database Syst Rev. 2004;(1):CD004104.
3. Alahmari MD. Noninvasive ventilation: Is a prehospital initiation an option? Saudi Crit Care J. 2017;1(1):47-8.
4. Coggins AR, Cummins EN, Burns B. Emerg Med J. 2016;33(11):807-11.
5. Schreiber A, Dominguez Petit AJ, Geoff P et al. Intra-hospital transport of patients on non-invasive ventilation: review, analysis and key practical recommendations by the International NIV committee. Eurasian J Pulmonol. 2017;19:124-9.
6. Ellis D, Hooper M. In: Cases in Pre-hospital and Retrieval Medicine. Netherlands: Elsevier. 2010.

Chapter 22

Noninvasive Ventilation during Intensive Care Unit Procedures

Sheila Nainan Myatra, Nishanth Baliga, Nirmalyo Lodh

▌ INTRODUCTION

Noninvasive ventilation (NIV), i.e. the delivery of assisted breaths without an invasive artificial airway, is a safe and effective means of improving gas exchange in patients. Traditionally NIV has been used for acute respiratory failure in the appropriate settings. This approach has advantages which include, avoiding complications associated with tracheal intubation, preserving airway defense mechanisms, speech and swallowing with a greater flexibility in instituting and liberating the patient from mechanical ventilation. NIV is also used to facilitate procedures in the ICU like preoxygenation before tracheal intubation, bronchoscopy, endoscopic procedures, transesophageal echocardiography, and procedural sedation.

▌ PREOXYGENATION

Preoxygenation or denitrogenation is a procedure done prior to tracheal intubation. During preoxygenation, the air present in the lungs is replaced with only oxygen to increase the reserve, leading to prolongation of the safe apnea time during tracheal intubation. This is particularly useful to prevent rapid arterial oxygen desaturation, when the tracheal intubation is difficult, and the intubation time is prolonged. Critically ill patients are considered to have a physiologically difficult airway, as they have a poor cardiopulmonary reserve and are prone to hypoxemia, hypotension, and cardiac arrest during tracheal intubation. As compared to the operating room, patient related factors, ICU related factors (infrastructure and equipment) and varying level of the operator skills at intubation, make tracheal intubation in ICU challenging, and a high risk procedure.[1] In addition, in critically ill patients, tracheal intubations are often performed in an emergency, leaving little time for preoxygenation.

Oxygen supply demand mismatch may exist in critically ill patients making them prone for cardiorespiratory complications during tracheal intubation. Hence preoxygenation is important in all critically ill patients. However, the usual preoxygenation methods using a non-rebreather bag valve mask may only be marginally effective, as the response to preoxygenation may be poor. A study compared a preoxygenation strategy of 4 minutes before tracheal intubation, using a non-rebreather bag valve mask in 34 unstable critically ill patients with 34 matched cardiac surgery patients. They found that after preoxygenation, the increase in arterial partial pressure of oxygen (PaO_2) was minimal in ICU patients (64.2 ± 3.5 to 86.8 ± 9.5) as compared to a significant increase in cardiac surgery patients (79 ± 12.3 to 403.6 ± 71.8).[2] This shows that preoxygenation before intubation in hypoxic patients, may not always be very effective.

Different methods to improve preoxygenation have been tried in critically ill patients. Positive pressure ventilation by continuous positive airway pressure (CPAP) was suggested to have potential benefit for preoxygenating patients.[3,4] This was proven by initial studies done in morbidly obese patients where application of CPAP for preoxygenation increased the time to hypoxia and reduced atelectasis during induction of anesthesia.[5] Following this, a study done on morbidly obese patients looked at application of pressure support ventilation along with positive end expiratory pressure (PEEP) for preoxygenation and found that it was feasible, safe, and efficient. They found that 95% of patients in NIV group attained target end expiratory oxygen fraction >90% compared to only 50% in oxygen group.[6]

Baillard et al. looked at NIV as a preoxygenation method to be more effective at reducing arterial oxyhemoglobin desaturation than usual preoxygenation in hypoxemic, critically ill patients requiring tracheal intubation for invasive ventilation in the ICU. This study recruited acute hypoxemic respiratory failure patients with PaO_2 <100 on 10 L/min flow of oxygen into two groups. One group received preoxygenation using non-rebreather bag valve mask with 15 L/min flow of oxygen. In the other group, pressure support ventilation was delivered by the ventilator, using a mask adjusted to obtain an expired tidal volume of 7-10 mL/kg FiO_2 of 100% and a PEEP of 5 cm of H_2O. The PaO_2 was significantly higher in the NIV group as compared to the control group (203 mm Hg vs. 60 mm Hg). This study concluded that NIV is safe and more effective in providing oxygenation and preventing arterial oxygen desaturation than the usual method of preoxygenation during tracheal intubation in critically ill patients. NIV in this study was used in a pressure limited mode, which allowed for precise control of the insufflations pressures, such that none of them received more than 20 cm of H_2O. Thus, the risk of pulmonary aspiration was reduced. They hypothesized that NIV probably increased FRC by recruiting collapsed alveoli and increasing lung volume, hence increasing oxygen reserves in the body.[7]

Following this study, NIV as method of preoxygenation was included as an integral component of an *"intubation bundle"* called the *"Montpellier-ICU intubation algorithm"* which consisted of 10 steps divided into preintubation, perintubation and postintubation bundles. In the preintubation section, it was suggested to preoxygenate patients with acute respiratory failure for 3 min with noninvasive positive pressure ventilation with 100% FiO_2 using pressure support ventilation between 5 and 10 cm H_2O and a PEEP of 5 cm of H_2O. This was validated by a multicenter before and after study, which found that the implementation of an tracheal intubation management protocol can reduce immediate severe life-threatening complications associated with tracheal intubation of ICU patients.[8]

High-flow nasal cannula (HFNC) oxygen can be used for preoxygenation and also provides apneic oxygenation. Frat JP et al. conducted a multicenter, randomized controlled trial (FLORALI 2) to study whether preoxygenation using NIV was more efficient than HFNC in reducing risk of hypoxemia during tracheal intubation. They found that preoxygenation with NIV or HFNC did not change the risk of severe hypoxemia. However, compared with HFNC, NIV might be better to prevent severe hypoxemia in patients with severe to moderate hypoxemia.[9]

Jaber et al. conducted a proof of concept study (OPTINIV trial) to assess whether adding HFNC to NIV was superior to NIV alone for preoxygenation during tracheal intubation in critically ill patients. They found lesser incidences of desaturation in NIV with HFNC group than NIV alone. However, further studies are needed to incorporate this into clinical practice.[10]

BRONCHOSCOPY

Bronchoscopy is a procedure usually performed for both diagnostic as well as therapeutic purposes in patients with respiratory disease. It helps to visualize upper airway and proximal divisions of the tracheobronchial tree. Samples from trachea, bronchi, mediastinum and lung parenchyma can be taken. Therapeutic procedures like clearing secretions, mucus plug removal, toileting, foreign body removal, tracheal intubation can also be done with bronchoscopes. Different bronchoscopes commonly used are rigid bronchoscope, flexible fiberoptic bronchoscope and ultrasound guided bronchoscopy (EBUS). In the ICU, the flexible fiberoptic bronchoscope is commonly used.

Bronchoscopy has been traditionally done in intubated patients or in patients who do not have hypoxemic respiratory failure. Bronchoscope can take up to 10% of the tracheal lumen reducing its caliber, which increases resistance of the airway. In critically ill patients with altered lung mechanics, this increased flow resistance can worsen respiratory failure. While performing bronchoscopy, application of suction can lower the end expiratory pressure leading to loss of PEEP and early airway closure. Overall, bronchoscopy can lead to reduction of PaO_2 by 10–20 mm Hg. This reduction in PaO_2 takes time to normalize in patients with lung disease, hence supplemental oxygen during procedure may be useful.[11]

A study done in critically ill hypoxemic patients found that bronchoscopy is often followed by an increase in ventilatory support and need for tracheal intubation.[12] Due to these factors, tracheal intubation and mechanical ventilation is usually opted in patients in whom bronchoscopy is deemed necessary in critically ill patients. However, this exposes the patient to complications related to tracheal intubation and mechanical ventilation, infections and liberation from mechanical ventilation. NIV is a useful alternative to perform bronchoscopy in ICU patients when feasible. Spontaneous ventilation maintained during the procedure helps balance the ventilation perfusion ratio and hemodynamic stability, facilitating the bronchoscopy.

Several studies have been conducted to look at the use of NIV during bronchoscopy. The first study which looked at bronchoscopy in patients on NIV was by Antonelli et al. who performed bronchoalveolar lavage in eight immunocompromised patients with severe hypoxemia and found that the use of NIV was associated with significant improvements in oxygenation during bronchoscopy which was well tolerated and none of the patients required mechanical ventilation.[13] A study was done in chronic obstructive pulmonary disease (COPD) patients without any signs of acute respiratory failure who required bronchoalveolar lavage. The feasibility and safety of noninvasive positive pressure ventilation (NIPPV) by facemask during fiberoptic bronchoscopy (FOB) was studied. It was found that SpO_2 significantly improved during bronchoscopy with no desaturation episodes.[14]

A CPAP device was used to facilitate performance of FOB in hypoxemic patients and was found to allow minimum alterations in gas exchange and prevented subsequent respiratory failure.[15] Subsequently, a randomized study compared noninvasive positive pressure ventilation with conventional oxygen in severe hypoxemic patients, and found that there was an increase in PaO_2/FiO_2 by 82% with NIV whereas in the oxygen therapy group PaO_2/FiO_2 declined by 10%. While the PaO_2/FiO_2 remained elevated in the NIV group, it fell by 10% in the oxygen therapy group an hour after the procedure. They concluded that in severely hypoxemic patient, NIV was superior to conventional oxygen supplementation as it prevented deterioration of gas-exchange during FOB and patients had better hemodynamic tolerance.[16]

One of the disadvantages of NIV during bronchoscopy is leaks and ineffective ventilation due to the passage of the bronchoscope through ventilating port in the mask. Hence other interfaces have been used. Chiner described nasal NIV, with FOB performed orally using a bite block sealed with an elastic glove finger. He concluded that FOB can be performed through the oral route without any increase in complications.[17] The helmet as an interface has been used for NIPPV in patients who required bronchoalveolar lavage. A specific sealed connector was used to insert the bronchoscope through the nasal route which was tolerated well by the patients. A full-face mask was used for delivery of positive pressure during diagnostic bronchoscopy, in patients with hypoxemia which was tolerated well by most patients.[18,19]

In a study of patients which compared the use of NIV with bronchoscopy in patients with decompensated COPD and hypercapnic encephalopathy due to community-acquired pneumonia with invasive ventilation, the use of NIV with therapeutic bronchoscopy was associated with similar improvement in PaO_2/FiO_2.[20]

A case series reported bronchoscopic lung biopsy in patients on NIV for obtaining diagnosis in hypoxemic patients with diffuse lung infiltrates. NIV was applied in patients with diffuse parenchymal infiltrates and PaO_2/FiO_2 <200 mm Hg who underwent bronchoscopic lung biopsy. FOB was well tolerated, and all 6 subjects maintained SpO_2 >92% during the procedure. One subject required tracheal intubation due to hemoptysis.[21]

All these studies showed that NIV can be used as a safe alternative for bronchoscopy, especially in patients in whom tracheal intubation and mechanical ventilation can be avoided. Common indications are acute hypoxemic respiratory failure, COPD with pneumonia, obstructive sleep apnea who need bronchoscopy, postoperative patients who require removal of mucus plug, tracheobronchomalacia, where NIV is found to be beneficial probably by pneumatic stenting. However, NIV does not provide definitive airway and patients are at a risk for aspiration. Hence only experienced bronchoscopists with expertise in airway management, should perform the procedure in such patients using NIV.

ENDOSCOPY AND TRANSESOPHAGEAL ECHOCARDIOGRAPHY

Endoscopic procedures such as gastroscopy, transesophageal echocardiography (TEE), endoscopic retrograde cholangiopancreatography (ERCP) are being routinely performed in ICU for diagnostic as well as therapeutic purposes. These procedures may require patients to be sedated and adequate analgesia needs to be provided. Patients who are not intubated are at risk of hypoxia and hypoventilation. Critically ill patients have a reduced respiratory and cardiovascular reserve which makes them vulnerable for deterioration while these procedures are performed.[22] NIV is particularly useful in this population as it provides an alternative to tracheal intubation and mechanical ventilation when feasible. NIV can be used for preoxygenation of the patient, during the procedure, and after the procedure to enhance recovery of patient.

Transesophageal echocardiography is being commonly done these days, not just for diagnostic purposes but also for interventions such as atrial appendage closure procedures, and transaortic valve implantation. Few case reports described periprocedural NIV application and TEE either through a hole in the NIV mask or special masks with connectors which allow TEE probe to be inserted. NIV allowed performance of continuous TEE examination in lightly sedated patients, avoiding tracheal intubation and general anesthesia.[23,24]

Gastrointestinal procedures like endoscopy, gastroscopy, ERCP are being increasingly performed in critically ill patients. The use of a face mask with a mask adaptor equipped with a port for ventilation and a port for the probe was successful in observational studies. Several other modifications of NIV mask have been used to perform these procedures. Heunks at al. have used a full face mask which was modified with a plastic cylinder secured in the mask which allowed introduction of bronchoscope through mouth and had a disposable cap from swivel connector which sealed cylinder and prevented air leakage.[25] Another device which was used is called a Janus mask. It is a full face mask with a hole covered by a membrane which allows insertion of endoscope and prevents interruption of pressure support.[26]

PROCEDURAL SEDATION

Certain painful procedures in awake patients like intercostal drain insertion, pleural tapping, ascites tapping, suprapubic cystostomy, cardioversion, and percutaneous nephrostomy may require sedation and analgesia. Due to their premorbid conditions, these patients are at risk for hypoventilation and airway obstruction after sedation, thus may require tracheal intubation and mechanical ventilation to increase the margin of safety. However, NIV can be used in these situations as an alternative. A small case series described use of nasal NIV in the emergency department in patients undergoing procedural sedation and analgesia. They reported that under supervised conditions, NIV can be used for procedural sedation and analgesia, thus avoiding hypoxia and hypoventilation.[27]

CONCLUSION

Preoxygenation before tracheal intubation using NIV, has been shown to be superior to preoxygenation using a non-rebreather bag valve mask in critically ill patients. NIV is being increasingly used for indications other than acute hypoxemic respiratory failure, such as for procedures like bronchoscopy, endoscopic procedures, transesophageal echocardiography and procedural sedation in the ICU. This approach has the advantages of avoiding complications associated with tracheal intubation, preserving airway defense mechanisms, speech, and swallowing etc. However, lack of definitive airway protection, risk of hypoventilation and hypoxia, mandates its use in expert hands. Further studies are required before strong recommendations can be made for its use in these settings.

KEY POINTS

- Preoxygenation with NIV is superior to preoxygenation using non-rebreather bag valve mask for reducing arterial oxygen desaturation during tracheal intubation of hypoxemic patients in ICU.
- Preoxygenation with NIV or HFNC does not change the risk of severe hypoxemia during tracheal intubation. However, compared with HFNC, NIV is better to prevent severe hypoxemia in patients with moderate to severe hypoxemia.
- Noninvasive ventilation is superior to conventional oxygen supplementation during FOB for preventing gas-exchange deterioration, with better hemodynamic tolerance in patients with severe hypoxemia.

- In patients in whom tracheal intubation can be avoided, NIV can be used as a safe alternative for performance of bronchoscopy, endoscopy, transesophageal echocardiography and ERCP, with modifications of interface to facilitate these procedures.
- In awake patients in ICU, NIV can be used to avoid the increased risk of hypoventilation and hypoxia during procedural sedation.

REFERENCES

1. Myatra SN, Ahmed SM, Kundra P, Garg R, Ramkumar V, Patwa A, et al. The All India Difficult Airway Association 2016 guidelines for tracheal intubation in the Intensive Care Unit. Indian J Anaesth. 2016;60(12):922-30.
2. Mort TC. Preoxygenation in critically ill patients requiring emergency tracheal intubation. Crit Care Med. 2005;33:2672-5.
3. Benumof J. Preoxygenation: best method for both efficacy and efficiency. Anesthesiology. 1999;91(3):603-5.
4. Reynolds S, Heffner J. Airway management of the critically ill patient: rapid-sequence intubation. Chest. 2005;127(4):1397-412.
5. Gander S, Frascarolo P, Suter M, Spahn DR, Magnusson L. Positive end-expiratory pressure during induction of general anesthesia increases duration of nonhypoxic apnea in morbidly obese patients. Anesth Analg. 2005;100(2):580-4.
6. Delay JM, Sebbane M, Jung B, Nocca D, Verzilli D, Pouzeratte Y, et al. The effectiveness of noninvasive positive pressure ventilation to enhance preoxygenation in morbidly obese patients: a randomized controlled study. Anesth Analg. 2008;107(5):1707-13.
7. Baillard C, Fosse JP, Sebbane M, Chanques G, Vincent F, Courouble P, et al. Noninvasive ventilation improves preoxygenation before intubation of hypoxic patients. Am J Respir Crit Care Med. 2006;174(2):171-7.
8. Jaber S, Jung B, Corne P, Sebbane M, Muller L, Chanques G, et al. An intervention to decrease complications related to endotracheal intubation in the intensive care unit: a prospective, multiple-center study. Intensive Care Med. 2010;36(8):248-55.
9. Frat JP, Ricard JD, Quenot JP, Pichon N, Demoule A, Forel JM, et al. Non-invasive ventilation versus high-flow nasal cannula oxygen therapy with apnoeic oxygenation for preoxygenation before intubation of patients with acute hypoxaemic respiratory failure: a randomised, multicentre, open-label trial. Lancet Respir Med. 2019;7(4):303-12.
10. Jaber S, Monnin M, Girard M, Conseil M, Cisse M, Carr J, et al. Apnoeic oxygenation via high-flow nasal cannula oxygen combined with non-invasive ventilation preoxygenation for intubation in hypoxaemic patients in the intensive care unit: the single-centre, blinded, randomised controlled OPTINIV trial. Intensive Care Med. 2016;42(12):1877-87.
11. Murgu SD, Pecson J, Colt HG. Bronchoscopy during noninvasive ventilation: indications and technique. Respir Care. 2010;55(5):595-600.
12. Cracco C, Fartoukh M, Prodanovic H, Azoulay E, Chenivesse C, Lorut C, et al. Safety of performing fiberoptic bronchoscopy in critically ill hypoxemic patients with acute respiratory failure. Intensive Care Med. 2013;39(1):45-52.
13. Antonelli M, Conti G, Riccioni L, Meduri GU. Noninvasive positive-pressure ventilation via face mask during bronchoscopy with BAL in high-risk hypoxemic patients. Chest. 1996;110(3):724-8.
14. Da Conceicao M, Genco G, Favier JC, Bidallier I, Pitti R. Fiberoptic bronchoscopy during noninvasive positive-pressure ventilation in patients with chronic obstructive lung disease with hypoxemia and hypercapnia. Ann Fr Anesth Reanim 2000;19(4):231-6.
15. Maitre B, Jaber S, Maggiore SM, Bergot E, Richard JC, Bakthiari H, et al. Continuous positive airway pressure during fiberoptic bronchoscopy in hypoxemic patients: a randomized double-blind study using a new device. Am J Respir Crit Care Med. 2000;162(3):1063-7.

16. Antonelli M, Conti G, Rocco M, Arcangeli A, Cavaliere F, Proietti R, et al. Noninvasive positive-pressure ventilation vs conventional oxygen supplementation in hypoxemic patients undergoing diagnostic bronchoscopy. Chest. 2002;121(4):1149-54.
17. Chiner E, Sancho-Chust JN, Llombart M, Senent C, Camarasa A, Signes-Costa J. Fiberoptic bronchoscopy during nasal non-invasive ventilation in acute respiratory failure. Respiration. 2010;80(4):321-6.
18. Antonelli M, Pennisi MA, Conti G, Bello G, Maggiore SM, Michetti V, et al. Fiberoptic bronchoscopy during non-invasive positive pressure ventilation delivered by helmet. Intensive Care Med. 2003;29(1):126-9.
19. Heunks LM, de Bruin CJ, van der Hoeven JG, van der Heijden HF. Non-invasive mechanical ventilation for diagnostic bronchoscopy using a new face mask: an observational feasibility study. Intensive Care Med. 2010; 36(1):143-7.
20. Scala R, Naldi M, Maccari U. Early fiberoptic bronchoscopy during non-invasive ventilation in patients with decompensated chronic obstructive pulmonary disease due to community-acquired-pneumonia. Crit Care. 2010;14(2):R80.
21. Agarwal R, Khan A, Aggarwal AN, Gupta D. Bronchoscopic lung biopsy using noninvasive ventilatory support: case series and review of literature of NIV-assisted bronchoscopy. Respir Care. 2012; 57(11):1927-36.
22. Pieri M, Landoni G, Cabrini L. Noninvasive ventilation during endoscopic procedures: rationale, Clinical Use, and Devices. J Cardiothorac Vasc Anesth. 2017; 32(2):928-34.
23. Guarracino F, Cabrini L, Baldassarri R, Cariello C, Covello RD, Landoni G, et al. Non-invasive ventilation-aided transesophageal echocardiography in high-risk patients: A pilot study. Eur J Echocardiogr. 2010;11(6):554-6.
24. Pisano A, Angelone M, Iovino T, Gargiulo S, Manduca S, De Pietro A. Transesophageal echocardiography through a non-invasive ventilation helmet. J Cardiothorac Vasc Anesth. 2013;27(6):e78-81
25. Heunks L, DeBruin C, van der Hoeven J, van der Heijden HJ. Non-invasive mechanical ventilation for diagnostic bronchoscopy using a new face mask: An observational feasibility study. Intensive Care Med. 2009;36(1):143-7.
26. Cabrini L, Landoni G. A novel non-invasive ventilation mask to prevent and manage respiratory failure during fiberoptic bronchoscopy, gastroscopy and transesophageal echocardiography. Heart Lung Vessel. 2015;7(4):297-303.
27. Strayer RJ, Caputo ND. Non-invasive ventilation procedural sedation in ED: a case series. Am J Emerg Med. 2015;33(1):108-22.

Chapter 23

Ambulation on Noninvasive Ventilation in Critically Ill Patients

Prashant Nasa, Aanchal Singh

INTRODUCTION

Young and healthy individuals can get skeletal muscle atrophy when they are immobilized for more than 72 hours, while older adults may exhibit greater loss of strength and muscle mass with prolonged bed rest.[1,2] Mechanical ventilation itself can cause atrophy and weakness of the diaphragm, also called ventilator-induced diaphragmatic dysfunction (VIDD).[3] The early initiation of physical therapy (PT) in patients on invasive mechanical ventilation (IMV) has been found to be associated with more rapid return to ambulation, and improved functional independence.[4,5] Even repeated daily passive mobilization has been shown to reduce and prevent muscle atrophy in mechanically ventilated patients.[6] Noninvasive ventilation (NIV) has revolutionized the mechanical ventilation in intensive care units (ICUs) by reducing the need of endotracheal intubation, length of stay in ICU, and even mortality. We reviewed advantages of NIV over IMV, and feasibility with efficacy of early ambulation with NIV in critically ill patients.

EFFECTS OF BED REST ON CRITICALLY ILL PATIENTS

The traditional concept of bed rest during an illness is not based on any scientific fact and the harmful effect of bed rest on critically ill patients has been reported in literature from late 19th century. In a controlled trial published in 1944, to evaluate the effectiveness of early mobility after major surgery, there was a trend of reduced complications, either local surgical or systemic, in the early mobility group.[7] The bed rest was challenged in many studies and in fact was found counterproductive by causing skeletal muscle deconditioning and even atrophy.[5,8]

There are many factors which are proposed for neuromuscular weakness in critically ill patients. The patients on invasive ventilation have risk of muscle deconditioning and disuse atrophy because of inability to mobilize. This risk is further increased by ventilation itself, which can cause atrophy and weakness of the diaphragm, known as VIDD. The effect on IMV on respiratory muscles was seen on muscle biopsy as necrosis and replacement of muscle fibers by adipose and connective tissue.[8,9] In a study among patients with acute respiratory distress syndrome (ARDS), all of who were ventilated and survived were found to have 3–11% relative decrease in muscle strength for each day of bed rest.[10] Sepsis further contributes to muscle weakness in the ICU and more specifically linked to respiratory muscle weakness.[11,12]

Intensive care unit-acquired weakness (ICUAW) is a term coined for new-onset clinically detectable weakness among patients in ICU with no other possible etiology other than their recent critical illness.[13] ICUAW is characterized by muscle weakness and/or wasting, nerve injury or damage which can start within few days of ICU stay.[8,13] The ICUAW has significant impact on ICU outcomes, with patients who develop ICUAW have been found to have increased duration of ventilator stay, ventilator-associated pneumonia recurrent respiratory failure, and higher mortality.[14,15] The effects on ICUAW is even seen postdischarge from ICU, as with increased mortality at day 90 and only one-third of survived patients were able to resume their work even after 6 months.[16]

The long-term sequelae seen with ICUAW are reduced strength of respiratory muscles, physical and psychological independence, and finally poor quality of life even months to years after ICU or hospital discharge.[15,16] The etiopathogenesis of ICUAW is multifactorial, with neuropathy myopathy, mixed neuromyopathy, and disuse atrophy, however immobility is the most important risk factor which may result in loss of strength, muscular endurance, and muscle bulk.[8]

■ MANAGEMENT OF INTENSIVE CARE UNIT-ACQUIRED WEAKNESS

There are unfortunately very few treatment options available once ICUAW sets in and patient may take either very long to become functionally independent or succumb to complications. The early mobilization of patients on mechanical ventilation and passive or active exercise while still being ventilated is a promising strategy which can attenuate ICUAW and improve outcome.[14,17,18] The early mobilization of critically ill patients on mechanical ventilation is a difficult task and logistic challenge for healthcare staff. The use of heavy sedation, safety aspect of cardiopulmonary dynamics, logistics of manpower, and fear of losing airway are some of the reasons which prevent healthcare staff from early mobilization of the patients.[19-21]

■ EARLY MOBILIZATION OF MECHANICALLY VENTILATED PATIENTS

The initial small pilot studies in last decade evaluated the safety aspect of mobilizing critically ill patients on IMV in ICU.[22,23] The effectiveness and safety of early mobilization of patients on invasive ventilator is then reviewed in controlled studies and found early mobilization of patients is not only safe in ICU, but may result in reduced ICU and hospital length of stay.[24-26] Recently, reviews and guidelines have become available for early mobilization of critically ill mechanically ventilated patients.[27,28] However, despite enough good quality evidence, the actual practices in ICU have not changed and there is reluctance among healthcare workers for early mobilization.[16,21,29]

The term "early mobilization" is used interchangeably in these studies for various things like early rehabilitation, early or progressive mobility, and actual early ambulation. This heterogeneity in definition effect the generalizability of studies, and actual bedside translation into practice.[16]

■ EARLY AMBULATION OF PATIENT ON NONINVASIVE VENTILATION

Vasilevskis et al. proposed "ABCDE bundle" which includes awakening and breathing coordination, delirium monitoring/management, and early exercise/mobility for preventing delirium and ICUAW.[30]

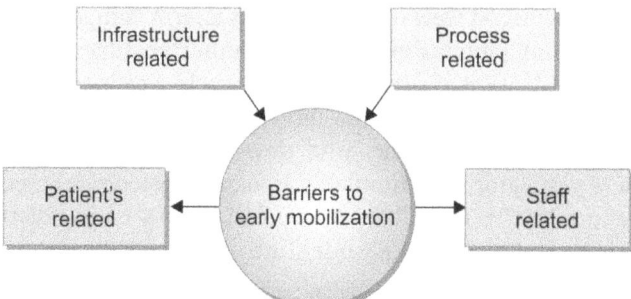

Fig. 1: Barriers in early mobilization of patients in ICU.

There are various barriers to prevent early mobilize patients in ICU (**Fig. 1**). In a clinical survey among healthcare professionals, the barriers to early mobilization can be due to—(1) Patients related (e.g. *delirium*, risk of musculoskeletal self-injury, and hemodynamic instability), (2) Infrastructure (insufficient healthcare professionals, equipment for safe mobilization), (3) ICU cultures (excessive sedations, overworked staff), and (4) Process (absence of standard operating procedures for safe mobilization).[31] In a point-prevalence study on early mobilization in Australia and New Zealand, the main barriers for early mobilization in mechanically ventilated patients were sedation and intubation.[32] In a point-prevalence study in Germany, 53% of patients on NIV were mobilized as compared to only 8% of patients on endotracheal tube.[21] Similar results were found in a Brazilian study with 50% patients on NIV were mobilized as compared to only 2% with endotracheal tube.[33] The main barriers in these studies were hemodynamic instability and sedation. In contrast to invasive ventilation, NIV has many advantages which may overcome these barriers like no sedation, and active patient with intact airway reflexes and can expectorate secretions. The absence of endotracheal tube and sedation with NIV, easy interface makes early mobilization possible. The patients on NIV are also better able to comprehend the instructions of staff which explain much higher mobilization.

The availability of adequate and appropriate professionals to form a multidisciplinary team is evaluated in studies as one of the barriers, especially attempting to make the patient walk with mechanical ventilation.[34,35] In a study, the increase in number of physiotherapists from one to three has significantly increased mobilization interventions during weekends.[35] However, it is common to find ICUs with inadequate manpower not only of physiotherapists, but also nursing staff which makes the early mobilization further challenging. The multidisciplinary team involving respiratory therapists, nurses, physiotherapists, and caregivers is integral in success of any mobilization strategy. The teams also should have been trained and supported adequately.

EARLY AMBULATION WITH NONINVASIVE VENTILATION

The recent availability of portable NIV has made early mobilization with NIV further feasible. These are standard NIV machines either mounted on mobile customized consoles. There are other new open interface which are compact and portable and user-friendly interface with better patient comfort and coordination.[36-38] The use of portable NIV machines with or without oxygen was used in these studies and found useful. The patients on high flow oxygen or NIV can easily communicate, understand, and comprehend healthcare staff instructions. The NIV machine can also be transported into different units of the hospital and/or home which can ensure continuation of ambulation and physiotherapy even after discharge. Patients on NIV are more comfortable and confident during periods of ambulation.

The issue of patient safety always deters physicians and other staff in early mobilization. In a single center study, the use of NIV with PT is found to be safe and effective, even in patients who have high oxygen requirements. There was positive trend noted toward length of stay, long-term functional outcome, and discharge disposition.[39] There are few other studies which explored use of NIV in early exercise training and ambulation of patients with chronic obstructive pulmonary disease (COPD) with limited success.[36,37] In comparison to standard oxygen therapy, these portable and open systems provided siginificantly increased daily activities, respiratory endurance time, and oxygenation with reduction of dyspnea, fatigue, and discomfort. The NIV has also been tried in rehabilitation of chronic respiratory failure with improvement in endurance time as compared to exercise alone.[38]

There are other studies which studied use of NIV in postoperative patients to reduce respiratory complications with physiotherapy and early ambulation. The combination of perioperative NIV and early postoperative mobilization can reduce postoperative pulmonary complications in high-risk upper abdominal surgery.[40] There is another study ongoing on combination of NIV plus early ambulation in upper abdominal surgery patients versus postoperative high flow nasal oxygen therapy.[41]

How to mobilize patient with noninvasive ventilation?

Early mobilization is considered when patients are first physiologically stable with reasonable fraction of inspired oxygen (FiO_2) (preferably less than 0.6). The mobilization protocol can start with initial testing of muscle strength which includes bed mobility exercises, sitting on the edge of the bed, standing, transferring to a chair, and gradual ambulation. Issues regarding equipment and specialized technological aids are important along with clear instructions to the team on mobilization process. The multidisciplinary team comprising of physiotherapist or nursing staff should be identified, trained, and using validated and customized clear protocol, a mobilization team can be made. The minimum equipment includes a portable cardiac monitor for hemodynamic monitoring and pulse oximeter to allow continuous monitoring of vital signs during ambulation, and a wheeled pole with infusion pumps for intravenous medications that cannot be temporarily stopped during mobilization. Early NIV and/or high flow oxygen nasal cannulas can be important component of rehabilitation equipment and standard physical medicine. Furthermore, NIV may be administered outside of the intensive care setting, allowing caregivers to more rationally utilize acute-care beds, and it greatly simplifies care for patients with chronic respiratory failure in the home.

COST-EFFECTIVENESS OF EARLY MOBILIZATION

The increased resources required for mobilization of patients are laborious and generally considered added cost. However in a study done in Medical ICU, study done in medical ICU of Johns Hopkins Hospital in United States, the financial model on early rehabilitation was found cost-saving.[42]

FUTURE DIRECTIONS

The portable light weight NIV equipment with oxygen cylinder or concentrator is being build which may help in mobilization of the patients. The physiotherapy or mobilization team driven simple interface models of NIV will be tested in future studies. The studies on early ambulation with use of NIV in postoperative patients after abdominal surgery are ongoing.[41] Similar studies in other subset of ICU patients like use of NIV to prevent extubation failure from invasive ventilation. The novel use of existing equipment and devices on mobile consoles may assist with early rehabilitation and can be considered in resource-limited settings.

SUMMARY

Noninvasive ventilation is a viable alternative to IMV in selected patients and has many advantages. The early mobilization with NIV is feasible, safe, and effective with early recovery of lung function and can reduce or prevent ICUAW. The patients on NIV should be mobilized at the earliest after initial stabilization. The locally developed protocol with involvement of all stakeholders and regular audits can be used as an initial tool for early mobilization.

REFERENCES

1. Iannuzzi-Sucich M, Prestwood KM, Kenny AM. Prevalence of sarcopenia and predictors of skeletal muscle mass in healthy, older men and women. J Gerontol A Biol Sci Med Sci. 2002;57:M772-7.
2. JiMorris PE, Goad A, Thompson C, Taylor K, Harry B, Passmore L, et al. Early intensive care unit mobility therapy in the treatment of acute respiratory failure. Crit Care Med. 2008;36:2238-43.
3. Hermans G, Agten A, Testelmans D, Decramer M, Gayan-Ramirez G. Increased duration of mechanical ventilation is associated with decreased diaphragmatic force: a prospective observational study. Crit Care. 2010;14:R127.
4. Bailey P, Thomsen GE, Spuhler VJ, Blair R, Jewkes J, Bezdjian L, et al. Early activity is feasible and safe in respiratory failure patients. Crit Care Med. 2007;35:139-45.
5. Kortebein P, Ferrando A, Lombeida J, Wolfe R, Evans WJ. Effect of 10 days of bed rest on skeletal muscle in healthy older adults. JAMA. 2007;297:1772-4.
6. Brahmbhatt N, Murugan R, Milbrandt EB. Early mobilization improves functional outcomes in critically ill patients. Crit Care. 2010;14:321.
7. Powers JH. The abuse of rest as a therapeutic measure in surgery: early postoperative activity and rehabilitation. JAMA. 1944;125:1079-83.
8. Puthucheary ZA, Rawal I, McPhail M, Connolly B, Ratnayake G, Chan P, et al. Acute skeletal muscle wasting in critical illness. JAMA. 2013;310:1591-600.
9. Derde S, Hermans G, Derese I, Güiza F, Hedström Y, Wouters PJ, et al. Muscle atrophy and preferential loss of myosin in prolonged critically ill patients. Crit Care Med. 2012;40:79-89.
10. Fan E, Dowdy DW, Colantuoni E, Mendez-Tellez PA, Sevransky JE, Shanholtz C, et al. Physical complications in acute lung injury survivors: a two-year longitudinal prospective study. Crit Care Med. 2014;42:849-59.
11. Herridge MS, Cheung AM, Tansey CM, Matte-Martyn A, Diaz-Granados N, Al-Saidi F, et al. One-year outcomes in survivors of the acute respiratory distress syndrome. N Engl J Med. 2003;348:683-93.
12. Herridge MS, Tansey CM, Matte A, Tomlinson G, Diaz-Granados N, Cooper A, et al. Functional disability 5 years after acute respiratory distress syndrome. N Engl J Med. 2011;364:1293-304.
13. Stevens RD, Marshall SA, Cornblath DR, Hoke A, Needham DM, De Jonghe B, et al. A framework for diagnosing and classifying intensive care unit-acquired weakness. Crit Care Med. 2009;37:S299-308.
14. Hermans G, Van Mechelen H, Clerckx B, Vanhullebusch T, Mesotten D, Wilmer A, et al. Acute outcomes and 1-year mortality of intensive care unit-acquired weakness: a cohort study and propensity-matched analysis. Am J Respir Crit Care Med. 2014;190:410-20.

15. Fan E, Cheek F, Chlan L, Gosselink R, Hart N, Herridge MS, et al. An official American Thoracic Society Clinical Practice guideline: the diagnosis of intensive care unit-acquired weakness in adults. Am J Respir Crit Care Med. 2014;190:1437-46.
16. TEAM Study Investigators, Hodgson C, Bellomo R, Berney S, Bailey M, Buhr H, et al. Early mobilization and recovery in mechanically ventilated patients in the ICU: a bi-national, multi-centre, prospective cohort study. Crit Care. 2015;19:81.
17. Wieske L, Dettling-Ihnenfeldt DS, Verhamme C, Nollet F, van Schaik IN, Schultz MJ, et al. Impact of ICU-acquired weakness on post-ICU physical functioning: a follow-up study. Crit Care. 2015;19:196.
18. Hermans G, De Jonghe B, Bruyninckx F, Van den Berghe G. Interventions for preventing critical illness polyneuropathy and critical illness myopathy. Cochrane Database Syst Rev. 2014;(1):CD006832.
19. Stiller K. Safety issues that should be considered when mobilizing critically ill patients. Crit Care Clin. 2007;23:35-53.
20. Zafiropoulos B, Alison JA, McCarren B. Physiological responses to the early mobilisation of the intubated, ventilated abdominal surgery patient. Aust J Physiother. 2004;50:95-100.
21. Nydahl P, Ruhl AP, Bartoszek G, Dubb R, Filipovic S, Flohr HJ, et al. Early mobilization of mechanically ventilated patients: a 1-day point-prevalence study in Germany. Crit Care Med. 2014;42:1178-86.
22. Stiller K. Physiotherapy in intensive care: towards an evidence-based practice. Chest. 2000;118:1801-13.
23. Stiller K. Physiotherapy in intensive care: an updated systematic review. Chest. 2013;144:825-47.
24. Winkelman C, Johnson KD, Hejal R, Gordon NH, Rowbottom J, Daly J, et al. Examining the positive effects of exercise in intubated adults in ICU: a prospective repeated measures clinical study. Intensive Crit Care Nurs. 2012;28:307-18.
25. Schweickert WD, Pohlman MC, Pohlman AS, Nigos C, Pawlik AJ, Esbrook CL, et al. Early physical and occupational therapy in mechanically ventilated, critically ill patients: a randomised controlled trial. Lancet. 2009;373:1874-82.
26. Hashem MD, Nelliot A, Needham DM. Early Mobilization and Rehabilitation in the ICU: Moving Back to the Future. Respir Care. 2016;61:971-9.
27. Li Z, Peng X, Zhu B, Zhang Y, Xi X. Active mobilization for mechanically ventilated patients: a systematic review. Arch Phys Med Rehabil. 2013;94:551-61.
28. Hodgson CL, Stiller K, Needham DM, Tipping CJ, Harrold M, Baldwin CE, et al. Expert consensus and recommendations on safety criteria for active mobilization of mechanically ventilated critically ill adults. Crit Care. 2014;18:658.
29. Fontela PC, Forgiarini LA, Friedman G. Clinical attitudes and perceived barriers to early mobilization of critically ill patients in adult intensive care units [Atitudesclínicas e barreiraspercebidas para a mobilizaçãoprecoce de pacientes graves emunidades de terapiaintensivaadulto]. Rev Bras Ter Intensiva. 2018;30:187-94.
30. Vasilevskis EE, Ely EW, Speroff T, Pun BT, Boehm L, Dittus RS. Reducing iatrogenic risks: ICU-acquired delirium and weakness—crossing the quality chasm. Chest. 2010;138:1224-33.
31. Clarissa C, Salisbury L, Rodgers S, Kean S. Early mobilisation in mechanically ventilated patients: a systematic integrative review of definitions and activities. J Intensive Care. 2019;7:3.
32. Berney S, Harrold M, Webb S, Seppelt IM, Patman S, Thomas P, et al. Intensive care unit mobility practices in Australia and New Zealand: a point prevalence study. Crit Care Resusc. 2013;15:260-5.
33. Fontela PC, Lisboa TC, Forgiarini-Júnior LA, Friedman G. Early mobilization practices of mechanically ventilated patients: a 1-day point-prevalence study in southern Brazil. Clinics (Sao Paulo). 2018;73:e241.
34. Barber EA, Everard T, Holland AE, Tipping C, Bradley SJ, Hodgson CL. Barriers and facilitators to early mobilisation in intensive care: a qualitative study. Aust Crit Care. 2015;28:177-82.
35. Duncan C, Hudson M, Heck C. The impact of increased weekend physiotherapy service provision in critical care: a mixed methods study. Physiother Theory Pract. 2015;31:547-55.
36. Ambrosino N, Xie L. The Use of Non-invasive Ventilation during Exercise Training in COPD Patients. COPD. 2017;14:396-400.

37. Gravier FÉ, Bonnevie T, Medrinal C, Debeaumont D, Dupuis J, Viacroze C. Noninvasive ventilation during pulmonary rehabilitation in COPD patients. Rev Mal Respir. 2016;33:422-30.
38. Vitacca M, Kaymaz D, Lanini B, Vagheggini G, Ergün P, Gigliotti F, et al. Non-invasive ventilation during cycle exercise training in patients with chronic respiratory failure on long-term ventilatory support: A randomized controlled trial. Respirology. 2018;23:182-9.
39. Halbert J, McGraw P, Gray C, O'Brien G, Maheshwari V, Caplan R, et al. Noninvasive Ventilation for Early Mobilization of Acutely Hypoxic Patients. Chest. 2016;150:215A.
40. Lockstone J, Parry SM, Denehy L, Robertson IK, Story D, Parkes S. Physiotherapist administered, non-invasive ventilation to reduce postoperative pulmonary complications in high-risk patients following elective upper abdominal surgery; a before-and-after cohort implementation study. Physiotherapy. 2018;9406:30651-5.
41. Lockstone J, Boden I, Robertson IK, Story D, Denehy L, Parry SM. Non-Invasive Positive airway Pressure therapy to Reduce Postoperative Lung complications following Upper abdominal Surgery (NIPPER PLUS): protocol for a single-centre, pilot, randomised controlled trial. BMJ Open. 2019;9:e023139.
42. Lord RK, Mayhew CR, Korupolu R, Mantheiy EC, Friedman MA, Palmer JB, et al. ICU early physical rehabilitation programs: financial modeling of cost savings. Crit Care Med. 2013;41:717-24.

Chapter 24

Sedation during Noninvasive Ventilation

Subhal Bhalchandra Dixit, Khalid Ismail Khatib

■ INTRODUCTION

Sedation practices during the use of noninvasive ventilation (NIV) are an understudied aspect, especially in patients with acute respiratory failure (ARF). Although agitation/delirium and inability to cooperate or tolerate the mask are relative contraindications for NIV, the judicious use of sedative drugs could lead to success of NIV therapy in patients at risk of NIV failure.[1,2] It will prevent the patient requiring endotracheal intubation (ETI). Different drugs have been used toward this end.

Though studies have demonstrated the safety of judicious use, patients may easily get oversedated and then require ETI. More randomized controlled trials (RCTs) are required for recommendations on ideal drug, its dose, and method of delivery.

■ INDICATIONS FOR SEDATION IN PATIENTS ON NONINVASIVE VENTILATION[3]

Patients on NIV may need to be sedated for one or more of the following reasons:
○ Inability to tolerate patient–ventilator interface
○ Patient–ventilator asynchrony. It is also informally termed as "patient fighting the machine"
○ Anxiety/delirium/agitation/disorientation in patients on NIV

It is postulated that anxiety associated with dyspnea generates high volumes on NIV and thus increases the transpulmonary pressure and ventilator-induced lung injury. This also explains the high mortality in patients with moderate-to-severe acute respiratory distress syndrome (ARDS) who failed NIV trial.[4,5] Thus, sedation during NIV may help to reduce the affective component of dyspnea, though care should be taken to avoid oversedation.

■ DRUGS USED FOR SEDATION DURING NONINVASIVE VENTILATION

The ideal sedative for use in patients on NIV should have the following properties:
○ It should be short acting
○ It should have no significant side effects on patient hemodynamics
○ It should not affect the patients' respiratory drive or airway patency

Evidence is available for the use of the following drugs for sedation in patients on NIV **(Table 1)**. There is no robust evidence that one or the other classes of the drugs used are better than the others. But the general consensus is that benzodiazepines are to be avoided in these situations.[6] The use of dexmedetomidine in these situations has been tested with two RCTs showing it to be superior to midazolam.[7,8] Even a careful study of the pharmacological effects of dexmedetomidine demonstrates all the positive effects of the drug in patients of ARF (very low risk of respiratory depression and no effect on airway patency). The use of propofol and remifentanil appears to be in the intermediate range.[9-11]

Table 1: Drugs used for sedation in patients on noninvasive ventilation (NIV).

Drugs	Initial dose	Route (SC/IM/ IV/PO)	IV bolus/continuous IV or SC infusion
Morphine	0.02 mg/kg/h	SC	Continuous SC infusion
Remifentanil	0.025 µg/kg/min	IV	Continuous IV infusion
Midazolam	0.03 mg/kg/h	IV	Continuous IV infusion
Propofol	0.3 mg/kg/h	IV	Continuous IV infusion
Haloperidol	2.5–5 mg	IV	IV Bolus
Risperidone	0.5 mg	PO	—
Dexmedetomidine	0.2 µg/kg/h	IV	Continuous IV infusion

(IM: intramuscular; IV: intravenous; SC: subcutaneous)

MONITORING DURING SEDATION FOR PATIENTS ON NONINVASIVE VENTILATION[12]

Patients on NIV who are candidates for sedation should be closely monitored. Evaluation of sequential and frequent arterial blood gas analysis, cardiopulmonary parameters (continuous heart rate, blood pressure either invasive or noninvasive, and SpO_2) and ventilator parameters [positive end-expiratory pressure (PEEP), FiO_2, and respiratory rate], adverse events (airway obstruction, respiratory depression, deep sedation, and seizures), and the level of sedation (by Richmond Agitation-Sedation Scale) is mandatory. One should lookout for signs of NIV failure (immediate and early NIV failure) and their presence should prompt ETI.

CONCLUSION

Sedation during NIV should be undertaken in only very selected patients and that too under strict supervision and monitoring of the patients. Patients failing NIV despite use of judicious sedation should undergo ETI without any delay.

REFERENCES

1. Nava S, Hill N. Non-invasive ventilation in acute respiratory failure. Lancet. 2009;374(9685):250-9.
2. Liesching T, Kwok H, Hill NS. Acute applications of noninvasive positive pressure ventilation. Chest. 2003;124(2):699-713.
3. Longrois D, Conti G, Mantz J, Faltlhauser A, Aantaa R, Tonner P. Sedation in non-invasive ventilation: do we know what to do (and why)? Multidiscip Respir Med. 2014;9(1):56.
4. Parshall MB, Schwartzstein RM, Adams L, Banzett RB, Manning HL, Bourbeau J, et al. An official American Thoracic Society statement: Update on the mechanisms, assessment, and management of dyspnea. Am J Respir Crit Care Med. 2012;185(4):435-52.
5. Muriel A, PenÃÉuelas O, Frutos-Vivar F, Arroliga AC, Abraira V, Thille AW, et al. Impact of sedation and analgesia during noninvasive positive pressure ventilation on outcome: A marginal structural model causal analysis. Intensive Care Med. 2015;41(9):1586-600.

6. Jakob SM, Ruokonen E, Grounds RM, Sarapohja T, Garratt C, Pocock SJ, et al. Dexmedetomidine for Long-Term Sedation Investigators: Dexmedetomidine vs midazolam or propofol for sedation during prolonged mechanical ventilation: two randomized controlled trials. JAMA 2012;307(11): 1151-60.
7. Senoglu N, Oksuz H, Dogan Z, Yildiz H, Demirkiran H, Ekerbicer H. Sedation during noninvasive mechanical ventilation with dexmedetomidine or midazolam: A randomized, double-blind, prospective study. Curr Ther Res Clin Exp. 2010;71(3):141-53.
8. Huang Z, Chen YS, Yang ZL, Liu JY. Dexmedetomidine versus midazolam for the sedation of patients with non-invasive ventilation failure. Intern Med. 2012;51(17):2299-305.
9. Constantin JM, Schneider E, Cayot-Constantin S, Guerin R, Bannier F, Futier E, et al. Remifentanil-based sedation to treat noninvasive ventilation failure: a preliminary study. Intensive Care Med. 2007;33(1):82-7.
10. Rocco M, Conti G, Alessandri E, Morelli A, Spadetta G, Laderchi A, et al. Rescue treatment for non-invasive ventilation failure due to interface intolerance with remifentanil analgo sedation: a pilot study. Intensive Care Med. 2010;36(12):2060-5.
11. Clouzeau B, Bui HN, Vargas F, Grenouillet-Delacre M, Guilhon E, Gruson D, et al. Target-controlled infusion of propofol for sedation in patients with non-invasive ventilation failure due to low tolerance: a preliminary study. Intensive Care Med. 2010;36(10):1675-80.
12. Ozyilmaz E, Ozsancak A, Nava S. Timing of noninvasive ventilation failure: causes, risk factors, and potential remedies. BMC Pulm Med. 2014;14:19.

Chapter 25

Humidification and Aerosol Therapy in Noninvasive Ventilation

Jayeshkumar Dobariya, Jigar Padalia, Milap Mashru

HUMIDIFICATION

INTRODUCTION

In a normal respiration, conditioning of respiratory gases takes place in upper respiratory tract (75%) and trachea (25%). Warming, humidification, and cleansing of respiratory gases are done by upper respiratory tract. Mucous membrane of mouth and nose moisturizes the passing respiratory gases during inspiration, due to which a normal healthy adult evaporates about 200–300 mL of water per day. The mucous membrane of upper respiratory tract cools down while inspiring through nose or mouth. During exhalation, this cooling effect causes moisture in air coming from lungs to condensate on mucous membrane; as a result, the mucous membranes are moisturized again. In this way, heat and moisture are maintained by upper airway and trachea. A temperature of 37°C and an absolute humidity of 44 mg H_2O/L corresponding to a relative humidity of 100% are required for optimum mucociliary clearance in lower respiratory tract, otherwise it hampers the mucociliary clearance and leads to bacterial colonization and infection.[1] So, proper heat and moisture of inspired respiratory gases are required.

In invasive mechanical ventilation, upper airway is bypassed, so humidification is must to avoid hypothermia, mucociliary dysfunction, bronchospasm, atelectasis, and airway obstruction. While in noninvasive ventilation (NIV), upper airway is not bypassed so whether additional heat and humidity are always necessary or not, there is no clear consensus on this **(Table 1)**.

Heat and humidification can be active or passive:
- Active (heated humidifier that uses water and external power source)
- Passive [heat and moisture exchanger (HME) which uses patients own heat and humidity].

POINTS THAT FAVOR HUMIDIFICATION DURING NONINVASIVE VENTILATION
- Extensive literature supports use of humidification for improving comfort and tolerance of nasal continuous positive airway pressure (CPAP) in sleep apnea patients.[2]
- For NIV success, comfort to the patient is very important. Humidification improves patient comfort and tolerance to NIV, so ultimately NIV success. This is one objective of early use of humidification during NIV.[3]

Table 1: Advantages and disadvantages of heat and moisture exchanger filter and heated humidifier systems during noninvasive ventilation

System	Advantages	Disadvantages
HME	Cost effective	Increased dead space
	Extended use in the ICU	Reduced efficacy in case of leaks
	Eliminates circuit condensation (hygroscopic models are recommended)	Efficacy depends on body and environmental temperatures
	A booster system applied to a hydrophobic HME may preserve AH capacity when incoming gases are delivered at a temperature lower than 26°C and at high flow	May lead to an increase in airway resistance in patients with heavy secretions and respiratory tract bleeding
	Dose not need electricity	
HH	Less work of breathing than with HME	Less efficacy with high environmental temperature
	Limited or no effect on dead space ventilation so CO_2 retention is minimal	Needs electricity
	Achieves RH and AH values sufficient for gas conditioning	Performance of different devices varies
	Clinically effective, especially in patients with mild to severe hypercapnic acute respiratory failure	

(AH: absolute humidity; HH: heated humidifier; HME: heat and moisture exchanger filter; RH: relative humidity.)

- In a patient of chronic obstructive pulmonary disease (COPD) and asthma, early use of humidification has shown good results.
- Few data are in favor of humidification in a patient of hypoxemic respiratory failure where fraction of inspired oxygen (FiO_2) requirement is >0.6 and those anticipated to require a prolonged use of NIV more than 2 hours.[4]
- Higher tidal volumes and high peak inspiratory flow rates increase the moisture loss. So in that condition, early humidification is beneficial.[5]
- In a disease like COPD and bronchiectasis, thick viscous bronchial secretions are present and due to low moisture, secretions become dry, causing serious problem of dryness of secretions and airway obstruction. So, in this situation, early humidification is very important.[5]
- Other conditions where an early implementation of humidification can be helpful are aged patients, mucociliary dysfunction, increased nasal resistance, medications causing dryness of mucosa, mouth breather, and bronchial hypersecretion.[5]

SOME POINTS AGAINST THE USE OF HUMIDIFICATION IN NONINVASIVE VENTILATION[6,7]

- Lack of consensus regarding appropriate patient and indication for early humidification
- Increased dead space which increases work of breathing, rebreathing problem, and sometimes causing a drop in inspiratory positive airway pressure

- Increased cost
- More chances of cross-infection.

CONCLUSION FOR HUMIDIFICATION IN NONINVASIVE VENTILATION

- There are no major guidelines or studies for best strategy of humidification in NIV.
- When you use NIV for acute respiratory failure, first identify factors that affect moisture loss and humidification.
- Other individual factors depend on patient's condition, settings of the ventilator, and type of interface used.
- Early use of humidifier is beneficial in patient of hypoxemic respiratory failure, COPD, asthma, bronchiectasis, diseases with secretions, high flow and high FiO_2 conditions, and those needing prolonged use of NIV.
- Proper education and protocols of humidification are very important for optimal results of humidification.

RECOMMENDATIONS

- Humidification is not required routinely (Grade D).[8]
- Heated humidification can be considered if the patient has mucosal dryness or if thick and tenacious respiratory secretions.[8]

AEROSOL THERAPY IN NONINVASIVE VENTILATION

INTRODUCTION

In last 2 decades, NIV has gained significant popularity in Indian intensive care units (ICUs). In last few years, NIV is widely used in non-ICU settings also such as in prehospital care, emergency department, home care, and for sleep apnea patients. The success and comfort of NIV depends on various factors, out of that humidification and aerosol therapy are very important. There is not much awareness about humidification and aerosol therapy during NIV. Aerosol therapy is integral part of almost every patient of respiratory disorders.

AEROSOL SYSTEM

- *Definition of aerosol*: Suspension of solid or liquid into a gaseous medium
- *Components of aerosol system*: The aerosol device, drug and patient's respiratory system, and NIV if the patient is on NIV
- *Factors determining the efficiency of the aerosol system*: Composite of the delivered drug, the dose delivered to respiratory system, and lung bioavailability.

AEROSOL DEPOSITION

- Size of molecule and gas velocity affect the aerosol deposition
- Deposition occurs by different mechanisms such as inertial impaction in large airways, gravitational sedimentation in medium-sized airways, and diffusion (Brownian motion) in very small airways or alveoli of very small aerosol particles of 2–5 µm **(Fig.1)**.

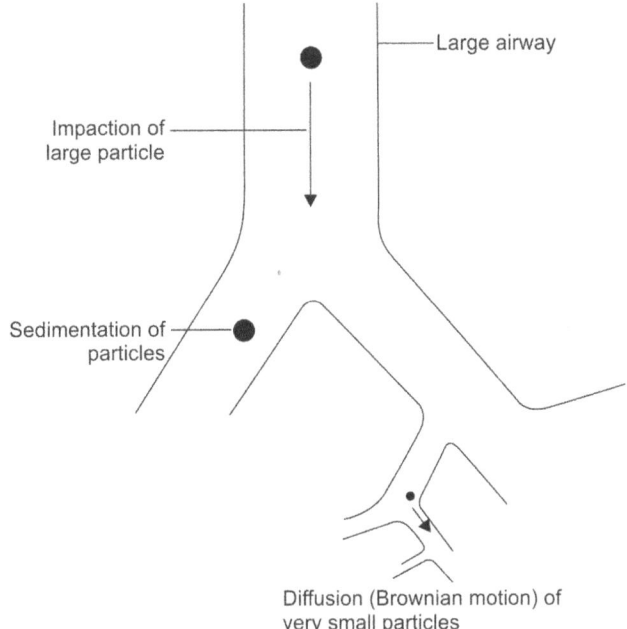

Fig. 1: Aerosol deposition.

FACTORS FAVORING DRUG DELIVERY BY AEROSOL SYSTEM (TABLE 2)[9]

Table 2: Factors favorable for effective aerosol drug delivery in the critically ill patient	
Mechanically ventilated	**Nonmechanically ventilated**
Patient ➤ Clear and patent airway i.e. minimal secretions	**Patient** ➤ Slow and deep breathing pattern
Drug ➤ Particle size 2–5 μm	**Drug** ➤ Particle size 2–5 μm
Aerosol device ➤ VMN for aqueous solutions ➤ If pMDI then with spacer (breath synchronized) ➤ Position-Adult: VMN/ultrasonic/pMDI—15 cm from Y-piece in inspiratory limb. Pediatric: Closer to ventilator	**Device** ➤ VMN for aqueous solutions ➤ If pMDI then use spacer (breath synchronized) ➤ DPI (breath activated) if adequate respiratory reserves ➤ Heliox may improve drug delivery
Ventilator parameters ➤ Slow flow (40 lpm better than 80 lpm) ➤ Long inspiratory time (duty cycle 0.5 better than 0.25) ➤ NIV with nebulizer ➤ PEEP	
Circuit and related factors ➤ Larger airway (Endotracheal tube or tracheostomy) ➤ For tracheostomy, use T-piece interface ➤ Humidification—remove HME and heated humidifier	

(VMN: vibrating mesh nebulizer; PMDD: pressurized metered dose inhaler; HME: heat and moisture exchanger filter; PEEP: positive end-expiratory pressure; DPI: dry powder inhaler; NIV noninvasive ventilation).

COMMON APPLICATIONS OF AEROSOL THERAPY IN CRITICAL CARE (TABLE 3)[9]

Table 3: Common applications of aerosol therapy in intensive care.

Feature	Drug class				
	Bronchodilators	Anti-inflammatory	Antimicrobial agents	Vasoactive agents	Heliox
Indications	Bronchospasm (e.g. acute asthma, COPD exacerbation)	Airway inflammation (e.g. actue asthma or COPD exacerbation, acute interstitial lung disease	MDR tracheobronchitis MDR pneumonia Aspergillus prevention (lung transplant)	Right ventricular failure Pulmonary hypertension	Asthma
Site of action	Airways	Airways or alveoil	Airways or alveoil	Alveoil	Airways
Preferred device	pMDI with spacer	pMDI with spacer	VMN	VMN	
Drugs	Beta-agonists (e.g. salbutamol, salmeterol) Anticholinergics (e.g. ipratropium, tiotropium)	Budesonide Fluticasone	Antibiotics (e.g. tobramycin, colistin, amikacin, ceftazidime, amphotericin B)	Epoprostenol Iloprost	Helium
Formulations available	Yes	Yes	Some	Yes	

(Heliox: helium and oxygen; COPD: chronic obstructive pulmonary disease; MDR: multidrug resistant; pMDI: pressurized metered dose inhaler; VMN: vibrating mesh nebulizer.)

FACTORS AFFECTING AEROSOL THERAPY IN NONINVASIVE VENTILATION[10]

- *Ventilator-related factors*:
  - Intensive care unit ventilators, dedicated NIV ventilators, and home care NIV, all are almost equally efficacious in aerosol delivery due to better and advanced functions.[11]
- *Mode of ventilation*:
  - In different modes of NIV, there is difference in pressure settings and airflow rates
  - Quantity of aerosol delivery is directly proportional to inspiratory pressure and inversely proportional to expiratory pressure **(Fig. 2)**
  - Higher airflow is associated with lower aerosol delivery.
- *Circuit-related factors*:
  - 40% or more aerosol drug is lost in humid circuit compared to dry circuit.
- Gas density—less density is better for effective aerosol drug delivery, e.g., inhalation of Heliox, which is less dense that makes airflow more laminar and less turbulent, so more drug delivery.[12,13]
- *Types of interface*:
  - Aerosol particle deposition in nasal passages reduces the drug delivery to lung which can be avoided by using a mouthpiece in nebulizer and in NIV also due to deposition of particles in nasal cavity.[14,15] Almost 40–99% of drug cannot reach the target site.[16,17]
  - Proper facemask fitting is must for maximum drug delivery, prevention of drug loss, and to decrease eye irritation by aerosol drug.[18]

Ventilator related
Critical care ventilator
NIPPV ventilator
Home care ventilator

Circuit related
Type of circuit
Position of leak port
Inhaled gas humidity
Inhaled gas density

Device related—pMDI
Type of spacer of adapter
used timing ok pMDI actuation
position of pMDI/spacer

Drug related
Dose
Aerosol particle size
Duration of action

Breathing parameters
Mode of ventilation
Tidal volume
Respiratory rate
Inspiratory air flow
Pressure settings

Type of interface
Facemask
Nasal cannula

Device related—nebulizer
Type of nebulizer used continuous/
intermittent operation duration
nebulization position in the circuit

Patient related
Severity of airway obstruction
Mechanism of airway obstruction
Presence of intrinsic PEEP
Patient-ventilator synchrony

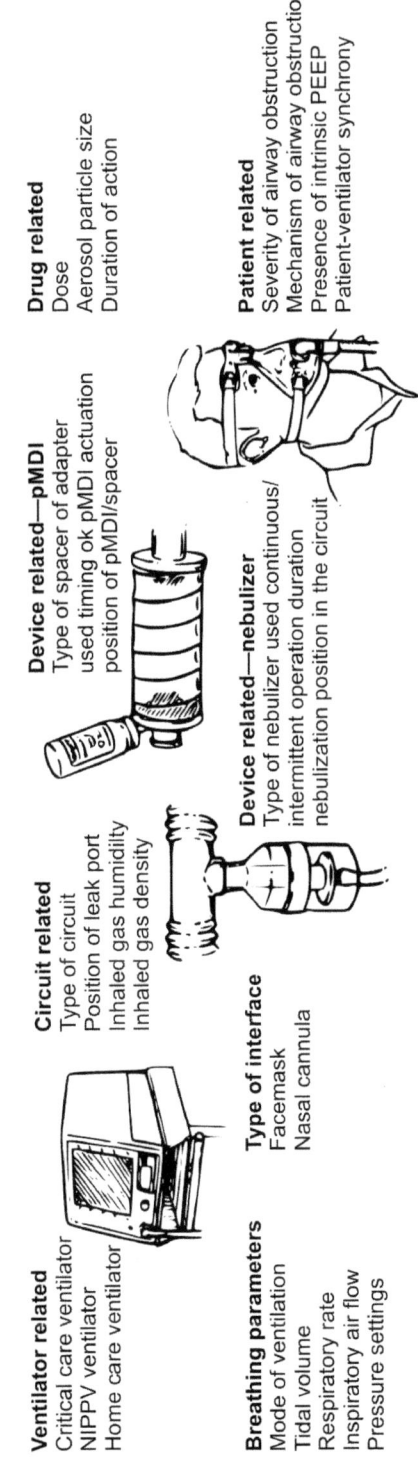

Fig.2: Schematic showing the various factors influencing aerosol delivery during noninvasive positive pressure ventilation (NIPPV).
(PEEP: positive end-expiratory pressure; pMDI: pressurized metered-dose inhaler.)

- Types of aerosol generator:
  - Pressurized metered-dose inhaler (pMDI) with spacer **(Fig. 3)**

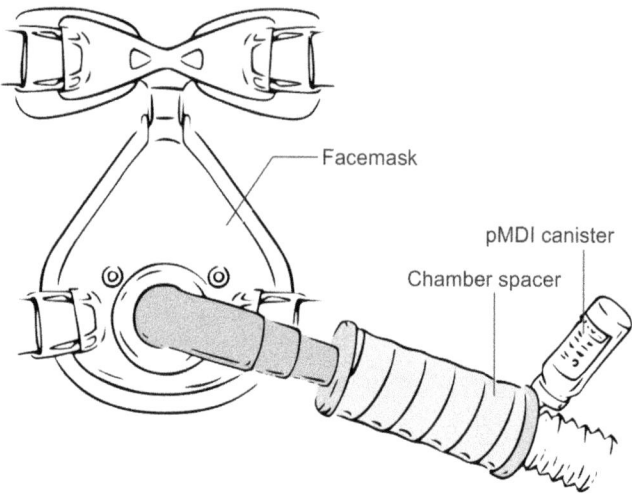

Fig. 3: Pressurized metered dose inhaler (pMDI) with spacer in NIV.

  - Nebulizer **(Fig. 4)**

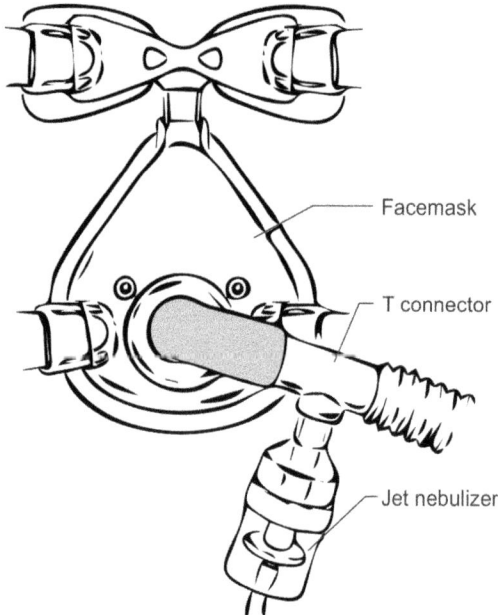

Fig. 4: Nebulizer in NIV.

- Drug related:
  - *Aerosol particles size*: Small enough to pass through the upper airway and large enough to avoid being carried out back by exhaled air.

Chapter 25: Humidification and Aerosol Therapy in Noninvasive Ventilation

- *Patient related*:
  - If the patient-ventilator synchrony is good, there is better aerosol deposition.
  - When the severity of airway obstruction is less, the gas flow is less turbulent, so more distal deposition of aerosol is possible. That is why, always bronchodilators are given before inhaled antibiotics.

How to use pMDI and spacer during NIV?[10]

- *Patient assessment*: Hemodynamic status, mask size and fitting, and patient-ventilator synchrony
- Minimize the leaks at the level of circuit and mask
- Apply spacer between circuit and mask
- Shake pMDI canister and then place in the adapter of the spacer
- Actuate pMDI at the beginning of inspiratory airflow
- Repeat actuations after every 15–20 seconds
- Administer desired number of doses
- Remove pMDI and spacer and then reconnect circuit
- Very important—if a HME filter is used, then it should not be placed between the facemask and pMDI because HME filter will trap the drug particles.

How to use a nebulizer during NIV?[10]

- *Patient assessment*: Hemodynamic status, mask size and fitting, and patient-ventilator synchrony
- Minimize the leaks at the level of circuit and mask
- Fill the nebulizer up to optimal volume (approximately 4–6 mL for jet nebulizer)
- Place nebulizer upright between the mask and circuit
- Use the nebulizer with a gas flow of 6–8 L/min
- Tap nebulizer until it sputters
- After completing nebulizer, remove it from circuit and clean with water and air dry and store in clean space.

CONCLUSION

- The pMDI, jet nebulizer, and mesh nebulizer should deliver a therapeutic dose to the mask
- Aerosol generator device should be in between the leak port and the mask for best results
- When the leak port is in the mask, the pMDI is more effective then nebulizer
- When using a nebulizer, more aerosol—with a higher level of pressure support and less aerosol—with a higher level of expiratory pressure
- In NIV, nebulizer should be placed near the mask rather than near the ventilator
- Aerosol drug delivery during inspiratory phase of NIV is still not available in the market.

RECOMMENDATIONS (GOOD PRACTICE POINTS)

- Aerosolized drugs should usually be administered during breaks from NIV.[8]
- If the patient is NIV dependent, aerosolized drugs can be given via a nebulizer attached into the ventilator circuit near the mask.[8]

REFERENCES

1. Wanner A, Salathé M, O'Riordan TG. Mucociliary clearance in the airways. Am J Respir Crit Care Med. 1996;154:1868-902.
2. Worsnop CJ, Miseski S, Rochford PD. Routine use of humidification with nasal continuous positive airway pressure. Intern Med J. 2010;40:650-6.
3. Nava S, Navalesi P, Carlucci A. Non-invasive ventilation. Minerva Anestesiol. 2009;75:31-6.
4. AARC clinical practice guideline. Humidification during mechanical ventilation. American Association for Respiratory Care. Respir Care. 1992;37:887-90.
5. Branson RD, Gentile MA. Is humidification always necessary during noninvasive ventilation in the hospital? Respir Care. 2010;55:209-16.
6. Esquinas AM, Al-Jawder SE, BaHammam AS. Practice of Humidification During Noninvasive Mechanical ventilation (NIV): Determinants of Humidification Strategies. Humid Intensive Care Unit. 2012;23:93-102.
7. Esquinas Rodriguez AM, Scala R, Soroksky A, BaHammam A, de Klerk A, Valipour A, et al. Clinical review: humidifiers during non-invasive ventilation—key topics and practical implications. Crit Care. 2012;16:203.
8. Davidson AC, Banham S, Elliott M, Kennedy D, Gelder C, Glossop A, et al. BTS/ICS guideline for the ventilatory management of acute hypercapnic respiratory failure in adults. Thorax. 2016;71:ii1-35.
9. Dhanani J, Fraser JF, Chan HK, Rello J, Cohen J, Roberts JA. Fundamentals of aerosol therapy in critical care. Crit Care. 2016;20:269.
10. Dhand R. Aerosol therapy in patients receiving noninvasive positive pressure ventilation. J Aerosol Med Pulm Drug Deliv. 2012;25:63-78.
11. Hill NS, Carlisle C, Kramer NR. Effect of a nonrebreathing exhalation valve on long-term nasal ventilation using a bilevel device. Chest. 2002;122:84-91.
12. Lellouche F, Maggiore SM, Lyazidi A, Deye N, Taille S, Brochard L. Water content of delivered gases during noninvasive ventilation in healthy subjects. Intensive Care Med. 2009;35:987-95.
13. Richards GN, Cistulli PA, Ungar GR, Berthon-Jones M, Sullivan CE. Mouth leak with nasal continuous positive airway pressure increases nasal airway resistance. Am J Respir Crit Care Med. 1996;154:182-6.
14. Chua HL, Collis GG, Newbury AM, Chan K, Bower GD, Sly PD, et al. The influence of age on aerosol deposition in children with cystic fibrosis. Eur Respir J. 1994;7:2185-91.
15. Everard ML, Hardy JG, Milner AD. Comparison of nebulised aerosol deposition in the lungs of healthy adults following oral and nasal inhalation. Thorax. 1993;48:1045-6.
16. Chen YS. Aerosol deposition in the extrathoracic region. Aerosol Sci Technol. 2003;37:659-71.
17. Kelly JT, Asgharian B, Kimbell JS, Wong B. Particle deposition in human nasal airway replicas manufactured by different methods. Part I: Inertial regime particles. aerosol sci technol. 2004;38:1063-71.
18. Nikander K, Agertoft L, Pedersen S. Breath-synchronized nebulization diminishes the impact of patient-device interfaces (face mask or mouthpiece) on the inhaled mass of nebulized budesonide. J Asthma. 2000;37:451-9.

Section 4

Monitoring and Weaning

26. Monitoring of Patients on Noninvasive Ventilation
27. Capnography in Noninvasive Ventilation: Clinical Implications
28. Weaning from Noninvasive Ventilation
29. Noninvasive Ventilation in Failure to Wean from Invasive Ventilation, Postextubation Failure, and Tracheostomy

Chapter 26

Monitoring of Patients on Noninvasive Ventilation

Neetu Jain, Satya Ranjan Sahu, GC Khilnani

INTRODUCTION

Noninvasive ventilation (NIV) has evolved over past two decades and is now widely accepted mode of ventilation in acute care setting for various indications like acute exacerbation of chronic obstructive pulmonary disease (COPD), acute respiratory failure (ARF) due to cardiogenic pulmonary edema, mild-to-moderate acute respiratory distress syndrome (ARDS), or immunocompromised patients.[1] If NIV is applied in proper setting, it can lower mortality and morbidity of patients and can be cost-effective as compared with invasive mechanical ventilation (IMV). It reduces the risk of complications related to IMV like ventilator-associated pneumonia (VAP), hence can shorten the intensive care unit (ICU) as well as hospital stay.[2] Despite these accepted indications and several advantages, NIV is used sparingly and failure rates are high. In-hospital mortality of COPD patients receiving NIV for ARF has shown to be higher in clinical settings than in randomized controlled trials (RCTs).[3] This mortality can be explained by inadequate patient selection and lack of close monitoring.

Noninvasive ventilation can do more harm than good, if it delays the application of more effective mode of treatment in critically ill patients like intubation and IMV.[4] Close monitoring is key to success of NIV in critically ill patients. Lack of monitoring can lead to late detection of NIV failure, delayed intubation, and eventually increased mortality.[4] Actions taken as a result of monitoring may be life saving for these patients. Close monitoring is only way to determine NIV failure and avoid delay in intubation. It has been shown by data that NIV application is beneficial only if it is carefully applied with adequate monitoring and treatment is escalated without delay in case of deterioration. Location and indications of NIV application will guide the parameters to be monitored. The parameters to be monitored would include clinical assessment and laboratory investigations. At bedside, clinical monitoring of utmost importance and should not be replaced by investigations. A trained nurse is primary requirement for adequate monitoring. A controlled environment of a dedicated NIV unit can be the best place of NIV application in term of monitoring and eventual success of NIV for patients. If such dedicated units are unavailable, intensive care unit (ICU) or high dependency unit (HDU) with facilities of invasive and noninvasive monitoring is the desired location for NIV application. Therefore, NIV for ARF should preferably be initiated in ICU/HDU and the subsequent monitoring may be continued in the respiratory wards where trained staff is available.

REQUIREMENTS FOR ADEQUATE MONITORING OF PATIENT ON NIV

Adequate monitoring of patient on NIV requires knowledge, technology, as well as commitment of the staff. It is important to provide NIV in appropriate setting, so as to ensure close monitoring of patient and successful application. Following are the basic requirements:[1]

- Location of initiation of NIV application should be ICU, HDU, or a dedicated NIV unit; however, it can be subsequently continued in wards
- There should be a documented plan of care and monitoring exclusively for patients on NIV, which should include all required parameter as well as frequency of monitoring
- A trained physician capable of selecting patients appropriately
- Trained staff
- Appropriate nurse-to-patient ratio preferably 1:1 or 1:2
- Dedicated respiratory therapist
- Multipara monitors with facility of continuous pulse oximetry
- Facility of blood gas analysis
- Availability of invasive mechanical ventilation

Monitoring Parameters

Clinical Parameters

The success of NIV depends on appropriate selection of patient and correct application interface (mask), mode, and pressure. Several clinical parameters such as patient comfort, adequate application of interface, dyspnea, vital parameters, and oxygen saturation should be monitored every 15 minutes for 1st hour of application, every half an hour for 1–4 hour period and at least hourly thereafter.[5]

Patient consciousness with the use of Glasgow coma scale (GCS), ability to cough out secretions, and maintain airways are important to assess before and after application of NIV. Kelly–Mathay score may also be applied to discern the level of consciousness. A score of more than 3 is suggestive of depressed consciousness leading to NIV failure.[6] Some patients may require mild sedation or analgesia to tolerate NIV; such patients require closer monitoring of conscious level using sedation scales like Ramsay sedation scale. Patients should also be assessed for delirium, as it can lead to decreased acceptability of NIV and eventual NIV failure.[7]

Patient should be clinically assessed for relief in dyspnea and tachypnea after about 30 minutes of appropriate NIV. The use accessory muscles of respiration may signify NIV failure or requirement of increase in pressure support.

Physiological/Gas Exchange Parameters

According to British Thoracic Society (BTS) guidelines, oxygen saturation should be measured continuously and invasive blood gas monitoring for pH and pCO_2 should be done intermittently.[1]

Pulse Oximetry

It is standard of care for any patient requiring ventilatory support. It requires a hemodynamically stable patient correct placement of probe. A target SpO_2 by pulse oximetry varies as per diagnosis hypercapnic or hypoxemic respiratory failure. Target SpO_2 should be between 88 and 92% for any patient with Type II respiratory failure.[8]

Transcutaneous CO_2

Transcutaneous CO_2 can very conveniently assess ventilatory response to NIV facilitating continuous NIV adjustment rather than intermittent in response to arterial blood gas (ABG). It underestimates the CO_2 level, especially in patients with severe hypercapnia. According to the recent BTS guidelines, transcutaneous CO_2 may facilitate weaning from NIV. It may replace frequent ABG monitoring because of feasibility but a baseline and intermittent ABG analysis (when transcutaneous values are >60 mm of Hg) should supplement it in view of questionable accuracy. Additionally, it does not give any information on pH values.[9]

End-tidal CO_2

Capnography is better established for intubated patients and has limited role in patients on NIV due to physiological dead space. It significantly underestimates $PaCO_2$. It is not recommended for monitoring of patients on NIV.[10]

Blood Gas Analysis

Arterial blood gas test is gold standard for diagnosis as well as monitoring of respiratory failure. Blood gas monitoring should be done at baseline, 1 hour after commencement of NIV or any change in setting and as per patient's clinical condition thereafter. A deterioration or nonimprovement in ABG after 4-6 hours is a poor prognostic feature. A decrease in CO_2 by 3 mm Hg and increase in pH by 0.03 should be considered a positive response.[11] ABG monitoring should be continued at least till the respiratory failure resolves and as per patient's condition thereafter. It can be done either by intermittent arterial puncture or by placing an arterial line to avoid frequent puncturing.

Ventilatory Parameters

Two types of NIV machines are usually used—one of which are home care NIV, which utilize single limb circuit and do not display any ventilatory waveforms, and others are acute care NIV/NIV module in invasive ventilators, which display ventilatory parameters and waveform on the screen of the machine. In acute care setting, second type of machines are recommended as these allow numerical monitoring of inspiratory (VTi) and expiratory (VTe) tidal volumes, minute ventilation, leak, I:E ratio, and respiratory rate. These machines should display flow and pressure waveforms in real time. Ventilatory parameters are based on in-built algorithm utilized by the machine and cannot replace other monitoring like ABG.

The most important parameter to be monitored is VTe, as it reflects patient's alveolar ventilation. Before starting NIV, desired VTe should be decided, which is a function of inspiratory pressure in pressure support mode. However, it is influenced by resistance of airways, compliance of ventilatory system of patient, his effort, and inspiratory time. Unlike IMV, NIV is a semi-open system and prone to leaks, which, if not compensated, lowers the effective VTe leading to NIV failure. Measurement of Rapid Shallow Breathing Index (RSBI) (RR/VTe) less than 105 can be good predictor of NIV success.[12]

Air leak is inevitable with use of NIV and adversely affects its successful application. Air leak should be continuously monitored both clinically and with help of VTe and VTi values provided by the ventilators (leak = VTi – VTe).[13]

The I:E ratio is another important parameter. In hypercapnic respiratory failure, expiratory time should be more, i.e., I:E ratio should be more than usual 1:2. In hypoxemic respiratory failure, inspiratory and expiratory time can be equal, i.e., I:E ratio can be close to 1:1.[8]

Intrinsic positive end-expiratory pressure (PEEPi) causes dynamic hyperinflation leading decrease compliance. External PEEP is applied in ventilators to counteract effect of PEEPi. The degree of PEEPi can be estimated in NIV by looking at expiratory flow–time curve. When expiratory flow–time curve does not touch the baseline, it is suggestive of presence of PEEPi.

Ineffective triggering and autotriggering are most important patient ventilator interactions that should be monitored. The most practical method of monitoring for asynchrony is looking at ventilatory waveforms. Clinically, it can be detected by observing patient and rhythm of respiration.[14]

Respiratory waveforms are very important in acute care setting. Pressure–time and flow–time curves provide information on quality of ventilation, asynchrony, leaks, and PEEPi. Constant monitoring of waveform is associated with improved outcomes.[15]

Cardiac Parameters

Continuous electrocardiography (ECG) monitoring is standard of care for patients on NIV, especially in cases with heart rate is more than 120, dysrhythmias, or pre-existing cardiomyopathy. Regular blood pressure monitoring should also be done for these patients.[1]

Monitoring for Adverse Effects of NIV

Interface-related Problems

Success of NIV is dependent upon choosing right interface. One of the most important problems with mask is pressure sore, which occurs in 20–34% patients. Loose positioning of mask leads to large leaks and failure of NIV. These problems can be circumvented by simple interventions like proper fitting mask, if patients are monitored continuously.[16]

Secretion Clearance

Presence of copious secretions is a relative contraindication to NIV and can lead to aspiration and subsequent NIV failure. Patient's Glasgow Coma Score (GCS) and ability to clear secretions should be carefully monitored, and in any patient with excessive secretions, NIV should be avoided. Physiotherapy and tracheal suction can help some of these patients.

Gastric Distension

It is common to have gastric distension due to aerophagy in patient on NIV. It increases the risk of vomiting and aspiration. Patients should be monitored for gastric distension and may be prescribed prokinetic agents. The use of nasogastric tube for decompression can be protective but there should be appropriate arrangements in mask for nasogastric tube to avoid leaks. If patient complains of nausea, mask should be removed immediately.[17]

Locations of NIV as per Level of Monitoring

Different locations of NIV application like ward, ICU, and HDU warrant different level of monitoring.[18] It should more intensive for patient with severe respiratory failure with imminent intubation in ICU as compared with ward. If there are set protocols for monitoring as per location, NIV can be less resource intensive and more successful. In patient with general wards, continuous nurse and clinical parameter monitoring is not required. These patients require less frequent blood gas analysis like every 8 hours initially and once in 24 hours in later stages. These patients do not require monitoring of ventilatory waveform and can be maintained on ambulatory NIV, which does not have such facility. However, all patients should be monitored for leaks, mask fit, and asynchrony.[12]

CONCLUSION

The NIV can be a life-saving intervention when applied properly. It can save patients from complications related to invasive mechanical ventilation like VAP. However, the success of NIV greatly depends upon proper patient selection and adequate monitoring. The level of monitoring depends upon clinical condition of the patient and location of NIV application. There is lack of data on optimal monitoring practices; hence, clinicians have to extremely cautious, especially in cases of ARF. Experienced and dedicated staff is key to success. Patient on NIV should be regularly monitored clinically, by non-invasive as well as invasive methods. Continuous SpO_2 and intermittent ABG are most important to predict the failure of NIV. Adequate and close monitoring not only improves success rate of NIV but also avoids delay in intubation leading to increased mortality.

REFERENCES

1. Rochwerg B, Brochard L, Elliott MW, Hess D, Hill NS, Nava S, et al. Official ERS/ATS clinical practice guidelines: noninvasive ventilation for acute respiratory failure. Eur Respir J. 2017;50(2): pii: 1602426.
2. Mehta AB, Douglas IS, Walkey AJ. Evidence-based Utilization of Noninvasive Ventilation and Patient Outcomes. Ann Am Thorac Soc. 2017;14(11):1667-73.
3. Titlestad I, Lassen, Vestbo. Long-term survival for COPD patients receiving noninvasive ventilation for acute respiratory failure. Int J Chron Obstruct Pulmon Dis. 2013;8:215-9.
4. Antonelli M, Conti G, Moro M, Esquinas A, Gonzalez-Diaz G, Confalonieri M, et al. Predictors of failure of noninvasive positive pressure ventilation in patients with acute hypoxemic respiratory failure: a multi-center study. Intensive Care Med. 2001;27(11):1718-28.
5. Nava S, Hill N. Non-invasive ventilation in acute respiratory failure. Lancet Lond Engl. 2009;374(9685):250-9.
6. Scala R, Naldi M, Archinucci I, Coniglio G, Nava S. Noninvasive positive pressure ventilation in patients with acute exacerbations of COPD and varying levels of consciousness. Chest. 2005;128(3):1657-66.
7. Charlesworth M, Elliott MW, Holmes JD. Noninvasive positive pressure ventilation for acute respiratory failure in delirious patients: understudied, underreported, or underappreciated? A systematic review and meta-analysis. Lung. 2012;190(6):597-603.
8. Davidson AC, Banham S, Elliott M, Kennedy D, Gelder C, Glossop A, et al. BTS/ICS guideline for the ventilatory management of acute hypercapnic respiratory failure in adults. Thorax. 2016;71 Suppl 2: ii1-35.

9. van Oppen JD, Daniel PS, Sovani MP. What is the Potential Role of Transcutaneous Carbon Dioxide in Guiding Acute Noninvasive Ventilation? Respir Care. 2015;60(4):484-91.
10. Lermuzeaux M, Meric H, Sauneuf B, Girard S, Normand H, Lofaso F, et al. Superiority of transcutaneous CO_2 over end-tidal CO_2 measurement for monitoring respiratory failure in nonintubated patients: A pilot study. J Crit Care. 2016;31(1):150-6.
11. Ram FSF, Picot J, Lightowler J, Wedzicha JA. Non-invasive positive pressure ventilation for treatment of respiratory failure due to exacerbations of chronic obstructive pulmonary disease. Cochrane Database Syst Rev. 2004;(3):CD004104.
12. Ergan B, Nasiłowski J, Winck JC. How should we monitor patients with acute respiratory failure treated with noninvasive ventilation? Eur Respir Rev. 2018;27(148):170101.
13. Doorduin J, Sinderby CA, Beck J, van der Hoeven JG, Heunks LMA. Automated patient-ventilator interaction analysis during neurally adjusted non-invasive ventilation and pressure support ventilation in chronic obstructive pulmonary disease. Crit Care Lond Engl. 2014;18(5):550.
14. Colombo D, Cammarota G, Alemani M, Carenzo L, Barra FL, Vaschetto R, et al. Efficacy of ventilator waveforms observation in detecting patient-ventilator asynchrony. Crit Care Med. 2011;39(11):2452-7.
15. Di Marco F, Centanni S, Bellone A, Messinesi G, Pesci A, Scala R, et al. Optimization of ventilator setting by flow and pressure waveforms analysis during noninvasive ventilation for acute exacerbations of COPD: a multicentric randomized controlled trial. Crit Care. 2011;15(6):R283.
16. Nava S. Behind a Mask: Tricks, Pitfalls, and Prejudices for Noninvasive Ventilation. Respir Care. 2013;58(8):1367-76.
17. Gay PC. Complications of noninvasive ventilation in acute care. Respir Care. 2009;54(2):246-57; discussion 257-58.
18. Plant PK, Owen JL, Elliott MW. Early use of non-invasive ventilation for acute exacerbations of chronic obstructive pulmonary disease on general respiratory wards: a multicentre randomised controlled trial. Lancet Lond Engl. 2000;355(9219):1931-5.

Chapter 27

Capnography in Noninvasive Ventilation: Clinical Implications

*Jacob George Pulinilkunnathil, Nirmalyo Lodh,
Swapna Chitra Vijayakumaran, Atul Prabhakar Kulkarni*

■ INTRODUCTION

In the early 20th century, oxygen supplementation and later iron lung ventilators were used for managing respiratory failure.[1] Later on, by the early 1950s mechanical ventilation emerged as the greatest invention to treat respiratory failure, leading to near extinction of the use of NIV. Soon the drawbacks of mechanical ventilation such as loss of airway defense began to be noticed, and there was a resurgence of NIV era which was aided by a refinement in technology and refinement in the interfaces.[2] NIV is currently used widely across hospitals to manage acute respiratory failure due to various causes and is the recommended treatment of choice for Type 2 respiratory failure associated with chronic obstructive pulmonary disease (COPD) exacerbation. It is also recommended as treatment of choice for select cases of Type 1 respiratory failure such as cardiogenic pulmonary edema, Type 1 respiratory failure in immunocompromised hosts, trauma, and also in palliative care.[3] NIV is also being increasingly used in domiciliary care for management of hypoventilation and Type 2 respiratory failure as in cases such as obesity hypoventilation syndrome, obstructive sleep apnea, etc.

■ NEED FOR CAPNOGRAPHY MONITORING DURING NONINVASIVE VENTILATION

Treatment failure with NIV has a wide range of incidence (5–60%) and is an important cause of increased mortality.[4] The important causes for treatment failure with NIV include an impaired cough reflex, increased tracheobronchial secretions, agitation, very severe disease, presence of multiorgan dysfunction syndrome (MODS), acute respiratory distress syndrome (ARDS), etc.[5] This treatment failure can be identified at the bedside by close monitoring of the patient and the early clinical signs include diaphoresis, worsening dyspnea, persistent tachycardia and tachypnea, hypotension, and cardiorespiratory arrest. In acute respiratory failure, supportive treatment with NIV aims to improve oxygenation and ventilation. Monitoring the oxygenation, ventilation, and serial quantification of dead space can be done invasively by blood gas analysis. The same information can be obtained noninvasively by monitoring both the oxygen saturation and carbon dioxide levels of blood, which will also give information regarding the adequacy of ventilation and quantification of dead space.

Constant monitoring of the carbon dioxide (CO_2) levels in body gives information regarding the disease severity, treatment efficacy, efficacy of the respiratory support provided.

It also helps in quantifying the alveolar ventilation and metabolic rate. This can be done by serial measurements of arterial blood gas (ABG) or serial/continuous measurement of end-tidal (ET) CO_2 **(Table 1)**. Blood gas measurements give an accurate estimate of CO_2 levels in the body and are considered the gold standard for CO_2 monitoring. They also give valuable information at the bedside regarding oxygenation, dead space, and acid–base status of the patient. However, this involves multiple arterial punctures or the requirement of invasive arterial lines, and provides only intermittent values. It cannot be used in conditions where NIV is used to treat sleep hypoventilation, as blood gas sampling will wake the patient up, leading to momentary albeit partial correction of hypoventilation.[6] On the other hand, ET CO_2 monitoring with NIV appears attractive in the ICU and also in domiciliary or hospice setting for the management of respiratory failure in view of its noninvasive nature, easy application, and the ability to provide a continuous monitoring of values.

Table 1: Comparison of arterial blood gas analysis and end-tidal carbon dioxide ($ETCO_2$) monitoring.

Arterial blood gas analysis	End-tidal carbon dioxide monitoring
Gold standard for assessing ventilation	Not the gold standard, as compared to blood gas analysis
Costly	Not as costly as blood gas analysis
Invasive, requiring multiple pricks and expertise	Noninvasive, and requires minimal expertise
Not continuous, and cannot track changes	Continuous, can track changes instantly
Provide information regarding oxygenation, dead space volume, and metabolic milieu	No information regarding oxygenation. Difficult to correlate with metabolic milieu
Values correspond to the clinical condition	Values may be falsely low or high depending upon the clinical situation, presence of bronchospasm, leaks in circuit, etc.

UNDERSTANDING THE CAPNOGRAPHY WAVEFORM (FIG. 1)

The capnography waveform can be broadly divided into four phases (phase 1 to phase 4 or phase 0 to phase 3).

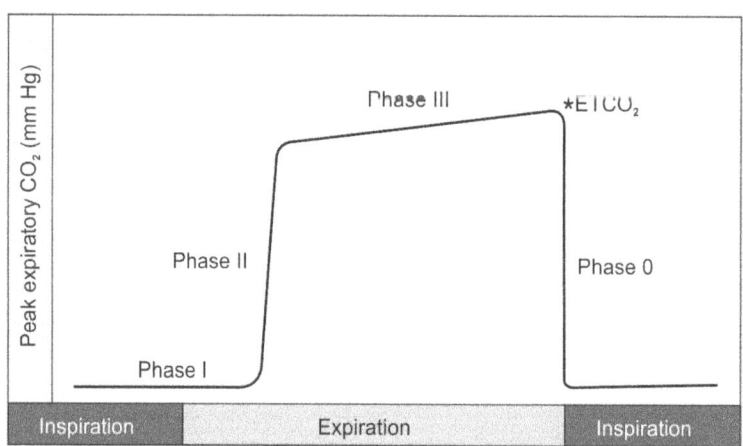

Fig. 1: The capnography waveform. ($ETCO_2$: end-tidal carbon dioxide)
Source: Adapted from Aminiahidashti H, Shafiee S, Zamani Kiasari A, Sazgar M. Applications of end-tidal carbon dioxide ($ETCO_2$) monitoring in emergency department; a narrative review. Emerg (Tehran). 2018;6(1):e5.

During inspiration, as no CO_2 passes the sampling port, the capnograph will not detect any CO_2 and a flat line is obtained unless due to rebreathing, ventilation circuit malfunction, etc. (phase 1). This is continued into the first part of exhalation, which contains gases in the anatomical dead space. A sudden build up in CO_2 that corresponds to mixture of gases from the anatomic dead space and gases from intermediate airways corresponds to phase 2. The CO_2 trace gradually builds up, corresponding to emptying of gases from the various alveoli and the slope depends upon their emptying pattern (phase 3). At the end of phase 3, the CO_2 measured will be highest and $PETCO_2$ is recorded. As inspiration starts, the expiratory gases are washed away from the sensor, which is shown as a rapid downstroke as the trace falls to baseline (phase 0 or phase 4), and the cycle continues with the next breath.[7]

END-TIDAL CAPNOGRAPHY AT THE BEDSIDE

Traditional capnography measures the CO_2 level at the end of the expiration and is a commonly used monitoring in patients who are invasively ventilated. The CO_2 levels are measured using either mainstream or the sidestream technology. Ideally, this should serve as a surrogate for the blood level of carbon dioxide ($PaCO_2$), if the metabolic rate, ventilation perfusion ratio, and dead space remain constant, but this may not be the case always. Among normal subjects, there is a difference of approximately 2-7 mm Hg between the end-tidal CO_2 values and blood CO_2 levels.[8,9] This difference can further vary depending upon various factors including patient-dependent factors and technical factors such as placement of the sensor, dead space ventilation, leaks, etc. $ETCO_2$ was found to underestimate CO_2 levels in COPD patients with dynamic hyperinflation and in spontaneously breathing subjects.[10] This may be due to the fact that in patients with airflow limitation, due to the prolonged expiration, a plateau in capnogram may not be achieved and the continuous flow during inspiration and expiration also makes $ETCO_2$ measurement technically difficult.[6] Other factors limiting the utilization of $PaCO_2$ levels are that the patients with respiratory failure often breathe with reduced tidal volumes, and these tidal volumes do not reach alveolar sacs and therefore this effectively becomes dead space ventilation. For those in whom nocturnal hypoventilation is present, the physiologic decrease in tidal volume and ventilation will result in increased CO_2 levels. These physiologic variations, along with ventilation and perfusion mismatch due to disease, can increase the $PaCO_2$-$ETCO_2$ gradient. Hence, after initiation of NIV, changes in the $ETCO_2$ may be due to changes in either disease, dead space or the physiological reasons already mentioned. Thus, the trend in the $PETCO_2$ values may be used as a surrogate for pCO_2 levels, only if the clinical assessment and judgment suggest that the dead space is constant. The dead space of the masks used for NIV is often considered a matter of concern, as it may affect both ventilation and sample measurement. However, studies have shown that the net physiological dead space as experienced by the patient is independent of the dead space of the mask. This is because during expiration, the expiratory flow washes out the CO_2 and reduces the dead space to even less than the mask volume.[11,12]

Monitoring $ETCO_2$ requires a closed system with no or minimal leaks to avoid losing the sample volume due to mouth breathing. $ETCO_2$ can be measured using either sidestream or mainstream technique. Mainstream capnographs have the infrared (IR) emitter/detector in the path of expiration gas flow. On the contrary, sidestream capnographs entrain a portion of expiratory gas via a sampling tube to the analyzer situated out of the path of expiratory gas flow.

A comparison of both techniques of capnography is given in **Table 2**. Mainstream monitoring requires the exhalation port of the mask to be located distal to the sampling location, as the CO_2 will be flushed out by the expiratory gas prior to its measurement. This is a serious limitation as a choice for $ETCO_2$ sampling during NIV. Sidestream assessment of $ETCO_2$ requires placement of the sensor either at the mask outlet or inside the mask or at the patient nares using nasal cannula **(Figs. 2 and 3)**. This minimizes the washout of CO_2 by the expiratory flow of gas but can lead to moisture condensation resulting in waveform distortion. This needs to be addressed separately by the use of dedicated filters or using specially designed tubings. Although promising, measuring $ETCO_2$ at the levels of nostrils by using a nasobuccal sensor during NIV was also shown to be inaccurate to predict both the absolute value of PCO_2 or the $PaCO_2$ variation over time.[13] Due to these constraints in measuring $ETCO_2$, the current interest is channeled to measure the cutaneous carbon dioxide ($PcCO_2$) as a surrogate for blood CO_2 levels.

Table 2: Comparison of mainstream and sidestream capnography.

Mainstream capnography	Sidestream capnography
CO_2 sensor is located prior to exhalation port and does not require a sampling port. Therefore, it is devoid of errors due to complications of the sampling tube such as delay in recording, obstruction, moisture condensation, and pressure drop. However, it can increase dead space.	Sensor is located outside the path of expiration gas flow. Does not affect dead space
As sensor is located in the exhalation path before expiration port, it is difficult to be used with NIV. It can cause significant traction on the endotracheal tubes. Sensor windows may be blocked in case of increased secretions	It is easier to use and can be used in non-intubated patients also. It has also been used with nasal prong, permitting their use with oxygen administration also. Associated with a delay in recording and is affected by complications such a sampling tube obstruction, moisture condensation, and pressure drop.

(NIV: noninvasive ventilation).

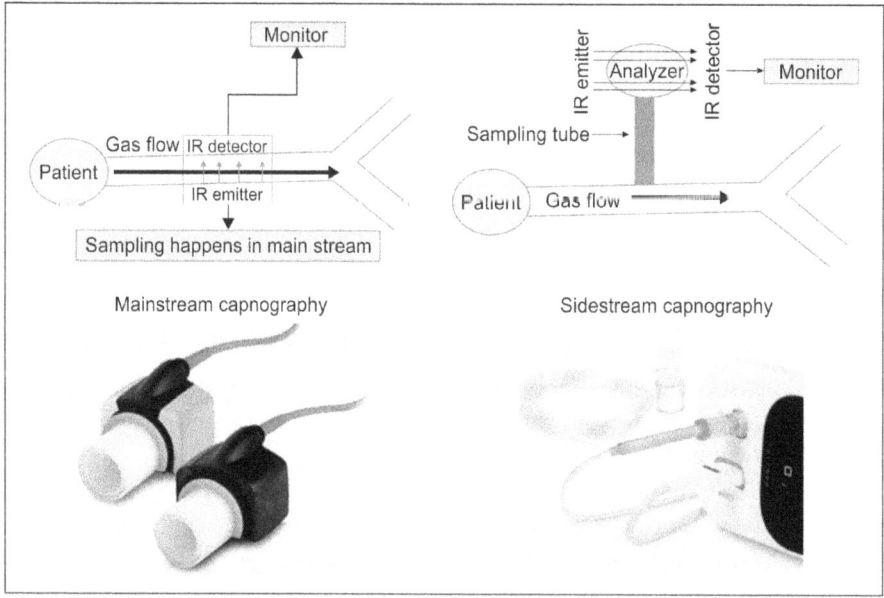

Fig. 2: Comparison of mainstream and sidestream capnography. (IR: infrared)

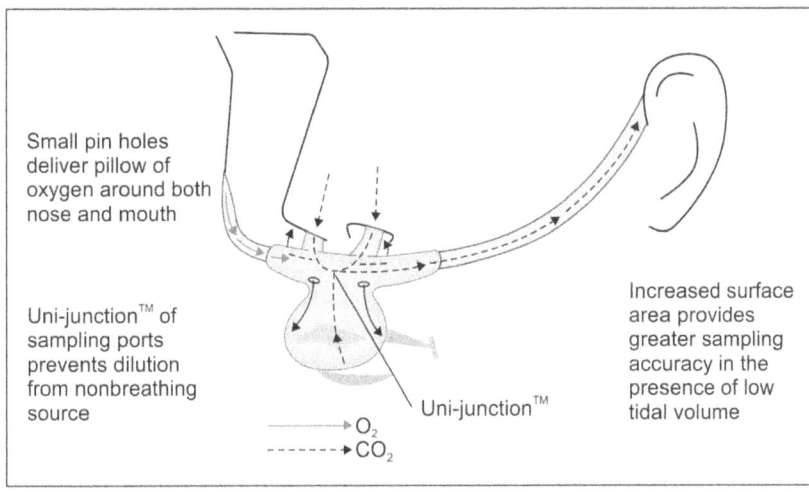

Fig. 3: Use of sidestream capnography with nasal prongs.

TRANSCUTANEOUS CO_2 MONITORING

Noninvasive monitoring of CO_2 levels can be done by electrochemical analysis of an electrolyte layer that is separated from the skin by a highly permeable membrane. Locally heated electrochemical sensors are applied to the epidermis, which increases the local vascularity by heating. CO_2 diffuses from the skin through the membrane into the electrolyte layer, reacts with water to form hydrogen and bicarbonate ions, which can be measured as a change in pH, and is proportional to the arterial PCO_2 value. The increase in vascularity and local temperature causes a rise in local CO_2 value, which is compounded by the CO_2 production from epidermal cells also. This is then adjusted and a rough estimate of arterial CO_2 levels can be reached.[14] As the transcutaneous CO_2 ($TcCO_2$) sensors require a temperature between 43° and 45°C, there is a hazard of thermal injury while measuring. The newer sensors require only a temperature of 42°C and are safe for application for a continuous period of up to 8 hours. The accuracy of cutaneous CO_2 measurement has been tried during polysomnography studies, during endoscopies and also in critically ill patients, and the results have been found satisfactory. Due to a high temperature generated at the probes (42–45° C), pCO_2 measurement will require change in monitoring site every 3–4 hours to prevent skin burn.[14] Another issue with cutaneous CO_2 monitoring is the development of sensor drift,[15] which is also an important and technically limiting factor for long-term continuous measurements. Thus although valuable in patient monitoring, $TcCO_2$ values can give false data due to improper calibration. The $PTcCO_2$ values may be spuriously low in the presence of air bubbles, leaks, in vasoconstricted states such as shock, vasopressor administration, in patients with increased dermal thickness or subcutaneous edema. Similarly, falsely high values may occur in cases of augmented capillary blood flow due to movement.[14] Currently, the guidelines suggest transcutaneous CO_2 monitoring with ABG correlation during the initiation of NIV, and to facilitate the discontinuation of NIV. Caution may be required in those with hypercapnia (transcutaneous CO_2 values (≥60 mm Hg), as it may underestimate the CO_2 values.[15,16]

USE OF CONTINUOUS CAPNOGRAPHY IN INTENSIVE CARE UNIT (ICU)

Continuous capnography appears to be promising in providing valuable information regarding ventilatory status in addition to the oxygenation status that is being routinely monitored. A systematic review of literature identified that continuous capnography enabled early identification of respiratory depression much before clinical examination or deterioration of clinical state. This is of particular importance in high-risk patients, especially the hypercapnic patients, currently requiring oxygen therapy or vulnerable patients requiring opioids for pain relief. Patients who are developing respiratory depression can be identified early and thus the drugs (oxygen/opioids) can be titrated accordingly. This not only improves patient safety but also improves the nurse's satisfaction and reduces treatment cost.[17]

INDICATIONS FOR USING CUTANEOUS MONITORING IN INTENSIVE CARE UNIT (ICU)

Transcutaneous capnometry monitoring (TCM) can be used in acutely ill patients who require continuous monitoring of oxygen and carbon dioxide with minimal blood usage. This helps in assessment of the adequacy of oxygenation and/or ventilation, and can influence patient treatment decisions such as weaning and extubation, and in other cases such as diabetic ketoacidosis. In diabetic ketoacidosis, monitoring of cutaneous values of CO_2 can aid in monitoring the treatment as $PTcCO_2$ correlates with serum HCO_3^- levels. Apart from these, $TcCO_2$ values are also used in wound care and hyperbaric oxygen therapy to monitor critical limb ischemia. The $PTcCO_2$ value of 30-40 mm Hg in the diseased limb is suggestive of adequate limb perfusion, while a value less than 30 mm Hg indicates poor perfusion and a value less than 10 mm Hg is considered incompatible with spontaneous healing process. A $PTcCO_2$ of 30 mm Hg is considered the critical dividing value that separates successful from unsuccessful amputation stump healing.[18]

FUTURE DIRECTIONS

Due to the high mortality associated with treatment failure of NIV, identifying those subsets of patients in clinical practice is of paramount importance. Currently, ABG analysis remains the gold standard for assessing adequacy of ventilation. However, owing to its noninvasive and continuous nature, CO_2 monitoring via exhaled gas or transcutaneous monitoring is gaining acceptance. We, at present, require more data from all patient subsets, along with data regarding variations due to measurement techniques, sensors of various companies, site of placement of sensor or probes before firm recommendations can be made. As more data emerges, a greater acceptance for the use of continuous volumetric capnography may ensue and may aid in better patient management. Application of this technology in clinical practice will always need correlation and clinical judgment regarding the physiologic variation of CO_2 levels and also regarding the influence of dead space due to disease and devices. As with any technology, misinterpretation of data may lead to inappropriate treatment of the patient. The future of capnography seems promising, as it is noninvasive and can give information regarding other dimensions of patient care including alveolar ventilation, acid-base status, resting energy requirements, and calorie requirements, and also in wound care.

REFERENCES

1. Pierson DJ. History and epidemiology of non-invasive ventilation in the acute-care setting. Respir Care. 2009;54(1):40-52.
2. Mehta S, Hill NS. Noninvasive ventilation. Am J Respir Crit Care Med. 2001;163(2):540-77.
3. Rochwerg B, Brochard L, Elliott MW, Hess D, Hill N, Nava S, et al. Official ERS/ATS clinical practice guidelines: non-invasive ventilation for acute respiratory failure. Eur Respir J. 2017;50(2):pii: 1602426.
4. Ozyilmaz E, Ugurlu AO, Nava S. Timing of noninvasive ventilation failure: causes, risk factors, and potential remedies. BMC Pulm Med. 2014;14:19.
5. Scala R, Pisani L. Noninvasive ventilation in acute respiratory failure: which recipe for success? Eur Respir Rev. 2018;27(149): pii: 180029.
6. American Association for Respiratory Care. Clinical practice guideline: Capnography/capnometry during mechanical ventilation–2003 revision and update. Respir Care. 2003;48(5):534-9.
7. Aminiahidashti H, Shafiee S, Zamani Kiasari A, Sazgar M. Applications of End-Tidal Carbon Dioxide (ET CO_2) Monitoring in Emergency Department; a Narrative Review. Emerg (Tehran). 2018;6(1):e5.
8. Ergan B, Nasiłowski J, Winck JC. How should we monitor patients with acute respiratory failure treated with noninvasive ventilation? Eur Respir Rev. 2018;27(148):pii:170101.
9. Saatci E, Miller DM, Stell IM, Lee KC, Moxham J. Dynamic dead space in face masks used with non-invasive ventilators: a lung model study. Eur Respir J. 2004;23(1):129-35.
10. Fraticelli A, Lellouche F, Taille S, Qader S, Brochard L. Comparison of different interface during NIV in patients with acute respiratory failure. Am J Respir Crit Care Med. 2003;167:A389.
11. Piquilloud L, Thevoz D, Jolliet P, Revelly JP. End-tidal carbon dioxide monitoring using a naso-buccal sensor is not appropriate to monitor capnia during non-invasive ventilation. Ann Intensive Care. 2015;5:2.
12. Chhajed PN, Gehrer S, Pandey KV, Vaidya PJ, Leuppi JD, Tamm M, et al. Utility of transcutaneous capnography for optimization of noninvasive ventilation pressures. J Clin Diagn Res. 2016;10(9):OC06-OC09.
13. Ruiz Y, Farrero E, Córdoba A, González N, Dorca J, Prats E. Transcutaneous carbon dioxide monitoring in subjects with acute respiratory failure and severe hypercapnia. Respir Care. 2016;61(4):428-33.
14. Restrepo RD, Nuccio P, Spratt G, Waugh J. Current applications of capnography in non-intubated patients. Expert Rev Respir Med. 2014;8(5):629-39.
15. Westhoff M, Schönhofer B, Neumann P, Bickenbach J, Barchfeld T, Becker H, et al. Non-invasive mechanical ventilation in acute respiratory failure. Pneumologie. 2015;69(12):719-56.
16. Davidson AC, Banham S, Elliott M, Kennedy D, Gelder C, Glossop A, et al. BTS/ICS guideline for the ventilatory management of acute hypercapnic respiratory failure in adults. Thorax. 2016;71 Suppl 2: ii1-35.
17. Lam T, Nagappa M, Wong J, Singh M, Wong D, Chung F. Continuous pulse oximetry and capnography monitoring for postoperative respiratory depression and adverse events: A systematic review and meta-analysis. Anesth Analg. 2017:125(6):2019-29.
18. Restrepo RD, Hirst KR, Wittnebel L, Wettstein R. AARC Clinical Practice Guideline: Transcutaneous Monitoring of Carbon Dioxide and Oxygen: Respiratory Care. 2012:57(11):1955-62.

Chapter 28

Weaning from Noninvasive Ventilation

Palepu B Gopal, Lakshmi Sasidhar Puvvula

■ INTRODUCTION

Noninvasive ventilation (NIV) is a provision of assisted mechanical ventilation without the need for an invasive artificial airway. NIV has seen increased popularity in past few decades in acute care setting. The increased popularity is related to a number of claimed advantages of NIV over invasive mechanical ventilation such as avoiding complications of intubation including aspiration of gastric contents, trauma to hypopharynx, larynx, trachea,[1] dental trauma, arrhythmias and hypotension[2] due to autonomic nervous stimulation, and ventilator associated pneumonia. Also, NIV is better tolerated than invasive ventilation and requires less or no sedation.

■ INDICATIONS FOR NONINVASIVE VENTILATION

Noninvasive ventilation is strongly recommended for chronic obstructive pulmonary disease (COPD) exacerbation,[3] COPD with failure to wean from invasive ventilation and acute cardiogenic pulmonary edema.[3] It may be considered in COPD in three settings: to prevent respiratory acidosis, to prevent endotracheal intubation in mild to moderate respiratory acidosis and as an alternate measure to invasive ventilation in severe acidosis.[4] Respiratory failure in acute cardiogenic pulmonary edema is associated with alveolar flooding and decreased respiratory system compliance and NIV in this setting improves respiratory mechanics, reduces left ventricular work load.[5,6] NIV is also indicated in acute respiratory failure (ARF) in immune compromised patients with an aim to prevent further respiratory deterioration and invasive ventilation related complications.[3,5] It can be used for treating postoperative respiratory failure[7] in patients with COPD and CHF, or as prophylaxis after high risk surgeries[8] in such patients. Other indications of NIV are carefully selected hypoxemic respiratory failure patients due to ARDS or community acquired pneumonia. Obesity hypoventilation syndrome, neuromuscular disorders, EOL patients with do-not-intubate status have also been candidates for NIV.[9]

■ MODES OF NONINVASIVE VENTILATION

Pressure support or bilevel is the most common mode used for NIV. Average volume assured pressure mode (AVAPS) is available on certain ventilators which has advantage over BiPAP in chronically hypoventilating patients such as obesity hypoventilation syndrome,[10] but has not been shown advantageous in acute care settings. Proportional assist ventilation uses inspiratory flow signal to determine how much flow and volume assistance to be provided to patient and it can function as NIV mode and can enhance patient comfort and synchronicity.[11-13]

Weaning from NIV is always a challenge and there have been attempts to formulate weaning protocols. Yet, there have not been strong evidence based studies in this field, as opposed to invasive ventilation. The reason for this might be the heterogeneous nature of indications for NIV and continuously evolving nature of this technology.

Criteria to Start Weaning from NIV (Readiness to Wean)

Weaning from NIV can be started once the patient becomes clinically stable. Protocol-based weaning strategies have found to be more successful with shorter duration of NIV requirement and shorter ICU length of stay.[14] The criteria to start weaning from NIV are shown in **Table 1.**

Table 1: Criteria to start weaning from noninvasive ventilation (NIV).

S. No.	Measure	Character
1.	Arterial pH	≥ 7.35
2.	SpO_2	> 90%
3.	Respiratory rate	≤ 25/min
4.	Heart rate	≤ 120/min
5.	Systolic blood pressure	≥ 90 mm Hg
6.	Signs of respiratory distress	No agitation, diaphoresis, anxiety

Strategies for weaning NIV[15]

- Stepwise reduction in NIV duration
- Stepwise reduction in NIV pressure support
- Immediate withdrawal of NIV after stabilization

Strategy 1: Stepwise Reduction in NIV Duration

This method involves progressively reducing the duration[12] of NIV over a period of 3-4 days once the patient satisfies the criteria for weaning. Initially weaning should be carried during day time.[12] The day time weaning can be divided into periods of 3 hours each and can be performed as follows[13]—during first 24 hours in each 3 hours, 1 hour without NIV (except during night period), in the second day in each 3 hours, 2 hours without NIV (except during night period) and in the 3rd day NIV can be used only during the night period. NIV may be discontinued on day 4 unless continuation is clinically indicated for example, few hours in day time and 6 hours or more overnight.[12]

Strategy 2: Stepwise Reduction in NIV Pressure Support

This strategy involves gradual reduction (2-3 cm of H_2O) of IPAP and EPAP over a period of 6-8 hours and removing NIV once the patient tolerates IPAP of 6-8 cm of H_2O and EPAP of 4-5 cm of H_2O.[15]

There are no studies comparing the effectiveness of stepwise reduction of duration versus stepwise reduction of pressure support, but both the strategies can be used in conjunction with each other.

Strategy 3: Immediate Withdrawal of NIV

This strategy involves immediate cessation NIV once the patient stabilizes. Though it has potential advantage of shortening the duration of weaning process, the rates of failure of weaning and reinstitution of NIV can be higher. A randomized control trial by Lun et al.[16] compared immediate withdrawal of NIV to stepwise reduction and found success rate of weaning to be 56% and 74% respectively, although the data is statistically not significant. Immediate withdrawal of NIV can be tried in patients who required NIV for a shorter duration of time and who have clinically recovered well.

Failure of Weaning from NIV

All the patients who are being weaned from NIV should be carefully monitored clinically and blood gas analysis should be done as and when necessary. Increase in respiratory rate, heart rate, use of accessory muscles of respiration, worsening pH and $PaCO_2$ may indicate failure of weaning process and warrant reinstitution of NIV or assessment for requirement of invasive ventilation. The predictors for failure[17] of weaning from NIV include elderly age group, obesity, patients who presented with more severe disease, presence of respiratory acidosis with low pH during admission, presence of multiple co morbid conditions including cardiovascular and renal disease.

CONCLUSION

Although NIV has become a common intervention in modern ICU there has been paucity of data regarding weaning from NIV. Nevertheless a careful identification of patient who is ready for weaning by clinical and laboratory criteria, a protocol-based weaning strategy and a close monitoring during process of weaning can result in successful weaning of most of the patients from NIV. Any deterioration after initiation of NIV or during weaning process should warrant the clinician to assess for requirement of invasive ventilation.

KEY POINTS

- A careful assessment with weaning criteria can help identify patients who can be successfully weaned.
- A protocol-based weaning strategy using stepwise reduction of duration or pressure support should be utilized.
- Patients should be carefully monitored during process of weaning, reinstitution of NIV or assessment for invasive ventilation should be undertaken if there is any deterioration in clinical or laboratory parameters.

REFERENCES

1. Alagoz A, Ulus F, Sazak H, Camdal A, Savkilioglu E. Two cases of tracheal rupture after endotracheal intubation. J Cardiothorac Vasc Anesth. 2009;23(2):271-72.

2. Anzueto A, Frutos-Vivar F, Esteban A, Alía I, Brochard L, Stewart T, et al. Incidence, risk factors and outcome of barotrauma in mechanically ventilated patients. Intensive Care Med. 2004;30(4): 612-9.
3. Rochwerg B, Brochard L, Elliott MW, Hess D, Hill NS, Nava S, et al. Official ERS/ATS clinical practice guidelines: noninvasive ventilation for acute respiratory failure. Eur Respir J 2017;50:1602426.
4. Nava S, Navalesi P, Conti G. Time of non-invasive ventilation. Intensive Care Med. 2006;32:361-70.
5. Squadrone V, Massaia M, Bruno B, Marmont F, Falda M, Bagna C, et al. Early CPAP prevents evolution of acute lung injury in patients with hematologic malignancy. Intensive Care Med. 2010;36: 1666-74.
6. D'Andrea A, Martone F, Liccardo B, et al. Acute and chronic effects of noninvasive ventilation on left and right myocardial function in patients with obstructive sleep apnea syndrome: a speckle tracking echocardiographic study. Echocardiography. 2016;33:1144-55.
7. Chiumello D, Chevallard G, Gregoretti C. Non-invasive ventilation in postoperative patients: a systematic review. Intensive Care Med. 2013;37:918-29.
8. Auriant I, Jallot A, Herve P, Cerrina J, Le Roy Ladurie F, Fournier JL, et al. Noninvasive ventilation reduces mortality in acute respiratory failure following lung resection. Am J Respir Crit Care Med. 2001;164:1231-5.
9. Nava S, Ferrer M, Esquinas A, Scala R, Groff P, Cosentini R, et al. Palliative use of non-invasive ventilation in end-of-life patients with solid tumours: a randomised feasibility trial. Lancet Oncol. 2013;14:219-27.
10. Storre JH, Seuthe B, Fiechter R, Milioglou S, Dreher M, Sorichter S, et al. Average volume-assured pressure support in obesity hypoventilation: a randomized crossover trial. Chest. 2006;130(3): 815-21.
11. Gay PC, Hess DR, Hill NS. Noninvasive proportional assist ventilation for acute respiratory insufficiency. Comparison with pressure support ventilation. Am J Respir Crit Care Med. 2001;164(9): 1606-11.
12. BTS/RCP London/Intensive Care Society. The use of noninvasive ventilation in the management of patients with chronic obstructive pulmonary disease admitted to hospital with acute type II respiratory failure. In Concise Guidance to Good Practice series, London, UK, 2008.
13. Plant PK, Owen JL, Elliott MW. Early use of non-invasive ventilation for acute exacerbations of chronic obstructive pulmonary disease on general respiratory wards: a multicentre randomised controlled trial. Lancet. 2000;355:1931-5.
14. Duan J, Tang X, Huang S, Jia J, Guo S. Protocol-directed versus physician-directed weaning from noninvasive ventilation: The impact in chronic obstructive pulmonary disease patients. J Trauma Acute Care Surg. 2012;72:1271-5.
15. Hadda V, Kumari R. Protocols for Weaning From NIV: Appraisal of Evidence. Insights Chest Dis. 2016;01.
16. Lun CT, Chan VL, Leung WS, Cheung AP, Cheng SL, Chu CM, et al. A pilot randomized study comparing two methods of non-invasive ventilation withdrawal after acute respiratory failure in chronic obstructive pulmonary disease. Respirology. 2013;18:814-9.
17. Moretti M, Cilione C, Tampieri A, Fracchia C, Marchioni A, Navaet S. Incidence and causes of non-invasive mechanical ventilation failure after initial success. Thorax. 2000;55:819-25.

Chapter 29

Noninvasive Ventilation in Failure to Wean from Invasive Ventilation, Postextubation Failure, and Tracheostomy

Khusrav Beji Bajan

"Life is pleasant. Death is peaceful. It is the transition that is troublesome."
Isaac Asimov

INTRODUCTION

A better understanding of the physiological merits of noninvasive ventilation (NIV) and its newer dimensions have expanded its horizons, from being indicated in acute exacerbation of hypercapnic respiratory failure and cardiogenic pulmonary edema to its use in palliative care, "Do not resuscitate" state, "Do not intubate" state, mild acute respiratory distress syndrome, viral pneumonia epidemics, *failure to wean from mechanical ventilation, postextubation respiratory failure*, and many more.

With better monitoring and technological advancements, more and more patients live longer in the critical care units, leading to woes of long stay in critical care arenas such as—inadequate nutrition, critical care neuromyopathies, prolonged ventilation, *weaning failure*, deep vein thrombosis, pulmonary embolism, and pressure ulcers to mention a few.

20–30% of mechanically ventilated patients fail their first attempted weaning, especially if ventilated for more than 24 hours. More than 40% of the total duration of mechanical ventilation is spent in the process of weaning. Studies have documented 27% mortality in the weaning failure and the reintubation group as against only 2.6% in the successfully weaned group.[1] In unselected patients with respiratory failure post-extubation, NIV has failed to show a difference in the reintubation rates or in reducing mortality.[2]

On one hand, we have associated risks of delayed *weaning/liberation* which encompass ventilator-associated pneumonia (VAP), ventilator-associated lung injury, prolonged sedation, gastrointestinal disturbances, etc., whereas on the other, *premature extubation* can lead to its own unique concerns like loss of airway protection (leading to aspiration), gas exchange failure, cardiovascular stress secondary to sympathetic discharge, respiratory muscle fatigue, and respiratory acidosis leading to events of *reintubation* and further increased morbidity and mortality. Thus, it is imperative to strike a balance on the timing for success of weaning/liberation.

Here, it is essential to note the distinction between weaning and liberation in the context of mechanical ventilation. The essential difference being—*weaning* is considered as gradual withdrawal of ventilatory support leading to extubation whereas *liberation* is direct or sudden withdrawal of ventilatory support leading to extubation.

Chapter 29: Noninvasive Ventilation in Failure to Wean from Invasive Ventilation...

To undertake a successful weaning, the primary indication for mechanical ventilation should be identified and corrected and the patient should be hemodynamically stable with being able to maintain adequate oxygenation and ventilation. However, despite essential and adequate care interventions, it is noted that one-third of the patients face the stigma of failure to wean in critical care settings.

Dissecting and assimilating the *weaning failure* diverges the term to—*difficult weaning and prolonged weaning*. *Difficult weaning* is termed when patients, who fail weaning, require up to three spontaneous breathing trials (SBTs) or up to 7 days from the first SBT to achieve successful weaning. According to the National Association for Medical Direction of Respiratory Care recommendations, *prolonged mechanical ventilation (prolonged weaning)* was defined as those patients who need mechanical ventilation for >6 hours per day for >21 consecutive days.[3]

There are multifactorial causes for weaning failure, the most important being—increased airway resistance, inspiratory muscle fatigue, acute cardiac dysfunction leading to pulmonary edema, critical care neuropathy, and so on.

All the above factors can be ameliorated by prompt application and utilization of NIV as seen in **Figure 1**.[4]

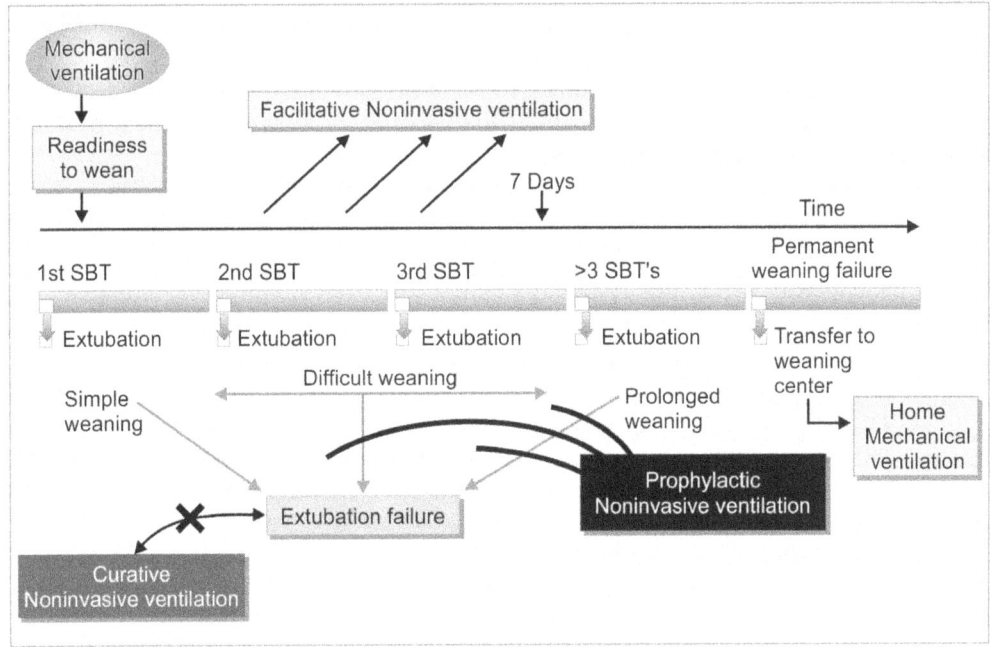

Fig. 1: Protocolized spontaneous breathing trial (SBT).
(MV: mechanical ventilation; NIV: noninvasive ventilation)

Nutrition, thyroid concerns, and hypophosphatemia also need attention and intervention in patient with failure to wean.

Noninvasive ventilation in weaning is not a *one-size-fits-all* solution. The key to success in preventing weaning failure is to identify the patients who are at *risk for weaning failure*, which includes patients more than 65 years of age, those with underlying cardiorespiratory disease, and those in whom arterial partial pressure of carbon dioxide ($PaCO_2$) persists to remain above 45 mm Hg even after adequate ventilation and while on an SBT.

Thus, umpteen strategies have been developed and studied to combat weaning failure from invasive ventilation like application of neurally adjusted ventilatory assist (NAVA), automatic tube compensation (ATC), proportional assist ventilation (PAV), protocolized weaning, computer-driven-closed-loop knowledge-based algorithm, Spontaneous Awakening trials (SATs), Awakening and Breathing Controlled (ABC) trials, and also *utilization of NIV*. Although these care interventions have proven to be beneficial for some groups of weaning failure patients, results from studies are controversial and hence the need to understand the evidence and physiology in averting weaning failure in patients.

Noninvasive ventilation improves oxygenation and work of breathing and is an exciting option to assist in circumventing weaning and extubation failure.

NONINVASIVE VENTILATION AS A WEANING ASSIST FROM INVASIVE MECHANICAL VENTILATION

Noninvasive ventilation is evidenced to be as effective as invasive mechanical ventilation in improving the work of breathing, reducing inspiratory workload, and maintaining adequate gas exchange during the weaning phase in certain patients intubated and ventilated for hypercapnic respiratory failure.

Since prolonged mechanical ventilation is beset with life-threatening infective and noninfective complications, NIV throughout the weaning process has opened avenues in shortening days on mechanical ventilation.

In a review by *Burns et al.*, 16 randomized controlled trials (RCTs) enrolling a total of 994 participants were identified which included nine studies on patients with chronic obstructive pulmonary disease (COPD), six studies on patients with a mixed group, and one study on patients with hypoxemic respiratory failure. The study findings on comparison with conventional weaning using either a progressive reduction of inspiratory support or SBTs noted that NIV was associated with a significant decrease in mortality [relative risk (RR): 0.53; 95% confidence interval (CI): 0.36–0.80; 994 patients], significant reductions in VAP (RR: 0.25; 95% CI: 0.15–0.43; 953 patients), intensive care unit (ICU) (mean difference 5.59 days; 95% CI: –7.90 to –3.28) and hospital length of stay (mean difference—6.04 days; 95% CI: –9.22 to –2.87), total duration of mechanical ventilation (mean difference—5.64 days; 95% CI: –9.50 to –1.77), and duration of invasive ventilation (mean difference—7.44 days; 95% CI: –10.34 to –4.55).[5]

As per the *European Respiratory Society (ERS)/American Thoracic Society (ATS) Clinical Practice Guidelines—2017*, use of NIV to facilitate weaning from mechanically ventilated patients with hypercapnic respiratory failure is recommended.[6] More studies on the use of NIV in hypoxemic patients being weaned are desirable.

NONINVASIVE VENTILATION TO PREVENT POSTEXTUBATION RESPIRATORY FAILURE

Extubation failure is an undesirable state in the patient care process and is further defined as the need for reintubation within 48 or 72 hours of extubation which is associated with significant deterioration in the patient's clinical condition.

Reintubation following extubation failure is as high as 23.5% in certain studies and has a worse prognosis and mortality, thus presenting as a major clinical problem.

The event carries a mortality rate of up to 50% and scores the highest for late reintubations due to clinical deterioration directly generated by extubation failure and respiratory distress of reintubation.

It stands for a clinician, an absolute mandate to redefine decisions with regard to extubation and postextubation management. Preextubation management involving patient optimization and addressing concerns with regard to fluid balance and cardiac dysfunction along with use of relevant biomarkers like pro-B-type natriuretic peptide (pro-BNP) is a routine and a norm.

One must identify patients at *high risk of extubation failure* and then stratify them into two groups.
1. *Extubate to NIV*—in which patients are placed onto NIV immediately after extubation in an attempt to prevent respiratory failure
2. Application of NIV postextubation after development of respiratory failure.

Extubate to Noninvasive Ventilation

As per a study conducted by *Jiang et al.* on *unselected patients* (high-risk group patients not identified), 93 consecutive patients following planned (60.2%) or unplanned (39.8%) extubation were enrolled and further randomized either to preventive NIV (treatment group) or standard treatment (control group), the study results of which noted no difference in the rate of reintubation between the two groups.[7] In a similar more recent study on *unselected patients* by *SU et al.*, it was noted that NIV provides no benefit compared with standard oxygen therapy.[8] Considering these two studies in unselected patients postextubation, NIV provides no benefit in the weaning process.

Nava et al. conducted a multicenter RCT on 97 *at high-risk patients* who were randomized 1 hour after extubation, following a successful SBT, to receive either NIV (minimum 8 hours per day for 2 days) or standard treatment (oxygen therapy). The NIV group was noted to have reduced rates of reintubation, which further resulted in a reduced ICU mortality.[9]

Another multicenter RCT on 162 *high-risk patients* conducted by *Ferrer et al.* showed in the NIV group, a decrease in the incidence of developing postextubation respiratory failure and ICU mortality; however, the rate of reintubation, ICU, hospital length of stay, and hospital mortality were not significantly different between the two groups. As per findings of the *post hoc* analysis on hypercapnic high-risk patients, the 90 days survival rate significantly improved. *Ornico et al.* found a reduction in reintubation and mortality in a group of patients with acute exacerbation of COPD who were ventilated for more than 72 hours.[10]

Application of Noninvasive Ventilation Postextubation After Development of Respiratory Failure

The use of NIV within 48 hours after development of respiratory failure postextubation has been shown to be ineffective in most studies. *Keenan et al.* conducted a single-center RCT and noted no beneficial effect of NIV on reintubation, mortality, or length of ICU stay.[11] In a multicenter RCT conducted by *Esteban et al.* on 221 patients with respiratory failure, postextubation also demonstrated no significant benefit in the NIV group. In fact, the researcher noted higher mortality in the NIV group probably due to the ill effects of delayed intubation.[2]

Thus, as per the *ERS/ATS Clinical Practice Guidelines—2017*, NIV use within after 48 hours to facilitate weaning in patients developing respiratory failure postextubation is not recommended.[6] A summary of the recommendations are shown in **Figure 2**.[12]

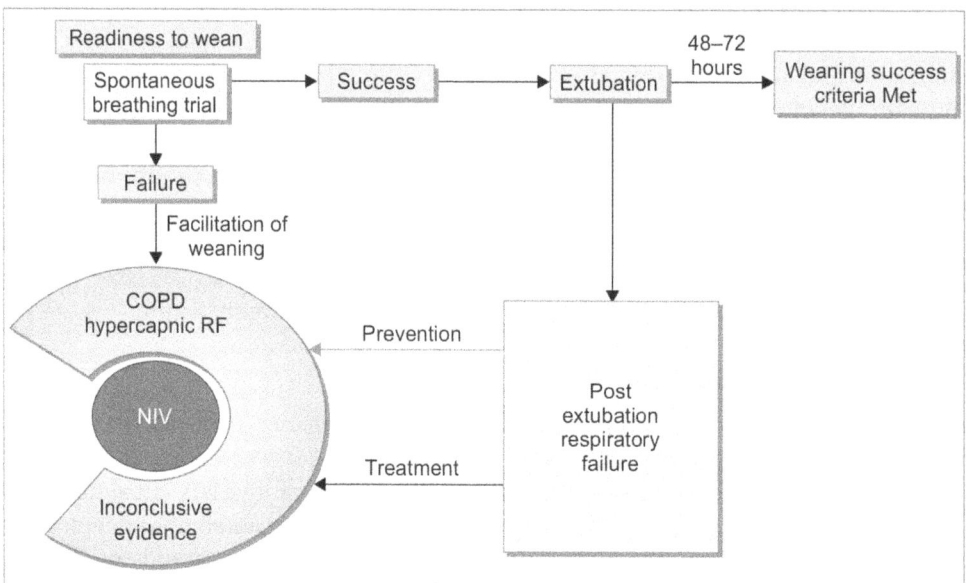

Fig. 2: Diagrammatic representation of the use of NIV in weaning. (COPD: chronic obstructive pulmonary disease; NIV: noninvasive ventilation; RF: respiratory failure; SBT: spontaneous breathing trial)

▌NONINVASIVE VENTILATION AND TRACHEOSTOMY

Though numerous studies in long-term mechanically ventilated patients comparing early versus late tracheostomy have been inconclusive, the practice of early tracheostomy to reduce the need for sedation and also to reduce dead space has found a niche as a weaning method in clinical practice.

Pu X et al. studied 50 patients with tracheostomies for weaning and further divided them into two groups—one with direct withdrawal of mechanical ventilation and second with sequential plugging of tracheostomy with intermittent use of NIV. The findings depicted a decrease in the incidence of VAP, duration of ventilation, hospital cost, and, in the other hand, an increased success rate of weaning.[13]

Thus, performing tracheostomy early or late is more an experience driven rather than an evidence-based decision.

▌CONCLUSION

The use of NIV in hypercapnia with COPD exacerbation and cardiogenic pulmonary edema is strongly recommended and unchallenged. Though, a newer therapy such as *high flow nasal oxygen (HFNO-AIRVO)* has been proven to be more effective in hypoxemic respiratory failure than NIV as per the *FLORALI study*.

Failure to wean is common, worsens mortality, and is nightmare for most clinicians. Protean modalities have been implicated in making weaning successful.

The *ERS/ATS Clinical Practice Guidelines—2017*:

- Recommends the use of NIV to wean *hypercapnic patients*
- Recommends the use of NIV prophylactically (*extubate to NIV*) in *high-risk patients*
- Recommends against the use of NIV for postextubation respiratory failure after it develops
- Recommends against the use of NIV in unselected patients who are not at high risk for extubation failure.[6]

Noninvasive ventilation, if used judiciously in select group of patients who are awake and with a patent airway, is a safe and effective ventilatory modality to combat the life-threatening perils of prolonged mechanical ventilation. Ventilation is lifesaving. Liberation is a success. It is the transition of weaning that is troublesome.

A thought can change a world and so weaning should be *thought* of, in all mechanically ventilated patients as soon as possible, to *change* the patient's outcome in a positive direction.

REFERENCES

1. Esteban A, Frutos-Vivar F, Ferguson ND, Arabi Y, Apezteguía C, González M, et al. Noninvasive positive-pressure ventilation for respiratory failure after extubation. N Engl J Med. 2004;350:2452-60.
2. Ferrer M, Valencia M, Nicolas JM, Bernadich O, Badia JR, Torres A. Early noninvasive ventilation averts extubation failure in patients at risk: a randomized trial. Am J Respir Crit Care Med. 2006;173:164-70.
3. Rochwerg B, Brochard L, Elliott MW, Hess D, Hill NS, Nava S, et al. Official ERS/ATS clinical practice guidelines: noninvasive ventilation for acute respiratory failure. Eur Respir J. 2017;50:1602426.
4. Talwar D, Dogra V. Weaning from mechanical ventilation in chronic obstructive pulmonary disease: Key to success. J Assoc Chest Physicians. 2016;4:43-9.
5. Burns KE, Meade MO, Premji A, Adhikari NK. Noninvasive ventilation as a weaning strategy for mechanical ventilation in adults with respiratory failure: a Cochrane systematic review. CMAJ. 2014;186:E112-22.
6. Sancho J, Servera E, Jara-Palomares L, Barrot E, Sanchez-Oro-Gómez R, Gómez de Terreros F, et al. Noninvasive ventilation during the weaning process in chronically critically ill patients. ERJ Open Res. 2016;2:00061-2016.
7. Jiang JS, Kao SJ, Wang SN. Effect of early application of biphasic positive airway pressure on the outcome of extubation in ventilator weaning. Respirology. 1999;4:161-5.
8. Su CL, Chiang LL, Yang SH, Lin HI, Cheng KC, Huang YC, et al. Preventive use of noninvasive ventilation after extubation: a prospective, multicenter randomized controlled trial. Respir Care. 2012;57:204-10.
9. Nava S, Gregoretti C, Fanfulla F, Squadrone E, Grassi M, Carlucci A, et al. Noninvasive ventilation to prevent respiratory failure after extubation in high-risk patients. Crit Care Med. 2005;33:2465-70.
10. Ornico SR, Lobo SM, Sanches HS, Deberaldini M, Tófoli LT, Vidal AM, et al. Noninvasive ventilation immediately after extubation improves weaning outcome after acute respiratory failure: a randomized controlled trial. Crit Care. 2013;17:R39.
11. Keenan SP, Powers C, McCormack DG, Block G. Noninvasive positive-pressure ventilation for postextubation respiratory distress: a randomized controlled trial. JAMA. 2002;287:3238-44.
12. Ferrer M, Sellarés J, Valencia M, Carrillo A, Gonzalez G, Badia JR, et al. Non-invasive ventilation after extubation in hypercapnic patients with chronic respiratory disorders: randomised controlled trial. Lancet. 2009;374:1082-8.
13. Pu X, Wang J, Yan X, Jiang X. Sequential invasive-noninvasive mechanical ventilation weaning strategy for patients after tracheostomy. World J Emerg Med. 2015;6:196-200.

Section 5

Problems with Noninvasive Ventilation

30. Skin Sore, Nutrition (RT Feeding), Gastric Insufflation, Physiotherapy: Lung Toileting, and Agitated Patients

Chapter 30

Skin Sore, Nutrition (RT Feeding), Gastric Insufflation, Physiotherapy: Lung Toileting, and Agitated Patients

Sachin Gupta, Deeksha Tomar

SKIN SORES

■ INTRODUCTION

The use of noninvasive ventilation (NIV) has almost tripled in the last 2 decades and has become the standard therapy for respiratory failure. However, this increased use has also increased the incidence of skin lesions at the site of device use. A recent review of 62 studies showed that the incidence of pressure ulcers (PUs) at the nasal bridge occurs in 5–50% after initial few hours and the incidence reaches to 100% by 48 hours.[1]

■ SKIN LESIONS

The most common skin lesions are redness, erythema, and skin peeling at the site of contact of interface with the nasal bridge or the contact of headgear with the cheeks. These are classified as device-related pressure necrosis and can be due to hypersensitivity or due to infection and generally responds to mask adjustments and skin protective techniques (**Fig. 1**).

The incidence of skin lesions is so high because of the lack of ideal interface (nontraumatic, nonallergenic, nondeformable with minimal leakage), lack of optimal fastening devices and techniques (easy to apply, breathable, reusable), and lack of consensus guidelines on what is the ideal technique to prevent PU.

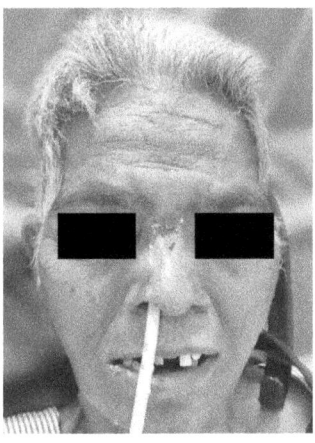

Fig. 1: Pressure ulcer at the nasal bridge due to NIV mask.

PATHOGENESIS

The tight contact of the mask on the skin causes local tissue ischemia and accumulation of metabolic substances. This gives rise to vasodilation at the local site and edema due to increase in vascular volume. This edema tightens the skin making it more fragile and prone to break and causing ulceration. The ulceration can appear even after a short duration of 2 hours of application of NIV mask.[2]

Secondly, the application of mask and harness causes sweating and accumulation of moisture at the contact surface. This leads to maceration of the skin. This increases the chances of friction and making the skin more susceptible for ulceration.[3]

RISK FACTORS

The most common risk factors for skin ulceration due to NIV are:
- Hemodynamic instability leading to poor perfusion and intense vasoconstriction due to vasopressors
- Poor nutritional status leading to hypoproteinemia and increased edema formation
- Increased duration of NIV therapy (more than 20 hours a day for 3 days)
- Patient's baseline condition like old age, hypothyroid status, anemia, low vitamin D levels, and on steroid therapy.[4]

STAGES OF PRESSURE ULCERS (FIG. 2)

- *Stage I*: Nonblanchable erythema that is painful and has temperature difference as compared to adjacent tissue
- *Stage II*: It is partial dermal loss like an intact blister
- *Stage III*: The subdermal contents are visible due to dermal loss
- *Stage IV*: Full-thickness tissue loss with visible underlying bone, muscle, or tendon.

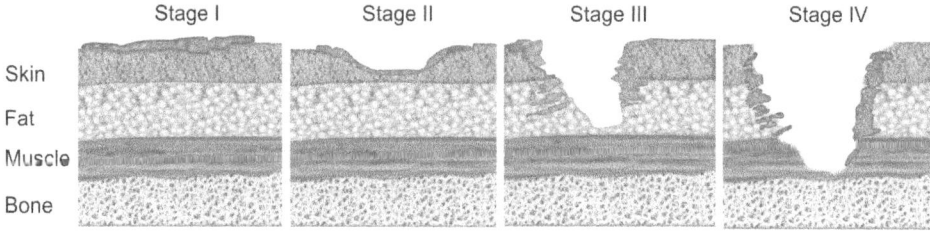

Fig. 2: Stages of pressure ulcers.

MEASURES TO PREVENT PRESSURE SORES

General Measures

Any patient who is on NIV is a potential candidate to develop pressure sores. Most of these PUs are developed because of lack of knowledge about application of mask and headgear and also by lack of understanding on how often the mask should be removed and when to inspect the skin. Twice daily inspection of the site in contact with the device should be done as per the European Pressure Ulcer Advisory Panel (EPUAP),[5] but as PUs develop more rapidly, the inspection period should be increased to 4–6 hours interval.[6,7] Moisture should be wiped gently with an absorbable material like cotton and the proper fitting of the mask and the harness should be ascertained.

Specific Measures

Proper Interface Material

The correct interface plays a major role in NIV success and in reduction of pressure sore development. The most common interface used in patients with acute respiratory failure is oronasal mask. The interface should be flexible and soft, so that it does not put pressure on skin. The structure of the interface should be rigid, so that it maintains its shape.[8] The dome of the mask should be transparent, so that the accumulation of oral secretions is visible and chances of skin maceration are decreased. The material of the interface should be soft and should ideally be made of hydrogel or even double spring air-filled cushions.

Proper Interface Fit

The most important strategy to decrease the incidence of pressure ulcer is to decrease the pressure required to inflate the mask. The ideal pressure of the mask should be at least 2–3 cm H_2O more than the inspiratory pressure to prevent leaks but such a measurement is difficult to ascertain, so the physician should take into account the patient's feedback about the fit of the mask. According to the British Thoracic Society (BTS) guidelines, the mask should be firm but not tight.[9] The mask fit should be such that there should be two fingers distance at the head strap, thus avoiding overtightening of head strap (**Fig. 3**).[10]

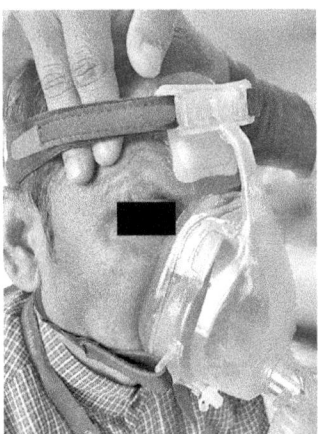

Fig. 3: The "Two finger rule" where two fingers can be inserted at the head strap to avoid over tightness.

Cushioning of Pressure Areas

In the study by Visscher et al.,[2] it was found that the PUs are more common in areas overlying the bone like nasal bridge, forehead, or the cheeks. According to the EPUAP guidelines,[5] the pressure areas should be cushioned with protective skin coverings like hydrocolloids, foam pads, transparent film, or silicone to prevent skin breakdown (**Fig. 4**).

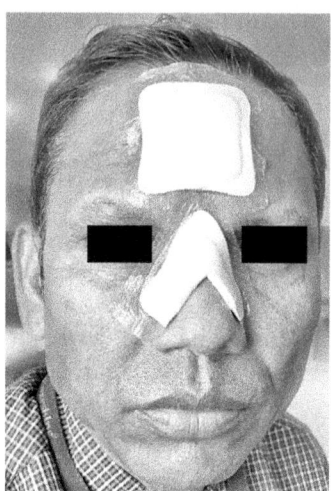

Fig. 4: The ideal technique to cushion the skin to prevent pressure ulcers due to NIV mask.

All high-risk patients should apply such protective coverings from the start of the therapy as the ulcer healing will be problematic in such patients. A recent study by Bishopp et al.[11] have shown the protective effect of hydrocolloid-based dressing on prevention of PUs due to NIV mask. Similar comparative studies of dressing versus no dressing have been done in past and have found that protective dressing decreases the incidence and severity of PUs.

Hyperoxygenated fatty acids (HOFAs) solution application on the skin in contact with the mask has shown to decrease the incidence of PU. Recently, Otero et al.[12] compared four strategies to prevent NIV-related facial ulcers. They compared direct mask application, mask with thin adhesive dressing, mask with thick adhesive dressing, and mask with HOFA and concluded that the incidence of facial ulcers was lowest with HOFA and should be included in daily protocol for NIV mask application. The proposed mechanism is that HOFA increases the inflammatory mediators at the local skin level resulting in better local tissue oxygenation, hence counteracting the impact of pressure and friction forces caused by mask application.[13]

Mask Rotation

This concept involves changing the type of mask used for NIV application, so that the pressure is distributed equally across the face. If the patient cannot tolerate even brief periods of discontinuation of NIV, the rotation of oronasal mask with total face mask (TFM) will relieve pressures on nasal bridge and thus help in decreasing the incidence of pressure sores.[7,14] Both the studies recommended using TFM in patients with expected prolonged NIV, as this approach decreases the ischemia-reperfusion injury and reestablishes blood flow to the pressure areas.

Change of Interface

Helmet is the only available device that can prevent the development of pressure sores on face, but the straps have to be applied properly to avoid sores in armpits. Helmet application should be done only in centers trained to handle it, as the incidence of claustrophobia and aspiration after vomiting is high in such patients.

Control of Humidity

Till date, as per the BTS,[9] there is no need for active humidification during NIV. The regular masks most commonly used decrease the absorption of moisture and hence cause accumulation of sweat under the interface. This along with humidification used during NIV causes the skin to macerate and becomes more fragile and prone for pressure sores.

NUTRITION

■ INTRODUCTION

Feeding the patients on NIV has always been an issue with no clear-cut guidelines. The fact that malnourished patients have high mortality has to be counterbalanced with the fact that the physicians are worried about aspiration on NIV.

■ REASONS FOR UNDERFEEDING PATIENTS ON NONINVASIVE VENTILATION

- Patients on NIV can deteriorate and require invasive mechanical ventilation any time during their initial few days and so keeping them nil-per-oral seems to be a safer strategy
- Placing a nasogastric (NG) tube will increase the leak through the mask and contribute to NIV failure
- Gastric insufflation during NIV application increases the diaphragmatic dysfunction and increases the risk of vomiting and aspiration
- Disconnection of NIV for oral feeding may result in failure of NIV therapy, as patients may have deterioration of their baseline condition.

In a recent French multicenter observation study,[15] more than 60% patients were starved for first 48 hours and less than 2.6% patients were fed enterally. In this study, enterally fed patients had higher mortality.

The use of NIV for prevention of reintubation after extubation is being used extensively in certain subset of patients. Macht et al.[16] showed that patients have some degree of swallowing dysfunction postextubation and this is a risk factor for aspiration, nosocomial infections, and increased mortality.

Approach to Feeding

- If the patients are not malnourished at the time of admission, then keeping them underfed or nil-per-oral is a feasible strategy for a maximum of 48 hours
- If the patient's nutritional status is poor at the time of admission, then attempts should be made to feed the patient. The route of feeding should be selected very carefully as certain studies have shown increased mortality after enteral route of feeding.
- The risk of gastric insufflation can be decreased by improving the patient ventilator synchrony and by titrating the pressures, so that the leak is reduced.
- Parenteral nutrition should not be started as the first choice of nutritional support, as it has been shown to increase mortality in intubated patients.
- Specialized NIV mask with NG tube hole can be used in a selected population, but they are costly and not easily available.

GASTRIC INSUFFLATION

■ INTRODUCTION

The incidence is varied and ranges from 5 to 40%[17] and is multifactorial in nature. The volume generated from a breath of NIV is distributed between lungs and stomach and is dependent on the compliance of the respiratory system and the tone of lower esophageal sphincter. It also depends on the position of the patient, the fitting of the mask, inspiratory flow rate, and the pressure settings.

Large tidal volumes, high inspiratory pressures, low inspiratory time, too tightly fit mask, and increased airway resistance increase the incidence of gastric insufflation. This causes gastric distension and pushing the diaphragm upward and compressing the lungs, demanding higher airway inspiratory pressures.[18] This all increases the incidence of aspiration and nosocomial pneumonia.

Smaller tidal volumes (around 500 mL) are safer as long as oxygenation is maintained. Patient should be nursed in sitting posture for at least 1 hour after the meal to decrease the effects of gastric insufflation. Airway pressures should ideally be maintained at 20–25 cm H_2O to avoid gastric distension.

PHYSIOTHERAPY

■ INTRODUCTION

The tracheobronchial mucosa is exposed to cool and dry air constantly during NIV therapy and this causes the secretions to desiccate. This leads to mucus plugging and atelectasis. This may be the reason for NIV failure and predisposing the patient to intubation and other serious airway obstruction complications.[19]

The physiotherapy technique should be based on assessment of patient's clinical condition, dependency on NIV, age and muscle strength, and consciousness status of the patient.

■ TECHNIQUES

Percussion and vibration strategies are done to mobilize the secretions from the peripheral to more central airways and then these secretions are taken out with the help of spontaneous coughing or manually-assisted coughing or huff. These therapies help in increasing the expiratory flow and should be carried out in patients with preserved cough reflex and muscle strength to throw out sputum.

Postural drainage involves positioning the patient in a head low posture, so that gravity helps in draining the periphery lobes of the lungs to the more central airways. This is better tolerated in patients on ventilator as patients may experience worsening of hypoxemia if they are spontaneously breathing as in NIV.

Mechanical-assisted cough can be either done by thoracic or abdominal compressions timed with expiration or by cough assist devices that are used in patients who have poor cough reflexes. As the chest expands during inspiration, the device is kept at the mouth just like a mouthpiece and the patient is asked to cough.[20] The machine has a suction-like phenomenon which promotes suctioning of the secretions when the patient attempts coughing. The ideal pressure applied should be +40 cm H_2O to –60 cm H_2O.

All NIV patients should be managed with a humidification system, as it dilutes the tenacious secretions and decreases the incidence of atelectasis and NIV failure although the BTS guidelines do not support it.[9] These diluted secretions can then be easily taken out by oral suction.

The oral or nasal suctioning is the last resort when the abovementioned measures fail. Suctioning should be done very carefully in patients with coagulopathy, nasal bone deviation or deformities, or in patients with recent upper airway surgeries.

AGITATED PATIENTS

INTRODUCTION

Patients with respiratory failure are generally agitated and restless due to air hunger, anxiety, psychosis caused by medications like steroids, and the claustrophobia of the mask. Sedation practices have no standard recommendations for such a situation and have been practiced as per the treating physician's comfort level. As per the web-based survey done by Devlin et al.,[21] it was found that less than 25% physicians use sedation or analgesia in NIV patients and the practice is very varied with no standardized protocol. Sedation helps to decrease the restlessness of the patient and may help in increasing NIV patient synchrony, but it may also lead to decrease in the respiratory drive and predisposing the patient toward mechanical ventilation.

Psychological counseling of the patients and confidence building should be the first step in making the patient comfortable with the device and also to allow better synchrony of the therapy. If this fails, then drugs like low-dose dexmedetomidine infusion or opioid infusion like fentanyl can help the patients in tolerating the NIV mask, but a close vigilance should be kept about the respiratory pattern of the patients when these infusions are given.

KEY POINTS

- The development of pressure ulcer at the site of mask application may give rise to pain and lead to NIV failure; hence, all precautions should be taken to prevent them.
- Malnourishment leads to increased mortality in critically ill patients and hence patients on NIV should be fed with the help of Ryle's tube, but can be kept starved for first 48 hours of admission if the baseline nutritional status is good.
- Careful attention should be paid to vomiting, gastric insufflation, and aspiration.
- Tracheobronchial toileting with the help of active and passive physiotherapy plays a very important role in preventing mucus plugging and decreases the intubation rate.
- Sedation should be titrated as per the patient's need and drugs like dexmedetomidine or fentanyl infusions should be preferred.

REFERENCES

1. Carron M, Freo U, BaHammam AS, Dellweg D, Guarracino F, Cosentini R, et al. Complications of noninvasive ventilation techniques: A comprehensive qualitative review of randomized trials. Br J Anaesth. 2013;110:896-914.
2. Visscher MO, White CC, Jones JM, Cahill T, Jones DC, Pan BS. Face masks for noninvasive ventilation: Fit, excess skin hydration, and pressure ulcers. Respir Care. 2015;60:1536-47.
3. Black J, Alves P, Brindle CT, Dealey C, Santamaria N, Call E, et al. Use of wound dressings to enhance prevention of pressure ulcers caused by medical devices. Int Wound J. 2015;12:322-7.

4. Munckton K, Ho K, Dobb G, Das-Gupta M, Webb S. The pressure effects of facemasks during noninvasive ventilation: A volunteer study. Anaesthesia. 2007;62:1126-31.
5. National Pressure Ulcer Advisory Panel, European Pressure Ulcer Advisory Panel, Pan Pacific Pressure Injury Alliance. (2014). Prevention and Treatment of Pressure Ulcers: Quick Reference Guide. [online] Available from https://www.epuap.org/wp-content/uploads/2016/10/quick-reference-guide-digital-npuap-epuap-pppia-jan2016.pdf. [Last accessed January, 2020].
6. Ahmad Z, Venus M, Kisku W, Rayatt SS. A case series of skin necrosis following use of non invasive ventilation pressure masks. Int Wound J. 2013;10:87-90.
7. Lemyze M, Mallat J, Nigeon O, Barrailler S, Pepy F, Gasan G, et al. Rescue therapy by switching to total face mask after failure of face mask-delivered noninvasive ventilation in do-not-intubate patients in acute respiratory failure. Crit Care Med. 2013;41:481-8.
8. Nava S, Navalesi P, Gregoretti C. Interfaces and humidification for noninvasive mechanical ventilation. Respir Care. 2009;54:71-84.
9. Davidson C, Banham S, Elliott M, Kennedy D, Gelder C, Glossop A, et al. British Thoracic Society/Intensive Care Society Guideline for the ventilatory management of acute hypercapnic respiratory failure in adults. BMJ Open Respir Res. 2016;3:e000133.
10. Schettino GP, Tucci MR, Sousa R, Valente Barbas CS, Passos Amato MB, et al. Mask mechanics and leak dynamics during noninvasive pressure support ventilation: a bench study. Intensive Care Med. 2001;27:1887-91.
11. Bishopp A, Oakes A, Antoine-Pitterson P, Chakraborty B, Comer D, Mukherjee R. The Preventative Effect of Hydrocolloid Dressings on Nasal Bridge Pressure Ulceration in Acute NonInvasive Ventilation. Ulster Med J. 2019;88:17-20.
12. Otero DP, Domínguez DV, Fernández LH, Magariño AS, González VJ, Klepzing JV, et al. Preventing facial pressure ulcers in patients under noninvasive mechanical ventilation: a randomised control trial. J Wound Care. 2017;26:128-36.
13. Lázaro-Martinez JL, Sánchez-Rios JP, Garcia-Morales E, Cecilia-Matilla A, Segovia-Gómez T. Increased transcutaneous oxygen tension in the skin dorsum over the foot in patients with diabetic foot disease in response to the topical use of an emulsion of hyperoxygenated Fatty acids. Int J Low Extrem Wounds. 2009;8:187-93.
14. Yamaguti WP, Moderno EV, Yamashita SY, Gomes TG, Maida ALV, Kondo CS, et al. Treatment-related risk factors for development of skin breakdown in subjects with acute respiratory failure undergoing noninvasive ventilation or CPAP. Respir Care. 2014;59:1530-6.
15. Terzi N, Darmon M, Reignier J, Ruckly S, Garrouste-Orgeas M, Lautrette A, et al. Initial nutritional management during noninvasive ventilation and outcomes: a retrospective cohort study. Crit Care. 2017;21:293.
16. Macht M, Wimbish T, Clark BJ, Benson AB, Burnham EL, Williams A, et al. Postextubation dysphagia is persistent and associated with poor outcomes in survivors of critical illness. Crit Care. 2011;15:R231.
17. Masip J, Betbesé AJ, Páez J, Vecilla F, Cañizares R, Padró J, et al. Noninvasive pressure support ventilation versus conventional oxygen therapy in acute cardiogenic pulmonary oedema: a randomised trial. Lancet. 2000;356:2126-32.
18. Luria O, Reshef L, Barnea O. Analysis of noninvasive ventilation effects on gastric inflation using a non-linear mathematical model. Resuscitation. 2006;71:358-64.
19. Wood KE, Flaten AL, Backes WJ. Inspissated secretions: a life-threatening complication of prolonged noninvasive ventilation. Respir Care. 2000;45:491-3.
20. Gosselink R, Bott J, Johnson M, Dean E, Nava S, Norrenberg M, et al. Physiotherapy for adult patients with critical illness: recommendations of the European Respiratory Society and European Society of Intensive Care Medicine Task Force on Physiotherapy for Critically Ill Patients. Intensive Care Med. 2008;34:1188-99.
21. Devlin JW, Nava S, Fong JJ, Hill NS. Survey of sedation practices during noninvasive positive-pressure ventilation to treat acute respiratory failure. Crit Care Med. 2007;35:2298-302.

Section 6

Home Ventilation

31. Home Ventilation: Essentials of Practice
32. Discharge Criteria of Noninvasive Ventilation Dependent Patients
33. Monitoring Accuracy of Home Ventilators and Telemonitoring of Patient on Home Bilevel Positive Airway Pressure
34. Home Ventilation in Long-term Noninvasive Ventilation Users

Chapter 31

Home Ventilation: Essentials of Practice

Sandesh Kumar, Yash Javeri, Rohit yadav

■ INTRODUCTION

The use of noninvasive ventilation (NIV) at home was introduced in the 1980s for the long-term management of sleep apnea. NIV has recently been used for the management of chronic respiratory failure. In last 2 decades, there is a revolution in the management of acute and chronic respiratory failure with NIV. NIV refers to a technique of increasing alveolar ventilation without the need for an invasive artificial airway. NIV is beneficial for managing full range of acute and chronic respiratory conditions. The best evidence comes for use in acute and acute-on-chronic respiratory failure. Home ventilation or long-term noninvasive ventilation (LT-NIV) refers to providing ventilator support using noninvasive interfaces for patients with chronic respiratory failure at the comfort of home or in long-term care centers.

There is ample evidence to suggest that NIV improves the quality of life and stabilizes the condition of many patients with chronic ventilatory failure. Home ventilation has now been widely accepted as a therapeutic option for patients with chronic respiratory failure due to restrictive lung diseases and patients with neuromuscular weakness. The application of NIV for acute exacerbation of chronic obstructive pulmonary disease (COPD) patients has strong evidence. However, the recommendations are equivocal regarding the use of NIV at home for patients with advanced chronic obstructive airway disease. Positive pressure ventilation with noninvasive interfaces is the most often prescribed mode for home ventilation.

■ EQUIPMENT

Standard equipment includes:
- *Portable ventilator with battery backup and modes as per requirement*: Continuous positive airway pressure (CPAP), pressure support (PS), pressure control (PC), and newer one, volume-targeted modes
- Ventilator tubing's
- *Patient ventilator interface*: Nasal, oronasal, or full face mask (**Fig. 1**)
- Straps to hold the interface.

Oxygen source/oxygen concentrator and monitoring equipment are also desirable. Without appropriate humidification, home ventilation leads to drying of nasal mucosa leading to increase in the resistance to flow of air causing patients discomfort. In the near future, telemonitoring will reinforce and improve home-NIV.

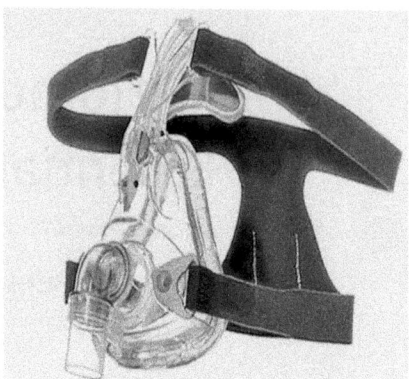

Fig. 1: Face mask.

INDICATIONS

Home ventilation is best suited for patients suffering from chronic respiratory failure due to these conditions:
- *Chronic obstructive pulmonary disease*: As mentioned earlier, the indication is not strongly supported by guidelines but based on current clinical practices. Many studies support use of home-NIV in COPD patients who are difficult to wean from mechanical ventilation or with persistent hypercapnia after acute exacerbation based on improved health-related quality of life (HRQL), numbers of readmissions, sleep quality, compliance, and gas exchange
- Neuromuscular and chest wall disease
- Obstructive sleep apnea (OSA).

Chronic Obstructive Pulmonary Disease

Home-NIV is thought to benefit patients with COPD and type II respiratory failure; these are the subgroup of patients who have an imbalance between respiratory muscle load and capacity.[1] Early physiological studies have explained the mechanism of action of home-NIV in stable COPD patients with type II respiratory failure.[2] However, randomized clinical trials failed to demonstrate significant benefit. The failure to translate sound physiological principles in randomized clinical trials into good outcomes can be attributed to wrong target population and low-intensity ventilator strategy.

Patients with severe COPD will have ventilation-perfusion mismatch due to injury to lung parenchyma. Initially, patients compensate by hyperventilation. However, hypercapnia will develop eventually owing to respiratory muscle weakness. Respiratory muscle dysfunction occurs due to several factors:[3]
- Protein loss due to catabolic activation and anabolic suppression
- Injury, damage, and inadequate repair of respiratory muscle
- Flattened diaphragm due to hyperinflation puts mechanical disadvantage on diaphragm
- Compromised nutrition leading to cachexia.

Noninvasive ventilation at night gives rest to respiratory muscles leading to improved respiratory function during daytime. Nocturnal NIV also leads to better gas exchange in daytime and improves respiratory muscle function which is sustained for longer duration sometimes over several years.[4]

The German guidelines recommend home-NIV therapy for COPD patients after prolonged weaning from mechanical ventilation if the patient's symptoms of hypoventilation and hypercapnia can only be controlled with continuous use of NIV following weaning from invasive mechanical ventilation.[5]

Most favorable outcome of home-NIV therapy in COPD patients observed when patient selection, timing of starting home-NIV, and ventilation strategy are optimized.

Patients with acute exacerbation of COPD with need of mechanical ventilation showed favorable outcome when home-NIV started after 2 weeks and high-intensity (PS > 20 cm) ventilation.[5]

Patients with end-stage COPD can present with hypoxemic and hypercapnic respiratory failure. Long-term oxygen therapy (LTOT) is a well-established therapy for hypoxemic respiratory failure.

Neuromuscular and Chest Wall Disease

Neuromuscular conditions that damage the respiratory muscles or their supplying nerves result in reduced lung volumes and may cause chronic respiratory failure.

Chest wall disorders like kyphoscoliosis, disease of the muscles, peripheral nerves, neuromuscular junction, and spinal cord lesions predispose patients to respiratory dysfunction due to mechanical failure. The underlying condition may itself be stable like spinal cord injury, or progressive like muscular dystrophies. Patients with these neuromuscular and chest wall diseases who have respiratory compromise can be treated by noninvasive positive pressure ventilation.

Home-NIV is associated with better survival, better gas exchange in daytime, improved quality of sleep, and improvement in other quality of life parameters. It is proposed that nocturnal NIV will reset chemoreceptor sensitivity leading to correction of hypercapnia.[6]

Obstructive Sleep Apnea

Obstructive sleep apnea is a pathological condition characterized by episodes of apnea and hypopnea due to obstruction of upper airway during sleep. OSA is the largest group of patients on domiciliary NIV. NIV prevents occlusion and apneic spells because it can be set to a constant pressure to keep the airway patent when the patient sleeps. Polysomnography studies are required to initiate and titrate therapy. Randomized controlled trials have consistently shown benefits with weight loss and home ventilation.

■ CONTRAINDICATIONS

Contraindications to home-NIV are few and relative. Increased secretions and poor sensorium are serious contraindications. Intolerance to interface can often be resolved with other options. Pressure-relieving dressings, particularly on the bridge of the nose, to avoid device-related pressure ulcers. Regular oral care and adequate hydration are important. Nasal decongestants can be effective for relieving nasal drying.

SELECTION OF PATIENT

- *Chronic obstructive pulmonary disease:*[6]
  - Not recommended for patients with stable COPD
  - Patients with partial pressure of carbon dioxide (pCO_2) more than 55 mm Hg and having repeated episodes of acute exacerbations
  - Difficult to wean from mechanical ventilation.
- *Chest wall and neuromuscular diseases:*[7]
  - Symptomatic patients with orthopnea
  - Daytime hypercapnia
  - Forced vital capacity less than 50% of predicted
  - Sniff nasal pressure (SNP)* less than 40 cm of H_2O.

*Sniff nasal pressure, a noninvasive measure of respiratory muscle strength.

INTERFACE

Quality of ventilation in NIV relies on good seal provided by an appropriate interface. An ideal interface will have a balance between minimizing leaks with good seal, addressing the patient discomfort by improving comfort, and also easy handling of mask by caregivers.

There are currently six different types of interfaces:
1. Oral mask
2. Nasal
3. Oronasal mask
4. Full face mask
5. Helmet
6. Nasal pillow.

With initial ventilatory strategies of low-pressure ventilation, nasal mask gained popularity, but over period of time, with high-intensity ventilation, strategies are proved beneficial in terms of better compliance, sleep quality, gas exchange, and readmission rates; oronasal or full face mask is interface of choice. In the long-term setting, nasal masks are rated to be more comfortable than other mask types.

VENTILATOR

Historically, both positive and negative pressure ventilators are used in home ventilation. Positive pressure ventilators are nowadays routinely used.

Selection of Ventilator Mode

Depending on the clinical needs of the patient, mode could be either CPAP or bilevel positive airway pressure. Pressure setting should be decided in a sleep laboratory after a polysomnography test.

Conventionally, CPAP, PS, and PC are modes of choice depending on patient requirement. Recently, hybrid modes with target-volume settings added to a pressure preset mode have become more popular over the last few years, studied in COPD patients. All of these studies investigated patients with chronic hypercapnic COPD who were subjected to higher levels of inspiratory positive airway pressure (IPAP), with respect to sleep quality measured by polysomnography, HRQL, compliance, or gas exchange monitoring and showed good outcomes. However, one advantage of target-volume NIV was that fewer titration days (secondary endpoint) were needed with this treatment approach. In light of this, target-volume NIV might serve as a means for faster establishment of home-NIV in chronic hypercapnic COPD patients, although this remains speculative and needs to be investigated further.

ASSESSMENT OF PATIENT SUITABILITY OF DOMICILIARY USE OF NONINVASIVE VENTILATION[8]

Full assessment at a specialist center is necessary to determine the exact form of respiratory support required. The patients should be initiated in the healthcare facility before discharge to home.

Comfort partially depends on the fit of the face or nose mask and the domiciliary team should do frequent reassessment.

PATIENT EDUCATION AND MONITORING

Monitoring of home-NIV is needed to assess the effectiveness of ventilation and compliance, negate adverse effects, reinforce patient knowledge, and provide maintenance of the equipment **(Figs. 2A to G)**. Clinical monitoring is must and titration of the ventilator settings is based on patient condition. Home care providers maintain ventilator and interface and educate patients for correct use. Patient's education should be initiated by respiratory clinician/therapist and supervised by domiciliary team.

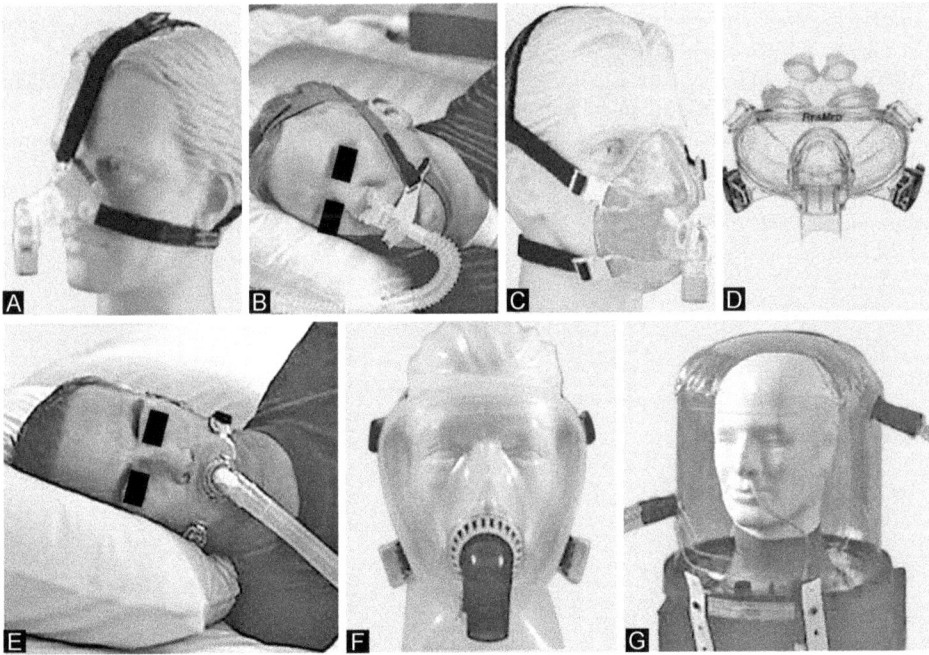

Figs. 2A to G: Various interfaces for noninvasive ventilation. (A) Nasal mask, (B) Nasal pillows, (C) Oronasal mask, (D) Hybrid mask, (E) Oral mask, (F) Total face mask, (G) Helmet.[9]

CONCLUSION

- Home ventilation is useful for a select subgroup of patients with COPD who have daytime hypercapnia and desaturation episodes during sleep.
- Home ventilation is not useful for stable COPD patients.
- Home ventilation with NIV support can be considered as a preferred option in patients with Neuromuscular weakness provided they have capacity to clear secretions.
- Home ventilation with CPAP using various interfaces has become the standard of care for patients with obstructive sleep apnea.

REFERENCES

1. Windisch W, Storre JH, Köhnlein T. Nocturnal non-invasive positive pressure ventilation for COPD. Expert Rev Respir Med. 2015;9(3):295-308.
2. Elliott MW, Mulvey DA, Moxham J, Green M, Branthwaite MA. Domiciliary nocturnal nasal intermittent positive pressure ventilation in COPD: mechanisms underlying changes in arterial blood gas tensions. Eur Respir J. 1991;4(9):1044-52.
3. Rochester DF, Braun NM, Arora NS. Respiratory muscle strength in chronic obstructive pulmonary disease. Am Rev Respir Dis. 1979;119(2 Pt 2):151-4.
4. Braun NM, Marino WD. Effect of daily intermittent rest of respiratory muscles in patients with severe chronic airflow limitation (CAL). Chest. 1984;85(6 Suppl):59S-60.
5. Storre JH, Callegari J, Magnet FS, Schwarz SB, Duiverman ML, Wijkstra PJ, et al. Home noninvasive ventilatory support for patients with chronic obstructive pulmonary disease: patient selection and perspectives. Int J Chron Obstruct Pulmon Dis. 2018;13:753-60.
6. Annane D, Quera-Salva MA, Lofaso F, Vercken JB, Lesieur O, Fromageot C, et al. Mechanisms underlying effects of nocturnal ventilation on daytime blood gases in neuromuscular diseases. Eur Respir J. 1999;13(1):157-62.
7. McKim DA, Road J, Avendano M, Abdool S, Cote F, Duguid N, et al. Home mechanical ventilation: a Canadian Thoracic Society clinical practice guideline. Can Respir J. 2011;18(4):197-215.
8. Crimi C, Noto A, Princi P, Cuvelier A, Masa JF, Simonds A, et al. Domiciliary non-invasive ventilation in COPD: An international survey of indications and practices. COPD. 2016;13(4):483-90.
9. Nava S, Navalesi P, Gregoretti C. Interfaces and humidification for noninvasive mechanical ventilation. Respir Care. 2009;54(1):71-84.

Chapter 32

Discharge Criteria of Noninvasive Ventilation Dependent Patients

Bharat Jagiasi, Archana Suraj Thakur, Tushar Sontakke

INTRODUCTION

The use of domiciliary noninvasive ventilation (NIV) has increased all over the world due to increased prevalence of various respiratory diseases causing chronic respiratory failure as well as to alleviate respiratory distress in patients on palliative care.

Chronic obstructive pulmonary disease (COPD), obstructive sleep apnea (OSA), various neuromuscular conditions such as Duchenne muscular dystrophy (DMD), amyotrophic lateral sclerosis (ALS), spinal cord injuries, etc. are the most common diseases which require NIV support on long-term basis.

As per Canadian prevalence study[1] and EUROVENT analysis,[2] prevalence of home ventilation per 1 lakh population was 12.9 and 6.6 respectively out of which 82–87% users were on NIV. There is lack of data regarding prevalence of home NIV in Indian population but according to the surveys, compliance is around 50%.[3]

The domiciliary NIV helps to reduce nocturnal hypoventilation, improves gas exchange, gives rest to respiratory muscles, and relieves associated symptoms.

Domiciliary NIV has shown to improve quality of life, relieving symptoms like dyspnea, etc. decrease in rate of recurrent hospitalizations as well as increasing life expectancy.[4]

Therefore, it is crucial for an intensivist to identify the patients who will benefit from long-term domiciliary NIV. For the success of home NIV, along with patient's primary disease other important factors to be considered are motivation of the patient and family, socioeconomic status, availability of resources, etc.

There is paucity of data about use of home NIV as well as selection of the patients needing the same. In this chapter, we have tried to simplify the criteria for discharging patients on NIV from ICU to home care so as to optimize the management and to achieve standardization of care.

GENERAL CRITERIA

Medically stable without constant or frequent monitoring, tests or treatment changes.
- Patient should be hemodynamically stable
- Glasgow coma scale (GCS) > 13
- Maintaining acceptable oxygen saturation on room air or minimal oxygen supplement
- Bulbar muscle weakness should be ruled out as it can increase chances of aspiration.

DEVICE CRITERIA

- Simple bi-level devices should be preferred in patients who need few hours of day time and overnight ventilation.[5]
- The use of volume targeted or hybrid devices should be reserved for patients who need longer hours (>18 hours/day) of ventilation or when bilevel devices are inadequate.[5]
- Full face mask should be the preferred initial interface.[6]
- There must be exhalation valve on the NIV circuit or exhalation port on the NIV mask so that exhaled air can be cleared adequately.[6]
- Titration of settings for long-term NIV should be done when patient is free from acute exacerbation and is chronically stable (pH > 7.35).[5]
- Adequate inspiratory positive airway pressure (IPAP) and expiratory positive airway pressure (EPAP) difference (minimum 4) should be maintained to mitigate hypoventilation.[5]
- Patients having difficulty in triggering will require flow triggered or volume cycled mandatory ventilation.[5]
- Initial settings should be done by the trained and experienced personnel in the ICU so that patient can be observed closely and troubleshooting can be done as and when needed.
- It is advisable to monitor SpO_2 with pulse oximeter whenever patient is shifted to wards or discharged home.
- Noninvasive ventilation machine should have alarm settings for "mask off, low pressure or power failure" and relatives/caretakers should be well versed with the same.[5]
- Inspiratory positive airway pressure should be increased to target the minute ventilation and as per patient's tolerance.
- Expiratory positive airway pressure should be increased so that each patient effort is triggered and work of breathing is reduced to minimal.
- Controlled mode of ventilation should be preferred in patients with neuromuscular diseases (NMD) in view of ineffective triggering.

DISEASE SPECIFIC CRITERIA

Chronic Obstructive Pulmonary Disease

- Chronic daytime hypercapnia with $PaCO_2$ > 50 mm Hg[7,8]
- Nocturnal hypercapnia with $PaCO_2$ > 55 mm Hg[7,8]
- Stable daytime hypercapnia (46–50 mm Hg) with rise in $PaCO_2$ > 10 mm Hg during sleep.[7]
- Patients who needed invasive ventilation for acute exacerbation and had difficult weaning.[5,9]
- Signs of nocturnal hypoventilation/hypercapnia while being on long-term oxygen therapy (LTOT)[5,9]
- Repeated hospitalizations at least more than twice in a year for frequent exacerbation.[7]
- Presence of symptoms of chronic respiratory failure like drowsiness, fatigability, dyspnea, morning headache, and decrease in quality of life.[8]

Neuromuscular Diseases

Special points to be considered:
- Inability to close the mouth secondary to oropharyngeal muscle weakness
- Hypersalivation

Chapter 32: Discharge Criteria of Noninvasive Ventilation Dependent Patients

- Ineffective cough
- Bulbar weakness leading to increase risk of aspiration

Following are the recommendations for discharging NMD patients on home NIV:
- Presence of symptoms of chronic respiratory failure like orthopnea, dyspnea, fatigability, daytime sleepiness, morning headache, cognitive dysfunction, etc.[5,7]
- In patients with NMD, NIV should be offered early; after documenting hypercapnia before acidosis sets in.
- Chronic daytime hypercapnia with $PaCO_2$ > 45 mm Hg[8]
- Nocturnal hypercapnia with $PaCO_2$ > 50 mm Hg[8]
- Daytime normocapnia with rise in $PaCO_2$ > 10 mm Hg during sleep[8]
- Forced vital capacity (FVC) < 50% of predicted[4]
- Sniff nasal inspiratory pressure (SNIP) < 40 cm H_2O. It is particularly helpful in patients having difficulty in closing mouth due to weakness of oropharyngeal muscles.[4]
- Maximum inspiratory pressure (MIP) < 40 cm H_2O[8]
- If vital capacity is <50%, patient should be evaluated with arterial blood gas (ABG) analysis and nocturnal oxymetry and should be discharged with home NIV if results show chronic hypoventilation[4]
- Oxygen should not be given without NIV support in NMD patients having ventilatory failure[10]
- Airway clearance ability should be assessed with peak cough flow. If peak cough flow (PCF) <270 L/min, then assisted coughing techniques, pharmacological measures and/mechanical cough assist devices should be used.[4,8]
- Patients with respiratory muscle weakness secondary to spinal cord injury should be discharged on home NIV if they have atelectasis, inability to clear secretions, lower-respiratory-tract infection (LRTI) or type I respiratory failure.[5]

Obstructive Sleep Apnea/Obesity Hypoventilation Syndrome
- Before discharge from ICU, patients with documented OSA/obesity hypoventilation syndrome (OHS) should be reassessed for clinical condition and home NIV settings.
- Thorough work-up for evaluation of clinically suspected OSA/OHS should be done after stabilization of the patient and accordingly should be discharged on overnight NIV [continuous positive airway pressure/bilevel positive airway pressure (CPAP/BiPAP).

SOCIAL CRITERIA

Since family plays crucial role in the overall care of the patient who is being discharged on home NIV, the counseling and education of the family members along with the patient is of prime importance. There is considerable physical, emotional, and financial stress to the patient as well as family. It is very important for the intensivist to assess, motivate, and counsel the family so that the patient can be managed optimally on domiciliary NIV. Help of the medical social worker/counselor should be taken for the same. There should be an easy access to technical person, respiratory therapist, and healthcare professionals if the need arises.

Intensivist should guide the family regarding equipment (other than NIV) needed at home as per patient's condition such as pulse oximeter, suction machine, cough assist device, oxygen, air bed and mechanical deep vein thrombosis (DVT) prophylaxis, etc.

Caretaker/family members should be educated to observe and report alarming signs such as fall in oxygen saturation, excessive drowsiness, labored pattern of breathing, change in character of secretions and fever, etc. They should also be guided well regarding patient's nutritional requirements and management for the same.

■ FOLLOW-UP CRITERIA

After discharging patient on home NIV, first follow-up should occur in 4–8 weeks with physician to assess improvement in symptoms, technical issues, NIV setting, compliance of the patient, and therapeutic success.[8]

■ NONINVASIVE VENTILATION IN PALLIATIVE CARE

Palliation is considered in patients having terminal illness like advanced malignancies, chronic end-stage diseases (COPD, neuromuscular disorders, chronic cardiac failure, advanced age with multiple comorbidities, etc.). NIV can be used as a "strictly palliative" as well as "palliative and probably curative" measure.[11]

The goal of palliative care is to make the patient as comfortable as possible and to alleviate distress and agony. Though the role of NIV in palliation is very popular, but certain controversies are there. Firstly, there may be issue with the intolerance of the patient to the NIV and secondly, regarding curative intent of NIV which may not be suitable as palliative measure.

Situations where NIV can be used as palliation:
- To relieve the respiratory distress associated with terminal illness
- To help maintaining consciousness, cognition so that terminally ill patients are able to communicate with their loved ones.
- To buy time in patients with impending respiratory failure till end-of-life care decision is made.
- To avoid intubation and invasive ventilation where patients/relatives have requested for *do not intubate* (DNI) in view of terminal illness with further futility of treatment.
- To help withdraw the endotracheal tube with the intent of palliation in patients who are already on invasive mechanical ventilation.

Help of pharmacological agents like opioids/benzodiazepines/analgesics can be taken along with NIV to decrease anxiety, pain, and distress (Doctrine of double effect).

Education of the patients/family is of utmost importance before discharge of the patient on home NIV as a means of palliative measure.

Noninvasive ventilation should not be used if it is not tolerated by the patient and causing distress by itself. In such situations, use of pharmacological agents alone is warranted for symptomatic relief.

■ KEY POINTS

- There is significant increase in the number as well as indications of domiciliary use of NIV.
- Common conditions in which patients are discharged from ICU with home NIV are COPD with chronic respiratory failure, obstructive sleep apnea, neuromuscular disorders (ALS, DMD) and patients who are difficult to wean due to critical illness neuromyopathy owing to prolonged ventilatory support.
- Domiciliary NIV has also evolved as a means to alleviate respiratory distress in patients on palliative care.

Chapter 32: Discharge Criteria of Noninvasive Ventilation Dependent Patients

- Device and interface selection, settings and home preparation should be done meticulously as per the need of the patient's clinical condition.
- Education and motivation of the patient and family is of paramount importance.
- While deciding the discharge of patient on home NIV, the intensivist should take into account evidences of chronic respiratory failure, ability to clear secretions, blood gas and PFT parameters, etc. as described above.
- Caution should be taken in patients with NMDs having bulbar involvement with poor cough reflex so as to avoid aspiration and help of cough assist device should be taken.

SUMMARY

General criteria	➢ Hemodynamic stability ➢ GCS > 13 ➢ Minimal oxygen requirement/on room air ➢ Rule out bulbar weakness.
Device criteria	➢ Volume targeted or hybrid devices should be reserved for patients who need longer hours (>18 hours/day) of ventilation ➢ Bilevel devices should be preferred in patients who need few hours of daytime and overnight ventilation. ➢ Full face mask should be the preferred initial interface. ➢ Adequate IPAP and EPAP difference (minimum 4) should be maintained. ➢ Flow trigger is preferred in case of difficult triggering. ➢ Home/ward monitoring of SpO_2 is advised. ➢ Adequate alarm settings should be ensured. ➢ Inspiratory positive airway pressure should be titrated to ensure minute ventilation. ➢ Expiratory positive airway pressure should be titrated to reduce work of breathing. ➢ Controlled mode of ventilation should be preferred in patients with NMD.
COPD	➢ Chronic hypercapnia; daytime $PaCO_2$ > 50 and nocturnal > 55 mm Hg ➢ Stable daytime hypercapnia (46–50 mm Hg) with rise in $PaCO_2$ > 10 mm Hg during sleep ➢ Signs of nocturnal hypoventilation/hypercapnia while being on LTOT ➢ Difficult weaning from invasive ventilation ➢ Repeated hospitalizations (>2/year) due to exacerbation ➢ Presence of symptoms of chronic respiratory failure
NMD	➢ Presence of symptoms of chronic respiratory failure ➢ Noninvasive ventilation (NIV) should be offered early; before acidosis sets in. ➢ Chronic hypercapnia; day time $PaCO_2$ > 45 mm Hg and nocturnal > 50 mm Hg ➢ Daytime normocapnia with rise in $PaCO_2$ > 10 mm Hg during sleep ➢ FVC < 50% of predicted ➢ SNIP < 40 cm H_2O ➢ MIP < 40 cm H_2O ➢ If vital capacity is <50% with documented chronic hypoventilation ➢ Oxygen should not be given without NIV support. ➢ Assisted coughing techniques, pharmacological measures and/mechanical cough assist devices should be used if PCF < 270 L/min.
Social criteria	➢ Counseling and education of the patient as well as family members ➢ Intensivist should guide the family regarding equipment needed at home.
NIV in palliative care	➢ To relieve the respiratory distress ➢ To avoid intubation and invasive ventilation

(COPD: chronic obstructive pulmonary disease; EPAP: expiratory positive airway pressure; FVC: forced vital capacity; GCS: Glasgow coma scale; IPAP: inspiratory positive airway pressure; LTOT: long-term oxygen therapy; MIP: maximum inspiratory pressure; NMD: neuromuscular diseases; PCF: peak cough flow; SNIP: sniff nasal inspiratory pressure)

REFERENCES

1. Rose L, McKim DA, et al; CANuVENT Group. Home mechanical ventilation in Canada: a national survey. Respir Care. 2015;60: 695-704.
2. Lloyd- Owen SJ, Donaldson GC, et al; Patterns of home mechanical ventilation in Europe: results from the Eurovent survey. Eur Respir J. 2005;25:1025-31.
3. Mir Shad Ali, Deepak Talwar; Compliance for domiciliary NIV in Indian patient's "issues and practices". European Respiratory Journal. 2014;44: P458.
4. Miller RG, Jackson CE, Kasarskis EJ, England JD, Forshew D, et al. (2009) Practice parameter update: the care of the patient with amyotrophic lateral sclerosis: drug, nutritional, and respiratory therapies (an evidence-based review): report of the Quality Standards Subcommittee of the American Academy of Neurology. Neurology. 73: 1218-26.
5. Respiratory Network Domiciliary Non-Invasive Ventilation Working Group. Domiciliary non-invasive ventilation in adult patients—a consensus statement. NSW Agency for Clinical Innovation; 2012. https://www.aci.health.nsw.gov.au/__data/assets/pdf_file/0008/159794/ACI-NIV-guidelines.pdf. Accessed on August 28 2017.
6. National Guideline C. BTS/ICS guideline for the ventilatory management of acute hypercapnic respiratory failure in adults. 2016.
7. Porte P. Clinical indications for noninvasive positive pressure ventilation in chronic respiratory failure due to restrictive lung disease, COPD, and nocturnal hypoventilation—A consensus conference report. Chest. 1999;116(2):521-34. PMID: 29382139.
8. Windisch W, Walterspacher S, Siemon K, et al. Guidelines for non-invasive and invasive mechanical ventilation for treatment of chronic respiratory failure. Pneumologie. 2010;64(10):640-52.
9. National Institute for H, Clinical E. National clinical guideline centre for acute and chronic conditions. Chronic obstructive pulmonary disease. Management of chronic obstructive pulmonary disease in adults in primary and secondary care. National institute for health and clinical excellence. 2010.
10. Hardinge M, Annandale J, Bourne S, et al. British thoracic society guidelines for home oxygen use in adults. Thorax. 2015;70:i1-i43. PMID: 608676290.
11. Perrin C, Jullien V, Duval Y, Defrance C. Noninvasive ventilation in palliative care and near the end of life. Rev Mal Respir. 2009; 26: e1-9.

Chapter 33

Monitoring Accuracy of Home Ventilators and Telemonitoring of Patient on Home Bilevel Positive Airway Pressure

Ganshyam Jagathkar, Divija Sannapareddy, Rahul Agrawal

■ INTRODUCTION

Evolution of medicine has thrown light on human health and disease for centuries. As a part of this evolution treatment of diseases reaches new heights every day to such an extent that what was once a treatment given in few medical centers has reached globally to more number of the centers and even more so to the homes of the diseased. Ventilatory support—an intervention of paramount importance is one such modality, which has reached homes in the form of various machinery. What once was a life-sustaining modality used in intensive care units alone with heavy machinery has now become more refined with home ventilation modalities. Thus, it necessitates one to understand how to and what to monitor on an interval basis and remote surveillance of such devices to tweak components for the best of medical care provision avoiding pitfalls.

■ INDICATIONS TO USE HOME NONINVASIVE VENTILATION

One of the earliest surveys dates to 1992 but only in 2005 did we get clearer picture of prevalence of use and common indications of home mechanical ventilation (HMV) through EUROVENT analysis.[1] This study categorized the indications to three categories: (1) Lung: chronic obstructive pulmonary disease (COPD), cystic fibrosis, bronchiectasis, pulmonary fibrosis, bronchopulmonary dysplasia; (2) Thoracic cage abnormalities: early-onset kyphoscoliosis, tuberculosis sequelae such as thoracoplasty, obesity hypoventilation syndrome/obstructive sleep apnea (OHS/OSA) and lung resection sequelae; (3) Neuromuscular diseases: muscular dystrophy, motor neurone disease including amyotrophic lateral sclerosis (ALS), central hypoventilation, spinal cord damage, and phrenic nerve paralysis. Monitoring the parameters set and utilization by the patient on an individualistic basis can only achieve customization to patient's condition.

■ WHAT TO MONITOR?

Home ventilator could be invasive versus noninvasive depending on the condition. Current article highlights monitoring of noninvasive ventilation (NIV) home ventilation. Accuracy of monitoring becomes important as many factors weigh in when a home device is being used for the simple fact that faults cannot be monitored by professionals on site and rely retrospectively or even if in real time on what is conveyed by the monitor. Thus an inaccurately monitored parameter can cause more harm as therapy modulations are based on them.

Monitoring involves two components: (a) machine and (b) patient.

Machine

Inspiratory Component[3]

Depending on the software and settings tidal volume is adjusted to an average of 8 mL/kg body weight. Variation in this usually indicates leaks or periodic breathing. Periodic breathing can be monitored in conjunction with respiratory rate. Increasing leaks underestimate tidal volume as seen in bench studies.[2] This can be overcome by mathematical algorithms, which estimate leaks at distal and proximal ends to improve accuracy.

The device has built in technology to measure and store breath pressures, volumes, flow, respiratory rate, number of apnea episodes and most important of all leaks and compensations. One important factor about HMV devices is the simplicity and size of the machine. This simplification includes using single limb circuits to avoid tube complications as tube disconnection was reported as one of most common events. However with single limb circuit it is mandatory to have an expiratory system (intentional leak port or active valve). Irrespective of number of limbs it is necessary for device to calculate total volume of gas exiting the ventilator to enter patient, intentional leak through port present ($V\text{-}IL$), and unintentional leaks related to suboptimal interface ($V\text{-}NIL$) and also compressible volume remaining in the tubing(s)-CV

$$\text{Total gas flow} = VT + V(IL) + V(NIL) = CV$$

Expiratory Component

That being the inspiratory system, expiratory system encompasses the leak port, which in fact has more resistance and thus more pressure than the tubing itself. This is calculated by "leak test". Here limb outlet is occluded and increasing pressures are calculated at each level of continuous airway pressure (CPAP). Problem with such a measurement is difficulty in measuring if the port is built in the mask, as the seal might be incomplete. At the same time as per Poiseuille's law as flow exiting ventilator increases, the pressure difference between the two points increases. Therefore overestimation of leak takes place. Hence a correction fraction is included based on tubing resistance following Poiseuille's law. All these pressures are calculated by pneumotachograph in the ventilator. This becomes a drawback in presence of active expiratory valve as the ventilator misses corresponding expiratory phase signal. This can be overcome by attaching the pneumotachograph between valve and interface.[3]

Unintentional Leaks

In bench studies unintentional leaks are measured using holes of different diameters punched out causing linear estimation of leak calculating differences in inspiratory, expiratory volumes, and pressures. However, in real life scenario leaks are nonlinear and have to be measured with an altogether different algorithm.[2] New modes of NIV such as dual control or volume targeted pressure support modes modify pressure support based on random leaks. One also needs to consider possible leak from mouth of patient on nasal mask. Such leaks reduce accuracy of monitored values.

Compressible Volume

Tubing's volume is calculated using the compliance of the tubing. Highly compliant tubing has higher volumes especially in pressure-limited modes while in volume-controlled modes the delivered volume to patient could be low due to higher compliance of tubing. Therefore while monitoring, tube compliance becomes an important factor. Most of the devices factor in compliance of tubing in calculation but errors key in when tubing is changed and CV not corrected.

Adjustment of interface and ventilator settings aims to maintain the 95th percentile of leak values under a predetermined threshold value. Bench studies are performed to understand the possible leak components and by adjusting the interface, the target is to achieve at least the 95th percentile during real time or remote monitoring.[4] Accuracy of monitoring of home ventilators very well depends on how each component is compensated for.

Monitoring Patient

Pulse Oximeter (SpO_2%)[4]

One of the most common indications for NIV is OSA where hypoxia is associated with 4% of hypopneas, which could be rectified using appropriate device and settings indicating importance of SpO_2 monitoring in-patient on NIV. Any SpO_2 above 80% seems accurate as seen in studies comparing arterial pO_2 to SpO_2. However recurrent desaturations may reflect: upper airway instability and residual obstructive events, or repetitive leaks interrupted by microarousals. Central events such as reduced respiratory stimulation with or without glottic closure may be residual events insufficiently corrected by NIV in subjects with central sleep apnea syndromes or induced by ventilator per se. During spontaneous breathing, prolonged desaturations may reflect ventilation/perfusion (V/Q) mismatch in severe obstructive or restrictive disorders, position-dependent V/Q mismatch in severe obesity or persistence of alveolar hypoventilation. Prolonged desaturations (10–30 min) coexisting acceleration of heart rate occurring approximately every 90–120 min during the night are also typical of rapid eye movement (REM) sleep hypoventilation. Therefore SpO_2 monitoring not only provides information on desaturation but also on sleep fragmentation by monitoring autonomic responses. It is to adjust ventilator settings to obtain a mean nocturnal SpO_2 of 90%. Less than 10% of the total recording time can have a SpO_2 < 90% after correction of leaks.[5] Oxygen supplementation should be provided only in case hypoxia is incompletely treated by NIV modulations.

CO_2 Monitoring

Measuring arterial CO_2 ($PaCO_2$) is a gold standard but is invasive and cannot be repeated more frequently at home. Thus, other modes become important like peak expired carbon dioxide ($PeCO_2$), which though not equalling to $PaCO_2$, can give a trend especially in invasively ventilated patients. However in NIV setting, ventilation is not homogeneous and CO_2 expired does not reach the plateau. Therefore, it is unreliable and technically difficult to measure in bilevel support mode due to continuous flow through mask.

Transcutaneous Measurement of Carbon Dioxide ($PtcCO_2$)[4]

Briefly, it consists of a pH-sensitive glass electrode, a silver/silver chloride reference electrode and a heater. The collar of the sensor heats the skin inducing a local hyperemia which improves the permeability of the skin to gas diffusion and "arterializes" the capillary blood to obtain

$PtCO_2$ readings closer to $PaCO_2$ values without causing local skin reactions or skin burns. CO_2 diffuses from the skin through the membrane. Postchemical reactions changes in pH are related to $PtCO_2$ according to the Henderson–Hasselbalch equation. Values of $PtCO_2$ reported by the sensor reflect correction factors used by the system software to compensate for patient and sensor temperature. $PtCO_2$ and $PaCO_2$ levels seem to have good correlation and it can be measured for straight 8 hours without recalibration. However drift has to be factored in which this might require measurement of $PaCO_2$. Though there is a lag of approximately 2 minutes, the $PtCO_2$ is reliable and useful.[6]

Respiratory Rate—Spontaneous versus Back-Up

Respiratory rate (RR) analysis allows an estimation of the difference between spontaneous RR and the pre-set backup RR. Ventilators usually detect breaths either triggered by the patient or by the ventilator (some inspiratory efforts may not be reported unless detailed flow curve analysis are provided). In many centers back-up RR is usually set at approximately two breaths below spontaneous RR; this can be easily adjusted using RR monitoring by ventilator. Importantly for patients with neuromuscular diseases, "capturing" the patient spontaneous RR is a common practice. Thus, monitoring respiratory rate especially number of breaths spontaneous or those delivered as back-up helps understand the needs of patient including trigger sensitivity of home ventilator.

Apnea–Hypopnea Index

Apnea: Cessation of airflow for ≥10 seconds during sleep, accompanied by persistent respiratory effort (obstructive apneas), or absence of respiratory effort (central apneas), hypopnea: A ≥ 30% reduction in airflow for at least 10 seconds during sleep that is accompanied by either a ≥3% desaturation or an arousal.[7] Although reported by ventilator software of several different devices, the effective meaning and reliability of the apnea and apnea–hypopnea indices has yet to be determined. In many cases, manufacturers use the same algorithms to recognize events that they developed for their auto-CPAP devices. This is probably inaccurate in patients during NIV.

■ TELEMONITORING

Telemonitoring is transmission of physiologic and other noninvasive data (i.e., biological storage data transfer) akin to monitoring discussed above. Depending on the modem used it can briefly be classified into first, second, and third generation. In first-generation systems, data from sensors are usually transferred via a telephone system to a database and relayed to the clinical team. Second-generation systems comprise a nonimmediate or analytical decision system in which the data transfer is synchronous with an automated algorithm. Response is delayed as the system is monitored only at certain times. Third-generation systems have a constant analytical and decision-making support in which monitoring centers are physician led and staffed by specialist nurses and have full authority to affect therapy round the clock. Thus, they are remote patient monitoring systems, which might be retrospective analysis of data stored in device or real time monitoring. Components of technology include synchronicity, network configuration, connectivity, and interoperability.

Telemonitoring is of great help to modify the settings appropriately in time to prevent hospitalizations especially in neuromuscular disorders such as amyotrophic lateral sclerosis with favorable implications on cost, survival, and functional status.[8] One study published recently commented about need for frequent checks for telemonitoring to be useful though they could not conclude how frequent is more appropriate.[9] In case of OSA as per one analysis every morning data is retrieved and if any of the following is present, patient is contacted and followed up regarding symptoms and issues: mask leak > 40 L/min or >30% of the night, < 4 hours use for two consecutive nights, machine measured apnea–hypopnea index (AHI) > 10 events/hour, and 90th percentile of pressure > 16 cm H_2O.[10]

Titration of CPAP in OSA is well-established, however titration of bilevel positive airway pressure (BiPAP) in patients with neuromuscular disorders is poorly understood. Monitoring with polysomnograph helps to identify nocturnal events like air leaks, ventilator–patient asynchrony, central events, and glottic closure leading to desaturations, arousals, impaired sleep architecture, and poor adherence which helps to accurately establish device settings to avoid these events. Telemonitoring provides good grounds for palliative care also, especially with the advent of video-contact though it should not replace actual visit.[11]

▌RECOMMENDATION

Based on the current evidence no recommendations can be made for or against telemonitoring.

▌CONCLUSION

Monitoring accuracy of home ventilators depends greatly on leak compensation, algorithms devised by manufacturers, interface used and also on the compliance of patients especially when apnea–hypopnea indices are monitored to assess disease severity in OSA. Telemonitoring though needs technical support can help in reducing hospital admission, though this factor is more studied in neuromuscular diseases, holds good even in COPD cases.[12] One needs to be cautious while interpreting the monitored parameters keeping in mind that different manufacturers have different strategies, therefore homogenization and standardization of data collected and transmitted is required. Though it looks encouraging, telemonitoring in clinical practice is still not common. One also needs to look into the medicolegal aspects which lack clarity currently thus making it more important to establish a body to oversee the process, formulate the recommendations, and guide clinicians and patients on the same platform.

▌REFERENCES

1. Lloyd-Owen SJ, Donaldson GC, et al. Patterns of home mechanical ventilation use in Europe: results from the Eurovent survey. Eur Respir J. 2005;25:1025-31.
2. Sogo A, Montanyà J, Monsó E, Blanch L, Pomares X, Luján M. Effect of dynamic random leaks on the monitoring accuracy of home mechanical ventilators: a bench study. BMC Pulm Med. 2013; 13:75.
3. Luján M , Pomares X , and Sogo A. Monitoring Accuracy of Home Mechanical Ventilators: Key Technical Elements and Clinical Implications.
4. Janssens JP, Borel JC, et al. Nocturnal monitoring of home non-invasive ventilation: the contribution of simple tools such as pulse oximetry, capnography, built-in ventilator software and autonomic markers of sleep fragmentation. Thorax. 2011;66:438e445.

5. Gonzalez C, Ferris G, Diaz J, et al. Kyphoscoliotic ventilatory insufficiency: effects of long-term intermittent positive-pressure ventilation. Chest. 2003;124:857e62.
6. Maniscalco M, Zedda A, Faraone S, et al. Evaluation of a transcutaneous carbon dioxide monitor in severe obesity. Intensive Care Med. 2008;34:1340e4.
7. Wellman A, Redline S. Sleep apnea. In: J Larry Jameson, Dennis L Kasper, Dan L Longo, Anthony S Fauci, Stephen L Hauser, Robert A Fishman, Loscalzo, et al., (eds). Harrisons principle of internal medicine. New York: Mc Graw Hill; 2018. Table 291-1.
8. Anabela P, Almeida P, José & Pinto, Susana & Pereira, João & Oliveira, Antonio & de carvalho, Mamede. Home telemonitoring of non-invasive ventilation decreases healthcare utilisation in a prospective controlled trial of patients with amyotrophic lateral sclerosis. Journal of neurology, neurosurgery, and psychiatry. 2010; 81:1238-42.
9. Young J, Ashforth N, Price K, Wilson A, Nickol A. Remote monitoring of home non-invasive ventilation: a feasibility study. Eur Respir J. 2018; 52: PA1669.
10. Ambrosino N. Tele-monitoring of ventilator-dependent patients: a European Respiratory Society Statement. Eur Respir J. 2016;48(3):648-63.
11. Chen CY, Thorsteinsdottir B, Cha SS, et al. Healthcare outcomes and advance care planning in older adults who receive home-based palliative care: a pilot cohort study. J Palliat Med. 2015;18:38-44.
12. Stoddart A, vanderPo LM, Pinnock H, et al. Telemonitoring for chronic obstructive pulmonary disease: a cost and cost-utility analysis of a randomised controlled trial. J Telemed Telecare. 2015;21: 108-18.

Chapter 34

Home Ventilation in Long-term Noninvasive Ventilation Users

Rajesh Pande, Maitree Pandey

INTRODUCTION

There has been an increase in number of patients receiving home ventilator care in recent years in India. Many home-care service providers are offering a variety of such services. However, in most cases ventilation is provided by mask noninvasive ventilation (NIV) and for those who are tracheostomized, ventilation is provided by NIV machines certified for such use. In fact, NIV remains the mainstay of home ventilation and most data from Europe and Canada shows that 70–80% of home ventilation is provided by NIV[1] and only 3–18% of patients received invasive ventilation via tracheostomy. In USA, single limb circuits with controlled leakage are labeled as respiratory assist devices (Bilevel or NIV devices). These devices have a passive exhalation port with or without a backup respiratory rate. These devices are also used via a tracheostomy tube. Such a distinction is not followed in Europe.

MAJOR INDICATIONS FOR HOME VENTILATION

- Chronic obstructive pulmonary disease (COPD)
- Obesity hypoventilation syndrome (OHS)
- Neuromuscular disease:
  - Amyotrophic lateral sclerosis (ALS)
  - Duchenne muscular dystrophy (DMD)
  - Kyphoscoliosis
  - Other neuromuscular diseases

Chronic Obstructive Pulmonary Disease

The aim of home ventilation in stable COPD patients generally is control of $PaCO_2$ and usually requires a high inspiratory positive airway pressure (IPAP) and back up rate. Major RCTs have shown variable results on home NIV use in severe COPD. A study by McEroy et al.[2] in 144 COPD patients with $PaCO_2$ > 54 mm Hg looked at survival with home NIV (mean IPAP 12.9 cm H_2O) and long-term oxygen therapy (LTOT) versus LTOT alone. Although NIV increased survival, but there was no improvement in $PaCO_2$ or health-related quality of life besides worsening of mood.

Another study[3] in 200 hypercapnic COPD patients ($PaCO_2$ > 52.5 mm Hg) compared mask NIV with LTOT. NIV was used with a high IPAP (21.9 cm H_2O) and a backup rate of

14 breaths per minute (bpm). Mask NIV use was associated with significant improvement in survival, 6-minute walk distance and disease-specific quality of life measures. Struik et al.[4] looked at impact of NIV home ventilation in 200 unstable COPD patients for >1 year (IPAP 19.2 cm H_2O, backup rate 15/min). These patients were unstable (hypercapnic) at 48 hours after stopping NIV for acute exacerbation. Despite improvement in $PaCO_2$, there was no difference in survival, acute admissions or quality of life, between NIV and those who did not receive it.

In a recent open label parallel RCT published in JAMA,[5] 116 severely hypoxic and hypercapnic COPD patients who continued to have persistent hypercapnia ($PaCO_2$ > 52 mm Hg) 2–4 weeks after resolution of respiratory acidosis were randomized to receive either home oxygen therapy (HOT) or home oxygen therapy with home mechanical ventilation (HOT-HMV-IPAP 24 cm H_2O, backup rate 14/min) to look at 1-year admission-free survival, readmission to hospital for any cause or death within 12 months after randomization. During hospital admission before randomization, these patients had required NIV for acute decompensated hypercapnic exacerbation of COPD. There was a 51% reduction in the risk of hospital readmission or death in the HOT-HMV arm compared to the HOT arm, along with three times increase in admission free survival time. The HOT-HMV trial concludes that among patients with persistent hypercapnia following an acute exacerbation of COPD, adding home NIV to HOT prolonged the time to readmission or death within 12 months.

From these major trials it can be inferred that high intensity (IPAP-22–24, backup rate > 14/min) home ventilation using NIV is associated with reduction in time to readmission or death within 12 months in patients with persistent hypercapnia following an acute exacerbation of COPD.

Obesity Hypoventilation Syndrome

Obesity hypoventilation syndrome patients are classified as having with body mass index (BMI) > 30 kg/m², with daytime hypercapnia. Patients with OHS and predominant obstructive sleep apnea (OSA) generally respond well to continuous positive airway pressure (CPAP) therapy but may need NIV when CPAP therapy fails. OHS patients with significant desaturation, hypercapnia, and worsening hypoventilation in REM sleep invariably need NIV support. Another patient subset is chronic lung disease (e.g., COPD) with OHS where hypoxemia and hypercapnia predominate, and NIV application has shown to improve survival.

The Spanish Sleep Network study[6] has shown significant improvement in daytime $PaCO_2$ over a 2-month period with NIV in OHS patients with severe OSA when compared to the control group with only lifestyle modifications. In a randomized controlled trial[7] of NIV in mild obesity hypoventilation syndrome (defined by BMI > 30 kg/m² and daytime PCO_2 > 45 mm Hg), the study group had NIV at home for 1 month whereas the control group received lifestyle counseling. NIV application was associated with reduced PCO_2, apnea–hypopnea index, and improved sleep architecture and nocturnal SaO_2, but the metabolic and cytokine markers were unremarkable.

Another long-term randomized trial[8] compared average volume assured pressure support (AVAPS) with standard pressure support in superobese patients (BMI: 50 kg/m²) and observed significant improvements in PaCO$_2$ and quality of life with no difference in sleep quality, adherence, and IPAP delivered. Although physiological parameters improve in OHS patient with HMV, but NIV use must be combined with other measures like rehabilitation, weight-loss support, and cardiovascular management.

Neuromuscular Disease

Noninvasive ventilation was first used in Duchenne muscular dystrophy many decades ago and is gradually being used in other chronic neuromuscular disorders with increased survival in inherited neuromuscular disease. Evidence suggests that nocturnal hypoventilation is a good indicator for initiation of NIV in these cases. NIV when combined with cough augmentation (physiotherapy, insufflation-exsufflation devices) and percutaneous gastrostomy feeding can delay tracheostomy and invasive ventilation. The symptoms suggestive of nocturnal hypoventilation in otherwise asymptomatic patients should be identified early. These symptoms include:

- Sudden awakenings from sleep
- Irregular respiratory pattern while asleep
- Early morning bifrontal headaches
- Excessive daytime sleepiness

These patients should be followed-up long term since the onset of ventilatory failure is often insidious. The mean survival following the development of diurnal hypercapnia in DMD is 9.7 months if ventilatory support is not provided. NIV should be initiated in symptomatic DMD patients with a daytime PaCO$_2$ of 6.0 kPa. Prophylactic NIV before development of diurnal hypercapnia has not been found to be effective. Although NIV is not very helpful in DMD patients with severe bulbar weakness, an initial trial of NIV can be given.

Patient selection

- Duchenne muscular dystrophy patients should receive respiratory outpatient follow-up once vital capacity or forced expiratory volume in one second (FEV1) is <40–50% predicted.
- Patients should be questioned about symptoms of nocturnal hypoventilation.
- Overnight monitoring of respiration should be considered once vital capacity is <30% predicted.
- A base excess of >4 mmol/L is predictive of significant nocturnal desaturation.
- Some patients develop obstructive sleep apnea/hypopnea syndrome before the appearance of overt nocturnal hypoventilation

A randomized control trial in 92 ALS patients with either daytime hypercapnia or orthopnea demonstrated that NIV improves the quality of life and increases survival in patients with more preserved bulbar function.[9] Early NIV seems to be beneficial but the right time to initiate ventilation is not well established as it is difficult to detect signs and symptom of respiratory impairment in these patients. Protocol-driven NIV has been shown to improve outcome in patients who do not have bulbar involvement. Cough-assist devices should be used as an adjunct as there is deterioration of both inspiratory and expiratory muscle strength, with significant reduction in peak cough flow which predisposes the patient to infections. Ventilatory failure may present as an emergency either during an acute illness, such as a chest infection, or following symptoms suggestive of nocturnal hypoventilation over the preceding weeks. Cough-assist devices may not offer much benefit if there is associated bulbar weakness.

Patient should be assessed for NIV if:
- Daytime arterial oxygen saturation (SPO_2) < 93%
- Forced vital capacity (FVC) < 70% predicted, or maximal inspiratory pressure < 60 cm H_2O
- There are symptoms of sleep-disordered breathing or orthopnea.

Indications for starting NIV in ALS are:
- Daytime hypercapnia, orthopnea, symptomatic sleep-disordered breathing, and rapidly deteriorating pulmonary function.
- If the vital capacity is <50% predicted, death is likely in 6–9 months.

CONGESTIVE HEART FAILURE

Traditionally, NIV has been used in acute respiratory insufficiency situations in heart failure patients with the objective of reversing pulmonary edema and acute respiratory failure. CPAP and BIPAP-NIV are considered level I-A recommendations in acute congestive heart failure. A recently published meta-analysis analyzing impact of incorporation of NIV in cardiac rehabilitation programs for heart failure patients (defined as nonpharmacological treatment emphasising physical exercise programs) reported that NIV was associated with increase in exercise tolerance (6-minute walk test) in these patients.[10]

Patients with congestive heart failure can suffer from central sleep apnea, OSA and Cheyne–Stokes respiration, which may affect the clinical outcome negatively. A Canadian randomized control trial[11] in 258 patients with heart failure and central apnea looked at survival benefit of CPAP therapy in these patients. CPAP application was not associated with any survival benefit but it attenuated central sleep apnea, improved nocturnal oxygenation, increased the ejection fraction, lowered norepinephrine levels, and increased the distance walked in 6 minutes.

The use of CPAP therapy is ineffective in case of central sleep apnea or Cheyne-Stokes breathing and has been found to offer no survival benefit in patients with central sleep apnea and heart failure. Studies looking at the impact of assisted servo ventilation (ASV) in this subset of patients have shown increased mortality[12] and do not recommend ASV therapy in heart failure patients with CSA and ejection fraction < 45%. A recently started trial (The ADVENT-HF trial[13]) will probably answer whether treating sleep disordered breathing (SDB) by ASV in patients with heart failure and reduced ejection fraction (HFrEF) improves morbidity and mortality.

Noninvasive ventilation home ventilation is a simple technique that controls PCO_2, improves survival, quality of life and exercise tolerance in many restrictive and obstructive diseases.[14] Identification of patients and timing for initiating NIV therapy may be challenging as the signs of respiratory failure may not be quite subtle. High IPAP and backup rate during NIV has been suggested in recent studies. There is absence of quality research on the subject and only few guidelines address the issue.

CONCLUSION

Home ventilation can be provided with a face mask or a tracheostomy tube. CPAP is a milder form of therapy, which is effective in mild congestive heart failure, obesity hypoventilation syndrome with obstructive sleep apnea. Bilevel form of NIV can be effectively used in moderate-to-severe form of CHF, OHS with OSA as well as in COPD and patients having amyotrophic lateral sclerosis with preserved bulbar function. Sicker patients with poor cough reflex and, or bulbar involvement may require tracheostomy and invasive ventilation using portable devices certified for such use. A pressure control or volume-assured pressure control form of ventilation can be used in such patients. FiO_2 control remains a major limitation in home ventilation therapy, and patients with continuous high oxygen requirement ($FiO_2 > 0.6$) cannot be managed at home.

REFERENCES

1. Rose L, McKim DA, Katz SL, Leasa D, et al. Home mechanical ventilation in Canada: a national survey. Respir Care. 2015; 60:695–704.
2. McEvoy RD, Pierce RJ, Hillman D, Esterman A, Ellis EE, Catcheside PG, et al. Nocturnal noninvasive nasal ventilation in stable hypercapnic COPD: A randomised controlled trial. Thorax. 2009;64: 561–6.
3. Köhnlein T, Windisch W, Köhler D, Drabik A, Geiseler J, Hartl S, et al. Noninvasive positive pressure ventilation for the treatment of severe stable chronic obstructive pulmonary disease: a prospective, multicentre, randomised, controlled clinical trial. Lancet Respir Med. 2014;2: 698–705.
4. Struik FM, Sprooten RT, Kerstjens HA, Bladder G, Zijnen M, Asin J, et al. Nocturnal noninvasive ventilation in COPD patients with prolonged hypercapnia after ventilatory support for acute respiratory failure: A randomised, controlled, parallel-group study. Thorax. 2014;69: 826–34.
5. P Murphy, et al. Effect of home noninvasive ventilation with oxygen therapy vs oxygen therapy alone on hospital readmission or death after an acute COPD exacerbation. A randomized clinical trial. JAMA. 2017;317:2177-86.
6. Masa JF, Corral J, Alonso ML, Ordax E, et al. Efficacy of different treatment alternatives for obesity hypoventilation syndrome. Pickwick study. Am J Respir Crit Care Med. 2015;192:86–95.
7. Borel J-C, Tamisier R, Gonzalez-Bermejo J, Baguet J-P et al. Noninvasive ventilation in mild obesity hypoventilation syndrome: a randomized controlled trial. Chest. 2012;14: 692–702.
8. Murphy PB, Davidson C, Hind MD, Simonds A, et al. Volume targeted versus pressure support noninvasive ventilation in patients with super obesity and chronic respiratory failure: A randomised controlled trial. Thorax. 2012; 67:727–34.
9. Bourke SC, Tomlinson M, Williams TL, Bullock RE, et al. Effects of non-invasive ventilation on survival and quality of life in patients with amyotrophic lateral sclerosis: A randomized controlled trial. Lancet Neurol. 2006; 5:140–7.
10. Bittencourt HS, Correia dos Reis HF, Lima MS, Neto MG. Noninvasive ventilation in patients with heart failure: A Systematic review and meta-analysis. Arq Bras Cardiol. 2017;108:161-8.
11. Bradley TD, Logan AG, Kimoff RJ, Series F, et al. Continuous positive airway pressure for central sleep apnea and heart failure. N Eng J Med. 2005;353:2025-33.
12. Cowie MR, Woehrle H, Wegscheider K, Angermann C, et al. Adaptive servo-ventilation for central sleep apnea in systolic heart failure. N Engl J Med. 2015; 373:1095–1105.
13. Lyons OD, Floras JS, Logan AG, Beanlands R, et al. Design of the effect of adaptive servo-ventilation on survival and cardiovascular hospital admissions in patients with heart failure and sleep apnoea: the ADVENT-HF trial. Eur J Heart Fail. 2017;19:579-87.
14. McKim DA, Jeremy Road J, Avendano M, Abdool S, et al. Home mechanical ventilation: A Canadian Thoracic Society clinical practice guideline. Can Respir J. 2011;18:197-215.

Section 7

High Flow Nasal Cannula

35. High Flow Nasal Cannula versus Noninvasive Ventilation
36. High Flow Oxygen Therapy: Disease Specific
37. Monitoring and Weaning in High Flow Nasal Cannula

Chapter 35

High Flow Nasal Cannula versus Noninvasive Ventilation

Susruta Bandyopadhyay, Ansuman Mukhopadhyay

INTRODUCTION

The mainstay of life support in patients with compromised respiratory functions in various situations, who were not stabilized with inhaled oxygen had been endotracheal intubation and mechanical ventilation. However, this invasive ventilation also comes with several collateral damages like trauma and damage to the vocal cords, general discomfort of endotracheal intubation, increased infections like ventilator associated pneumonia, etc. Hence there has been always a search for life support systems which will avoid intubation. Noninvasive ventilation has developed over the last few decades to a very useful tool in the ICU. Its advantage over conventional invasive ventilation was in being less invasive, avoiding intubation related trauma, reducing the incidence of ventilator associated pneumonia, etc. It has been well proven in managing acute exacerbations of chronic obstructive pulmonary disease (COPD), cardiogenic pulmonary edema [mostly as continuous positive airway pressure (CPAP)], some postoperative patients, in planned extubation, etc. However, its use in hypoxemic respiratory failure remained unproven. A new technique namely high flow nasal cannula oxygen (HFNO) has recently drawn the attention of the intensivists in managing such patients. HFNO will deliver a higher fraction of inspired oxygen (FiO_2), than all conventional oxygen delivery masks, with a higher flow rate which will reduce the work of breathing. Although devices like venturi mask theoretically delivers an FiO_2 >60%, in practice, in a very dyspneic patient this capacity is offset by the high respiratory efforts of the patient. This air hunger and excessive effort entrains air from the atmosphere, bypassing the relative low flow of the oxygen delivery system and dilutes the delivered oxygen. HFNO overcomes this limitation and hence is suitable even for a very dyspneic patient. If the patient keeps his mouth closed, it may also generate a positive end expiratory pressure (PEEP) up to 7.4 cm of water, if the patient keeps his mouth closed. Thirdly, a humidified and heated oxygen will help in clearing the airways from secretions. In comparison to noninvasive ventilation (NIV), HFNO has advantages like; a free mouth and no interruption of the support during feeding or even during doing procedures like intubation, it allows the patient to speak, there are no facial abrasions due to tight masks, the patients do not feel claustrophobic, etc. Of course HFNO does not have the provisions for higher PEEP and back up rate like the NIV.[1] We, in this article, will give an overview of the comparison between the uses, advantages and disadvantages of HFNO when compared to NIV.

■ HYPOXEMIC RESPIRATORY FAILURE

High flow nasal cannula oxygen seems to be an attractive option for the treatment of acute hypoxemic respiratory failure. HFNO supplies oxygen at a much higher flow rate than conventional oxygen therapy. When used in a patient who keeps his mouth closed, HFNO also provides a certain amount of PEEP, further improving oxygenation. Moreover, NIV has not been proven well for this situation. However, the data about the use of HFNO in acute hypoxemic respiratory failure has been conflicting. HFNO has been studied in comparison with NIV in several studies. Mortality benefit, need for invasive ventilation, ventilator free days, ICU length of stay (LOS), patient comfort, etc. have been various end points in these studies. Some trials have directly compared HFNO and NIV. Some have also included conventional oxygen therapy (COT).

In one of the largest studies in hypoxemic patients, HFNO showed mortality benefit and less need for invasive ventilation than the patients treated with NIV in the patients with acute hypoxemic respiratory failure. This benefit was more prominent in the patients who were more hypoxemic (PaO_2: FiO_2 ratio <200). The patient comfort was also more with HFNO. However, there was no difference in ICU LOS. There were two meta-analyses which compared HFNO to NIV. Both did not show any difference in the rate of intubation between NIV and HFNO patients. There was also no mortality benefit. The ICU LOS were similar, only the patient discomfort was less in the HFNO groups. So, HFNO remains a treatment option in hypoxemic respiratory failure. The treatment is less uncomfortable for the patient than NIV. There is a trend towards less need of intubation and less mortality with HFNO in such patients than NIV.[2,3]

■ CARDIOGENIC PULMONARY EDEMA

The evidence for HFNO in heart failure is not strong. There are some ADHF patients included in the studies of HFNO in hypoxemic respiratory failure mentioned above. However, studies comparing HFNO with NIV solely in ADHF remains a few with very small number of patients. The number of patients with heart failure in studies comparing HFNO to NIV in hypoxemic patients is also low. Small studies on HFNO in ADHF mostly demonstrated relief from dyspnea. A larger study of 128 patients comparing HFNO to NIV in ADHF, also demonstrated relief from dyspnea, which was the main advantage of HFNO. There was no change in mortality nor the number of patients requiring intubation and mechanical ventilation.[4,5]

■ IN POSTEXTUBATION PATIENTS

Noninvasive ventilation is an accepted therapy after planned extubation after weaning from mechanical ventilation. HFNO has been compared to NIV in this situation, in the high risk patients. High risk was defined by, the presence of heart failure or COPD, ventilation more than 7 days, difficult weaning, APACHE II score more than 12, BMI more than 30, airway maintenance problem, etc. Although ICU LOS was less in the HFNO group, the difference in the rate of reintubation in these two groups was statistically nonsignificant. Hence HFNO can be an alternative to NIV in high risk patients who have been weaned from the mechanical ventilation and extubated. Of note, HFNO has not been superior to even COT, in low risk postextubation patients.[6]

PREINTUBATION APNEIC OXYGENATION

Complications may arise in patients with AHRF, when trying to intubate them. 20–25% of such patients may become severely hypoxemic and this may cause cardiac arrest in 2–3%. One of the main reasons for this may be severe hypoxemia during orotracheal intubation, particularly if sedation and paralysis are induced during rapid sequence intubations. The norm has been to preoxygenate these patients before the intubation and continue the supplemental oxygen during the procedure. NIV, with an adjustable FiO_2, has been proven to be a better option than conventional oxygen therapy, with added benefits like addition of PEEP. The PEEP keeps the alveoli patent and provides back up ventilation during the apneic phase after the induction of paralysis. The disadvantage of NIV is that the facial mask needs to be removed during the intubation, which transiently stops the oxygen delivery. HFNO may have some advantages in this regard. It provides a higher FiO_2 than normal nasal cannulas and masks, it may produce a PEEP like the NIV (although only when the mouth is kept closed) and it keeps the mouth free for the procedure and can be continued during the procedure. It was thought that these advantages will translate into better oxygenation during the procedure and therefore less complications like intubation related infections, cardiac arrhythmias, death, etc. With this in mind, two trials were conducted comparing HFNO with NIV in preintubation apneic oxygenation. The larger trial of these two called FLORALI-2 showed better oxygenation, (i.e. less incidence of severe hypoxemia) with NIV than HFNO, in patients whose initial $PaO_2 : FiO_2$ was <200. There was no difference in other patients in the degree of hypoxemia during the procedure. The other outcomes like the incidence of pneumonia, mortality, cardiac arrhythmias, ICU LOS, etc. did not show any difference. The other trial, OPTINIV, was done on similar lines. It compared minimum SpO_2 during the procedure. The primary outcome in this case was better with HFNO. The secondary outcomes like intubation related complications, ventilator associated pneumonia (VAP), ICU LOS, 28 days mortality were similar in the two groups.[7,8]

IN " DO NOT INTUBATE" PATIENTS

Many patients who are terminally ill, or of advanced age may require high oxygen support. Sometimes it is decided not to intubate these people. Traditionally, when they could not be managed with conventional oxygen therapy (COT), they were managed with NIV. In these situations, HFNO may offer some advantages over NIV, like easier food and drink intake and ability to speak while on the ongoing therapy. 50 such patients were studied in an observational study and only 18% required a crossover to NIV. So, HFNO remains a feasible treatment option in these patients.

POST-CARDIAC SURGERY RESPIRATORY FAILURE

Post-cardiac surgery patients who remain hypoxemic require low level pressure support ventilation. A large multicenter trial, (BiPOP trial) was done on such post cardiothoracic surgery high risk, hypoxemic patients. The patients were considered in high risk, when they had a high BMI, poor left ventricular ejection fraction (LVEF) or earlier failed extubation. 416 and 414 patients were randomized to NIV and HFNO respectively. The primary outcome was treatment failure. The secondary outcomes were respiratory variables, comfort score, dyspnea score, need for bronchoscopy, etc. HFNO had a noninferior primary outcome to NIV. SPO_2 was higher with NIV and surprisingly CO_2 washout was earlier with HFNO.[9]

OTHER INDICATIONS

High flow nasal cannula infection has been used with some success in long-term home oxygenation in COPD patients, and in immunocompromised patients, etc. However, as they have not been compared with NIV, these are beyond our scope of discussion.

CONCLUSION

The main advantage of HFNO over NIV remains comfort. It also needs less supervision, as the setting and control of HFNO is much simpler. So, it may be preferred over NIV, in places with low intensity nursing or at home. It is an acceptable treatment option in hypoxemic patients. It can also be a better alternative than NIV in high risk post-extubation patients. It can also replace NIV in the patients who have undergone cardiothoracic operations. It can also be used in the place of NIV in preprocedure apneic oxygenation. It will be easier to handle than NIV, when used in "do not intubate" patients, particularly when they are out of the ICU. Its use however has not been proven in situations like acute exacerbation of COPD. NIV, though slightly uncomfortable, and requires more trained staff to handle, has some inherent advantages over HFNO. NIV allows one to set a higher PEEP, which may be helpful in severe hypoxemic patients, it also ensures a better minute ventilation. Most of the NIV machines now can have a backup rate, which may be necessary for the patient with poor respiratory drive. Moreover, concerns have been raised that its use HFNO may create some false sense of security, delay necessary intubation, and worsen the outcomes.[10]

Indications	Evidence	Outcomes	Recommendations
1. Acute hypoxemic respiratory failure	Observational studies, open labeled studies, RCTs and meta- analysis of RCTs	Lesser intubation rates, improved comfort, no difference in LOS, no mortality advantage	Level of evidence II Grade of recommendation C (Weak)
2. Postextubation hypoxemia	RCTs	No difference in reintubation rates	Level of evidence II Grade of recommendation C (Weak)
3. Preintubation oxygenation	RCTs	NIV better in severely hypoxemic patients No difference in final outcomes	Level of evidence II Grade of recommendation C (Weak)
4. Postcardiac surgery postextubation hypoxemia	RCT	HFNO noninferior to NIV	Level of evidence III Grade of recommendation C (Weak)
5. Acute decompensated heart failure	Observational studies, open label studies	Improved RR, no difference in requirement for NIV, MV, mortality	Level of evidence III Grade of recommendation C (Weak)
6. Acute hypercapnic respiratory failure	Only studied in chronic hypoxemia in the COPD patients		No recommendation
7. Patients with do not intubate orders	Small observational studies, no clear endpoints	Comfort, feeding, communication better	Level of evidence III Grade of recommendation C

(COPD: chronic obstructive pulmonary disease; HFNO: high flow nasal oxygen; LOV: length of stay; NIV: noninvasive ventilation; RCT: randomized controlled trial)

REFERENCES

1. Renda T, Corrado A, Iskandar G, Pelaia G, Abdalla K, Navalesi P. High-flow nasal oxygen therapy in intensive care and anaesthesia. Br J Anaesth. 2018;120(1):18-27.
2. Sztrymf B, Messika J, Mayot T, Lenglet H, Dreyfuss D, Ricard JD. Impact of high-flow nasal cannula oxygen therapy on intensive care unit patients with acute respiratory failure: A prospective observational study. J Crit Care. 2012;27(3):324.e9-324.e13.
3. Frat J-P, Thille AW, Mercat A, Girault C, Ragot S, Perbet S, et al. High-flow oxygen through nasal cannula in acute hypoxemic respiratory failure. N Engl J Med. 2015;372(23):2185-96.
4. Carratalá Perales JM, Llorens P, Brouzet B, Albert Jiménez AR, Fernández-Cañadas JM, Carbajosa Dalmau J, et al. High-flow therapy via nasal cannula in acute heart failure. Rev Española Cardiol (English Ed). 2011;64(8):723-5.
5. Makdee O, Monsomboon A, Surabenjawong U, Praphruetkit N, Chaisirin W, Chakorn T, et al. High-flow nasal cannula versus conventional oxygen therapy in emergency department patients with cardiogenic pulmonary edema: A Randomized Controlled Trial. Ann Emerg Med. 2017;70(4):465-72.e2.
6. Hernández G, Vaquero C, Colinas L, Cuena R, González P, Canabal A, et al. Effect of postextubation high-flow nasal cannula vs noninvasive ventilation on reintubation and postextubation respiratory failure in high-risk patients a randomized clinical trial. JAMA. 2016;316(15):1565-74.
7. Frat J-P, Ricard J-D, Quenot J-P, Pichon N, Demoule A, Forel J-M, et al. Non-invasive ventilation versus high-flow nasal cannula oxygen therapy with apnoeic oxygenation for preoxygenation before intubation of patients with acute hypoxaemic respiratory failure: a randomised, multicentre, open-label trial. Lancet Respir Med. 2019;2600(19):1-10.
8. Jaber S, Monnin M, Girard M, Conseil M, Cisse M, Carr J, et al. Apnoeic oxygenation via high-flow nasal cannula oxygen combined with non-invasive ventilation preoxygenation for intubation in hypoxaemic patients in the intensive care unit: the single-centre, blinded, randomised controlled OPTINIV trial. Intensive Care Med. 2016;42(12):1877-87.
9. Stéphan F, Bérard L, Rézaiguia-Delclaux S, Amaru P. High-flow nasal cannula therapy versus intermittent noninvasive ventilation in obese subjects after cardiothoracic surgery. Respir Care. 2017;62(9):1193-202.
10. Kang BJ, Koh Y, Lim CM, Huh JW, Baek S, Han M, et al. Failure of high-flow nasal cannula therapy may delay intubation and increase mortality. Intensive Care Med. 2015;41(4):623-32.

Chapter 36

High Flow Oxygen Therapy: Disease Specific

Sameer Jog, Jaikumar D Mulchandani, Carol D'silva

■ INTRODUCTION

Oxygen therapy is the first-line therapy for hypoxemic respiratory failure. Oxygen delivery devices include low-flow systems (nasal cannula, simple facemask, non-rebreathing reservoir mask) and high-flow systems (Venturi mask).[1] In patients with acute respiratory failure, the peak inspiratory flow rate is high and often exceeds the oxygen flow delivered by these traditional oxygen devices. The contrast between patient inspiratory flow and delivered flow results in a fraction of inspired oxygen (FiO_2), which is both inconstant and often lower than expected.[2] In addition to the limitation of the FiO_2, conventional devices have other drawbacks that restrain their efficacy and tolerance, such as insufficient humidification and insufficient warming of the inspired gas at high flows which cause patient discomfort. Oxygen therapy with a high-flow nasal cannula (HFNC) overcomes these limitations, and allows for delivering up to 60 L/min of heated and fully humidified gas with a FiO_2 ranging between 21 and 100%.[1]

■ EQUIPMENT

Several devices are available for the provision of high flow nasal oxygen (HFNO) therapy. The apparatus includes the following: high pressure sources of oxygen and air, an air-oxygen blender, a flow meter, a sterile water reservoir, an active heated humidifier for conditioning the gas to optimal temperature (37°C) and humidity (44 mg H_2O/L), a heated non-condensing circuit, and a silicon nasal cannula **(Fig. 1)**.[3]

Depending on the device used, HFNC offers maximum gas flow rates of between 40 and 60 L/min. The flow rate (ranging from 5 to 60 L/min) and FiO_2 (0.21 to 1) are set at the air/oxygen blender. The gas admixture is heated to 37°C, humidified to 100% relative humidity at the active humidifier and then delivered through the heated circuit to the nasal cannula.[4]

Humidity can be provided by a disposable vapor transfer cartridge, a heated plate humidifier or a bubble humidifier.
- The vapor transfer cartridge, a patented device, surrounds the gas flow. Water diffuses through the cartridge, heats up, and passes as vapor into the gas flow.
- The heated plate humidifier has a water chamber over which gas flows and is humidified up to 100% relative humidity.
- The bubble humidifier used in high-flow nasal oxygen delivery devices is designed for use at higher flows than a conventional bubble humidifier. Gas is directed into a water bottle where small bubbles are formed. These gain humidity as they rise to the surface of the water.[3]

Chapter 36: High Flow Oxygen Therapy: Disease Specific

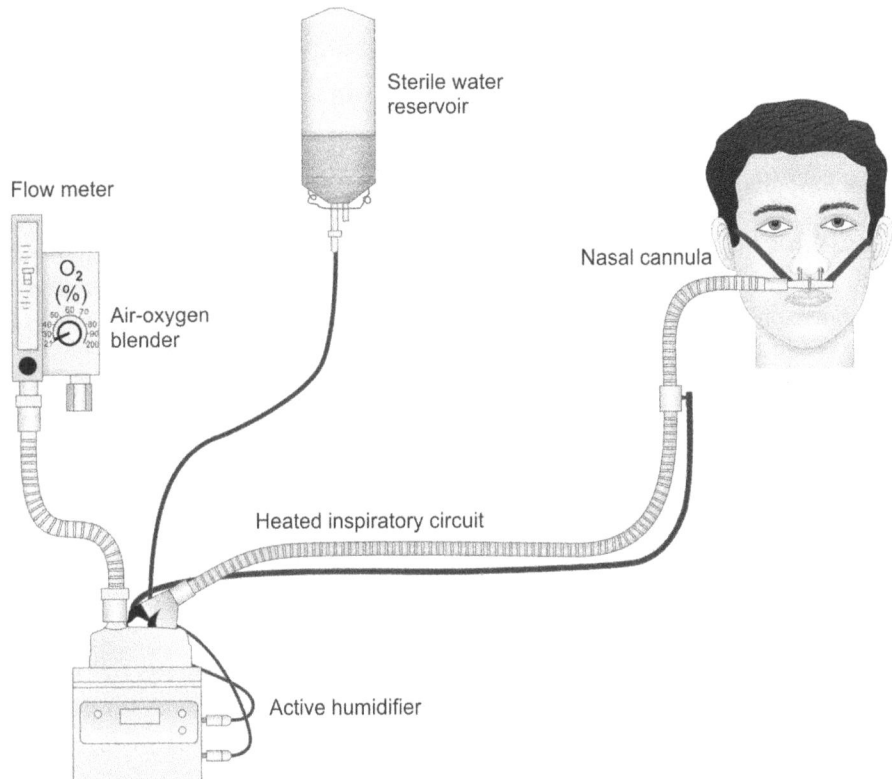

Fig. 1: Set-up of high-flow nasal cannula. An air/oxygen blender, allowing from 0.21 to 1.0 FiO_2, generates up to 60 L/min flow. The gas is heated and humidified through an active heated humidifier and delivered via a single-limb heated inspiratory circuit. The patient breathes the heated and humidified gas through nasal wide bore cannulas.

Some devices provide insulation with a water jacket delivery system surrounding the breathing circuit, while others provide warm breathable tubing to reduce condensation build up.

Nasal cannulas are available in different sizes with adaptations for tracheostomized patients. Most interfaces have wide-bore, soft contoured nasal prongs designed to reduce gas jetting.[3]

PHYSIOLOGICAL EFFECTS AND MECHANISMS OF ACTION

Mechanisms by which oxygen delivered via HFNC offers benefit include the following **(Table 1)**:
- *High flow rates*
    - HFNC flow rates can be adjusted to meet or exceed the patient's inspiratory flow rate demands, so that there is less entrainment of room air, thus resulting in a more reliably delivered FiO_2.
    - It has also been shown that high flow rates result in an improved breathing pattern by decreasing respiratory rate and increasing tidal volume.[4]
- *Flushing of anatomic dead space*: HFNC provides an anatomical oxygen reservoir in the nasopharynx and oropharynx due to a CO_2 washout effect as a result of the high oxygen flow. This reduces dead space and the work of breathing in turn.

- *Positive end-expiratory pressure (PEEP)*
  - The continuous delivery of high flow, which impedes expiratory flow, generates a degree of PEEP. This PEEP effect results in increased end-expiratory lung volume, and thus alveolar recruitment.
  - The splinting of the upper airway also has the effect of reducing airflow resistance in the nasopharynx, thereby reducing the work of breathing.
  - Expiratory pressures vary depending on the amount of flow delivered (the higher the flow, the higher the pressure generated), and on whether the mouth is open or closed (higher pressures with a closed mouth). Flow rates of around 35–60 L/min generate mean expiratory pressures of 2–3 cm H_2O with the mouth open and 5–7 cm H_2O with the mouth closed.[4]
- *Effects of optimal gas conditioning*: As the gas is optimally conditioned before delivery in HFNC therapy, the metabolic load associated with warming and increasing the humidity of inspired gas is averted. This likely impacts the oxygen need and CO_2 production by reducing this energy requirement.
  Furthermore, conditioned gas prevents airway desiccation, improves mucociliary function, facilitates clearance of secretions, and is associated with less atelectasis.[5]
- *Effects on tolerance and comfort*: Conventional oxygen devices delivering dry and unwarmed gas are associated with mask discomfort, claustrophobia, oronasal dryness, eye irritation, nasal and eye trauma, gastric distension, and aspiration.
  Patients with acute hypoxemic respiratory failure (AHRF) experience better comfort and tolerance with HFNC than conventional low-flow oxygen delivery devices and noninvasive ventilation (NIV), and are less likely to interrupt or discontinue therapy.[4]

Table 1: Summary of the physiological benefits provided by high flow nasal cannula (HFNC).

Feature of HFNC	Physiological effect
High flow rates	Carbon dioxide washout Reduction in anatomical dead space Provides an oxygen reservoir Reliable delivery of FiO_2 Improved breathing pattern
Positive end-expiratory pressure (PEEP)	Alveolar recruitment Enhanced oxygenation Decrease work of breathing Unload auto-PEEP (if present)
Warmed humidified gas	Reduced airway surface dehydration Improved secretion clearance Decreased atelectasis Decreased work of breathing

INDICATIONS

- *Acute hypoxemic respiratory failure*: The main use of HFNO is to provide a relatively high FiO_2 to patients with acute hypoxemic respiratory failure (AHRF). HFNO has successfully been used in AHRF due to severe influenza, ARDS, congestive heart failure, hematologic malignancies and organ transplant.

HFNO has been shown to improve oxygenation, comfort, respiratory rate and heart rate in patients with AHRF. However, it has not shown a consistent and convincing benefit in intubation rates and survival.[4]

- *Heart failure:* HFNC can also be used in patients with cardiogenic pulmonary edema, where HFNC-based application of PEEP leads to improved dyspnea and arterial oxygen tension.[3]
- *Preoxygenation before endotracheal intubation:* HFNC is an acceptable way of providing oxygen to patients both before (preoxygenation) and during (to prevent desaturation) endotracheal intubation.
  NIV for preoxygenation must be stopped during laryngoscopy, and thus does not enable oxygenation during intubation. In contrast, HFNO therapy can be continued uninterrupted throughout.[4]
- *Postcardiac surgery and postextubation support:* In the postcardiac surgery population, HFNC can reduce respiratory rate, and increase end-expiratory lung volume. It has been shown to reduce the requirement for continuous positive airway pressure (CPAP) and reintubation rates but has not been consistently shown to improve other respiratory parameters such as PaO_2/FiO_2 ratios or basal atelectasis.
  Following extubation, HFNO is also useful as an adjunct support measure and can been used successfully in prevention and treatment of postoperative respiratory failure.[2,4]
- *During invasive procedures:* Invasive procedures such as fiberoptic bronchoscopy may be associated with hypoxemia, particularly in critically ill patients and during bronchoalveolar lavage. Hypoxemic patients undergoing fiberoptic bronchoscopy can successfully be oxygenated with HFNC.[1,4]
- *Chronic obstructive pulmonary disease (COPD):* Domiciliary HFNO therapy may be useful in stable hypercapnic COPD patients, and in the acute setting for patients intolerant of NIV. Although it does not reduce frequency of COPD exacerbations, it may reduce the duration of these events.[3]
- *End-of-life care:* HFNO can be used in some patients deemed not suitable for intubation, or patients requiring palliative care. Both economic considerations (justice) and ethical considerations (beneficence) justify the use of HFNC in setting. The justice to be considered is the cost of care. The benefit to be considered is alleviation of suffering.[6]
- *Immunocompromised patients:* Use of HFNC is feasible and safe in selected groups of immunocompromised patients with acute hypoxemic respiratory failure. Studies have demonstrated equipoise between HFNC, NIV, and standard oxygen therapy in this setting.[2]

CONTRAINDICATIONS

Contraindications to HFNC are much the same as for NIV.[3,5] These include:
- Abnormalities or surgery of the face, nose, or airway which preclude an appropriate-fitting nasal cannula
- Blocked nasal passages/choanal atresia, epistaxis and airway obstruction
- Uncooperative patients, reduced levels of consciousness and patients at risk of aspiration
- Unstable hemodynamics (shock, post-cardiopulmonary resuscitation, intractable arrhythmias)
- Respiratory arrest

COMPLICATIONS

High flow nasal cannula is usually well tolerated and complications are rare in adults.

Complications include local trauma, discomfort and pressure areas, epistaxis, blocked cannulae due to secretions, abdominal distension, aspiration, and, rarely, barotrauma (e.g., pneumothorax). In addition, failure of HFNC may result in delayed intubation and worse clinical outcomes in patients with respiratory failure.

ESSENTIALS OF PRACTICE

Initial Settings and Adjustments

- *Flow rate*:
  - First, the flow rate must be adjusted to match or exceed the patient's inspiratory flow rate, to achieve a target oxygen saturation. Increases in FiO_2 should then be made if the target oxygen saturation is not reached.
  - HFNC can be initiated with flow rates of around 30–50 L/min.
  - Flow rates should be increased in 5–10 L/min increments, aiming to reduce respiratory rate, or until further increases are not tolerated.
  - Patient discomfort is usually due to the velocity of gas rather than the flow itself, and can be mitigated by using a large-bore cannula.
  - In case of persistent discomfort, the flow can be decreased down to a minimum of 30 L/min.
- *FiO_2*:
  - The FiO_2 (range 21–100%) is next set to target a desired oxygen saturation.
- *Dew point temperature:*
  - Dew point should be maintained close to body temperature at 37°C to optimize the humidification effect.
  - Temperature may be reduced if the patient complains that the gas is too warm.

Monitoring

High flow nasal cannula therapy should be delivered in an intensive care, intermediate care facility, or emergency department, with close monitoring for signs of respiratory failure that necessitate intubation and mechanical ventilation.

These include failure to adequately improve oxygenation within an hour of HFNC initiation, additional elevations of respiratory rate and presence of thoracoabdominal asynchrony.

HFNC can be delivered in a less controlled environment once the patient is improving and is on a trajectory of reduced oxygen requirements (e.g., 50 L/min at 60% FiO_2).

Weaning from HFNC

- After clinical improvement, weaning should begin with FiO_2, while maintaining a steady flow rate. Once FiO_2 is <0.5, flow rate can be reduced.
- Patients can be weaned to conventional low-flow oxygen once the flow rate reaches ≤20 L/min and $FiO_2 \leq 0.5$.

Chapter 36: High Flow Oxygen Therapy: Disease Specific

Other Practice Essentials
- Careful patient selection is essential for the success of HFNC, as patients most likely to benefit are those with mild-to-moderate forms of AHRF.
- HFNC devices should be cleaned and disinfected before use in a new patient. Consumables need to be replaced for every new patient.
- For prolonged treatment, the breathing tube and humidifying chamber kit should be replaced every 14 days, and the patient interface every 7 days.
- It should be ensured that nasal cannulae snuggly fit into the patients' nares, in order to prevent entrainment of room air around the cannula.
- In most cases, nebulized medication is given directly by mouthpiece and not delivered through HFNC equipment. However, aerosol delivery may not be guaranteed at high flows.

HIGH FLOW NASAL CANNULA IN CLINICAL PRACTICE: EVIDENCE

High flow nasal cannula has garnered much interest in patients with hypoxemic failure due to its physiological advantages of providing heated humidified oxygen of up to 60L/min in a noninvasive manner, decreasing dead space and providing a positive end expiratory pressure, albeit minimal, but can help to improve alveolar ventilation and increase end expiratory lung volume. HFNC has been studied in the last two decades in various populations of patients with acute respiratory failure, postextubation, preoxygenation, in patients with COPD and obstructive sleep apnea (OSA), each with varying results.

High Flow Nasal Cannula in Hypoxemic Respiratory Failure

Physiological studies using electrical impedance tomography, has shown that HFNC in acute hypoxemic patients improves oxygenation, work of breathing, lesser respiratory rates and improves compliance with a more homogenous distribution of ventilation.[7]

Prior to use in adults HFNO has been studied in neonates compared to CPAP especially in patients with respiratory distress syndrome.[8]

In the FLORALI trial by Frat et al.,[9] patients with acute hypoxemic respiratory failure with a PaO_2/FiO_2 ratio of less than 300, were subjected to oxygen supplementation via HFNO, NIV or standard oxygen therapy. Although the primary outcome of rate of intubation was not significantly different among the three groups, patients who had received HFNC had significantly lesser ventilator free days and lower mortality compared to the other groups. An additional post hoc analysis showed lower rates of intubation in patients receiving HFNO with PaO_2/FiO_2 ratios of less than 200. In spite of its limitations of being underpowered and patients in NIV group additionally receiving HFNO intermittently, this trial highlighted HFNC as a potential option in treatment of patients with non-hypercapnic acute respiratory failure.

Systematic reviews and meta-analysis have also showed conflicting results with respect to benefits of HFNC in acute respiratory failure.

A meta-analysis of six trials of HFNC versus NIV or COT showed that no differences were found between use of NIV and HFNC with respect to pH, $PaCO_2$ levels and rates of intubation. However, compared to conventional oxygen therapy, there was a benefit with respect to intubation rates and respiratory rates in favor of HFNC.[10]

A meta-analysis by Thalia et al.[11] comprising of 14 studies (including FLORALI) and over 2,000 patients of acute respiratory failure attempted to compare HFNC with usual care (conventional oxygen therapy and/or NIV). There was no overall difference in mortality and rate of intubation as compared to usual care in patients with acute respiratory failure. However, use of HFNC in these patients was met with improved patient comfort and lower dyspnea scores.

Acute Respiratory Distress Syndrome (ARDS)

A single center observational study done in patients studied the outcomes in patients receiving HFNC as a modality in treatment of ARDS. 87 of 560 patients received HFNC either as first line therapy or in supplementation with other methods. The rate of intubation in these patients was 40%. Failure of HFNC was seen in patients with Higher Simplified Acute Physiology Score II, lower PaO_2/FiO_2 ratios, presence of organ failure and higher respiratory rates.[12]

It is also important to note that delay in intubation and waiting for failure of HFNC has been associated with poor outcomes. In a propensity-adjusted and matched analysis, early intubation, that is within 48 hours, was associated with better overall ICU mortality.[13] Delay in intubation due to failure of HFNC had a higher mortality in patients with respiratory failure.

High Flow Nasal Cannula for Procedures

High flow nasal cannula has also been attempted in patients with acute hypoxemic respiratory failure undergoing invasive procedures involving the airway. In a study by Simon et al.,[14] NIV was compared with HFNC in patients undergoing flexible bronchoscopy and incidence of hypoxemia was not different among the two groups. The postoperative pulmonary complications also were not different among the two groups. Hence stronger evidence is needed to define the role of HFNC in these cases.

Postextubation

High flow nasal cannula in earlier smaller studies has been associated with lower heart rates, respiratory rates and dyspnea postextubation when compared to non-rebreathing masks.[15]

Stefan et al. have shown that HFNC is noninferior to NIV in patients who developed or were at risk of developing acute respiratory failure post cardiothoracic surgeries.[16] The rate of treatment failure in terms of reintubation and stopping therapy prematurely was higher in the NIV group, with no differences in ICU mortality between the two groups.

In yet another multicenter randomized control trial (RCT),[17] patients at a low risk of intubation failure were randomized to receive either conventional oxygen therapy or HFNC for 24 hours postextubation. It was seen that patients who received HFNC had a lower reintubation rate with lower rates of postextubation failure.

Similar benefits were not demonstrated in all postoperative cases following extubation however.

The OPERA trial by Futier et al.[18] attempted to see if HFNC scores over conventional oxygen therapy in patients at moderate risk of postoperative pulmonary complications following major abdominal surgeries. There was no difference reported in the incidence of hypoxemia and postoperative complications between the two groups.

In 155 postoperative cases of coronary artery bypass grafting (CABG) surgery, patients with BMI of >30 were prophylactically put on HFNC postextubation to prevent postoperative atelectasis.[19]

In comparison to standard care no difference was seen with HFNC in this RCT with respect to atelectasis, mean P/F ratios and mean respiratory rates postextubation. Dyspnea levels alone were found to be lower in patients who had received HFNC.

Preoxygenation in Hypoxemic Respiratory Failure Patients

High flow nasal cannula has an added advantage of providing continuous oxygen even during laryngoscopy and this apneic oxygenation technique has been postulated to prevent hypoxemia during endotracheal intubation.

Keeping this in mind, Jaber et al. attempted use HFNC + NIV versus NIV alone for preoxygenation in hypoxemic patients needing intubation.[20] In terms of the primary outcome which was lowest SpO_2 recorded during the procedure. It was noted that the minimal SpO_2 values were significantly higher in the interventional group compared to the reference group (NIV alone).

In the PROTRACH study recently published by Guitton et al.,[21] HFNC was compared with standard bag and mask ventilation for preoxygenation. This was a negative trial, in the sense that the primary outcome of lowest pulse oximetry (SpO_2) throughout the intubation procedure showed no statistically significant difference between the two groups. However, HFNC showed a benefit with regards to secondary outcomes like fewer intubation related adverse outcomes and lesser events of desaturations below 95%.

FLORALI 2, a more recent study by Frat et al.,[22] wherein they attempted to compare the effect of NIV and HFNC for preoxygenation during intubation of critically ill patients for acute hypoxemic respiratory failure. In this open label randomized controlled trial, it was seen that severe hypoxemia occurred more in the HFNC group as compared to the NIV group, in the patient subset who had a PaO_2/FiO_2 ratio <200 to begin with. Serious adverse events and the 28-day mortality did not differ between the two groups. They concluded in patients with acute hypoxemic respiratory failure, NIV when compared with high-flow oxygen therapy, did not change the risk of severe hypoxemia during intubation.

HFNC in Obstructive Sleep Apnea

The main pathophysiology in OSA is that of upper airway collapse during sleep leading to spells of hypopnea and apnea spells with intermittent hypoxemia. Over a period of time this may lead to significant changes leading to right ventricular dilatation and cor pulmonale.

Use of CPAP is the recommended treatment in these patients, however due to issues of interface, claustrophobia, airway dryness, the compliance with CPAP remains poor.

HFNC acts as a means to continuous positive airway pressure, and thus preventing airway collapse during sleep. Parke et al. have shown that in comparison to CPAP, high flow nasal oxygen at flows of 30, 40 and 50 L, can increase the expiratory pressures by 1.5 ± 0.6, 2.2 ± 0.8, and 3.1 ± 1.2 respectively, with the subjects mouth closed.[23]

An RCT by McGinley et al. showed lesser AHI scores and a lesser respiratory arousal in patients treated with HFNC with flows of 20 L/min.[24]

HFNC has also been shown to decrease the apnea hypopnea index and improve the nadir oxygen saturation in a small cohort of children without adenotonsillar hypertrophy.[25]

HFNC in Hypercapnic Respiratory Failure

Although NIV is the cornerstone for the initial management of acute exacerbations of COPD, HFNC is now being studied as an alternative in patients with hypercapnic failure.

Earlier physiological studies done by Braunlich et al.[26] in healthy volunteers and patients with COPD and IPF showed that nasal high flow oxygen has been shown to improve mean airway pressures, improve tidal ventilation and reduced respiratory rates in patients of COPD. They attributed these changes to the reduction of anatomical dead space and CO_2 washout from the nasopharyngeal space. However, this study was done in stable patients.

To further this study, Braunlich et al. also demonstrated a small flow dependent decrease in capillary $PaCO_2$ levels in patients with severe COPD.[27]

Hill et al. also demonstrated similar findings in patients with stable severe COPD (GOLD class 3-4) showing lower diaphragmatic work of breathing and lower RR with better Vt at HFNC flows of > 30 L/min.[28]

These findings based on physiological studies and in noncritically ill patients of COPD have not been translated in the clinical scenarios.

Lee et al. showed that there was no mortality benefit with HFNC when compared to NIV inpatients with moderate hypercapnic failure due to AECOPD. Amongst 92 patients of AECOPD having P/F ratios of less than 200, $PaCO_2$ >45 mm Hg and pH between 7.25-7.35, there was no difference found in the 90 day mortality rate or the rate of intubation with HFNO and NIV.[29]

▌KEY POINTS

1. HFNC therapy is an innovative and powerful modality for the early treatment of adults with respiratory failure associated with diverse underlying diseases.
2. Advantages of HFNC compared with conventional oxygen delivery systems include enhanced comfort, increased humidification, high flow rates with reliable FiO_2 delivery, washout of nasopharyngeal dead space, and provision of a small PEEP effect.
3. HFNC is more effective than conventional oxygen therapy in improving oxygenation in patients with hypoxemic ARF. HFNC improves safety in patients undergoing elective intubation, and it may help in limiting hypoxemia during invasive diagnostic procedures.
4. Indications of HFNC are not absolute, and much of the proven benefit of HFNC is subjective and physiologic. HFNC is an alternative to other high-flow systems and NIV. The choice between these systems depends on patient and clinician preference, need for ventilation and PEEP, severity of hypoxemia and institutional availability.

▌REFERENCES

1. Renda T, Corrado A, Iskandar G, Pelaia G, Abdalla K, Navalesi P. High-flow nasal oxygen therapy in intensive care and anaesthesia. Br J Anaesth. 2018;120:18.
2. Papazian L, Corley A, Hess D, Fraser JF, Frat JP, Guitton C, et al. Use of high-flow nasal cannula oxygenation in ICU adults: a narrative review. Intensive Care Med. 2016;42:1336-49.

3. Ashraf-Kashani N, Kumar R. High-flow nasal oxygen therapy. BJA Education. 2017;17(2):63-7.
4. Hare A. High-flow nasal cannula therapy in adults. Clinical Pulmonary Medicine. 2017;24(3): 95-104.
5. Nishimura M. High-flow nasal cannula oxygen therapy in adults. J Intensive Care. 2015;3:15-23.
6. Helviz Y, Einav S. A systematic review of the high-flow nasal cannula for adult patients. Critical Care. 2018;22(1):71.
7. Mauri T, Turrini C, Eronia N, Grasselli G, Volta CA, Bellani G, et al. Physiologic effects of high-flow nasal cannula in acute hypoxemic respiratory failure. Am J Respir Crit Care Med. 2017;195:1207-15.
8. Robert MD. Nasal continuous positive airway pressure (CPAP) for the respiratory care of the newborn infant. Respir Care. 2009;54(9):1209-35.
9. Frat JP, Thille AW, Mercat A, Girault C, Ragot S, Perbet S, et al. High-flow oxygen through nasal cannula in acute hypoxemic respiratory failure. N Engl J Med. 2015;372:2185.
10. Ou X, Hua Y, Liu J, Gong C, Zhao W. Effect of high-flow nasal cannula oxygen therapy in adults with acute hypoxemic respiratory failure: a meta-analysis of randomized controlled trials. Canadian Med Assoc J. 2017;189(7), E260-7.
11. Monro-Somerville T, Sim M, Ruddy J, Vilas M, Gillies MA. et al. The effect of high-flow nasal cannula oxygen therapy on mortality and intubation rate in acute respiratory failure: A systematic review and meta-analysis. Crit Care Med. 2017;45:e449.
12. Messika J, Ben Ahmed K, Gaudry S, Miguel-Montanes R, Rafat C, Sztrymf B, et al. Use of high-flow nasal cannula oxygen therapy in subjects with ARDS: A 1-Year observational study. Respir Care. 2015;60(2):162-9.
13. Kang BJ, Koh Y, Lim CM, Huh JW, Baek S, Han M, et al. Failure of high-flow nasal cannula therapy may delay intubation and increase mortality. Intensive Care Med. 2015;41:623.
14. Simon M, Braune S, Frings D, Wiontzek AK, Klose H, Kluge S. High-flow nasal cannula oxygen versus non-invasive ventilation in patients with acute hypoxaemic respiratory failure undergoing flexible bronchoscopy–a prospective randomised trial. Crit Care. 2014;18(6):712.
15. Rittayamai N, Tscheikuna J, Rujiwit P. High-flow nasal cannula versus conventional oxygen therapy after endotracheal extubation: a randomized crossover physiologic study. Respir Care. 2014;59(4):485-90.
16. Stéphan F, Barrucand B, Petit P, Rézaiguia-Delclaux S, Médard A, Delannoy B, et al. High-flow nasal oxygen vs noninvasive positive airway pressure in hypoxemic patients after cardiothoracic surgery: A randomized clinical trial. JAMA. 2015;313(23):2331-9.
17. Hernández G, Vaquero C, González P, Subira C, Frutos-Vivar F, Rialp G, et al. Effect of postextubation high-flow nasal cannula vs conventional oxygen therapy on reintubation in low-risk patients: A Randomized Clinical Trial. JAMA. 2016;315(13):1354-6.
18. Futier E, Paugam-Burtz C, Godet T, Khoy-Ear L, Rozencwajg S, Delay JM, et al. Effect of early postextubation high-flow nasal cannula vs conventional oxygen therapy on hypoxaemia in patients after major abdominal surgery: a French multicentre randomised controlled trial (OPERA). Intensive Care Med. 2016;42(12):1888-98.
19. Corley A, Bull T, Spooner AJ, Barnett AG, Fraser JF. Direct extubation onto high-flow nasal cannulae post-cardiac surgery versus standard treatment in patients with a BMI ≥30: a randomised controlled trial. Intensive Care Med. 2015;41(5):887-94.
20. Jaber S, Monnin M, Girard M, Conseil M, Cisse M, Carr J, et al. Apnoeic oxygenation via high-flow nasal cannula oxygen combined with non-invasive ventilation preoxygenation for intubation in hypoxaemic patients in the intensive care unit: the single-centre, blinded, randomised controlled OPTINIV trial. Intensive Care Med. 2016;42:1877-87.
21. Guitton C, Ehrmann S, Volteau C, Colin G, Maamar A, Jean-Michel V, et al. Nasal high-flow preoxygenation for endotracheal intubation in the critically ill patient: a randomized clinical trial. Intensive Care Med. 2019;45(4):447-58.

22. Frat JP, Ricard JD, Quenot JP, Pichon N, Demoule A, Forel JM, et al. Non-invasive ventilation versus high-flow nasal cannula oxygen therapy with apnoeic oxygenation for preoxygenation before intubation of patients with acute hypoxaemic respiratory failure: A randomised, multicentre, open-label trial. Lancet Respir Med. 2019;7(4):303-12.
23. Parke RL, McGuinness SP. Pressures delivered by nasal high flow oxygen during all phases of the respiratory cycle. Respir Care. 2013;58:1621.
24. McGinley BM, Patil SP, Kirkness JP, Smith PL, Schwartz AR, Schneider H. A nasal cannula can be used to treat obstructive sleep apnea. Am J Respirator Crit Care Med. 2007;176(2):194-200.
25. Joseph L, Goldberg S, Shitrit M, Picard E. High-flow nasal cannula therapy for obstructive sleep apnea in children. J Clin Sleep Med. 2015;11:1007-10.
26. Bräunlich J, Beyer D, Mai D, Hammerschmidt S, Seyfarth H-J, Wirtz H. Effects of nasal high flow on ventilation in volunteers, COPD and idiopathic pulmonary fibrosis patients. Respiration. 2013;85:319-25
27. Bräunlich J, Seyfarth HJ, Wirtz H. Nasal high-flow versus non-invasive ventilation in stable hypercapnic COPD: a preliminary report. Multidiscip Respir Med. 2015;10(1):27.
28. Hill NS. High flow nasal cannula: Is there a Role in COPD? Tanaffos. 2017;16(Suppl 1):S12.
29. Lee MK, Choi J, Park B, Kim B, Lee SJ, Kim SH. (2018). High flow nasal cannulae oxygen therapy in acute-moderate hypercapnic respiratory failure. Clin Respirator J. 2018;12(6):2046-56.

Chapter 37

Monitoring and Weaning in High Flow Nasal Cannula

Simran Singh

■ INTRODUCTION

High flow nasal cannula (HFNC) was historically developed to improve gas exchange in neonatal and pediatric patients. But now there is good-quality evidence for its successful use in critically ill adult patients as well.

High-flow nasal cannula oxygen therapy comprises an air/oxygen blender, an active humidifier, a single heated circuit, and a nasal cannula.

The device delivers gas (37 °C containing 44 mg H_2O/L [100% relative humidity] using a heated humidifier and a heated inspiratory circuit) through a wide-bore nasal cannula at very high flow rates at a predetermined oxygen concentration (21–100%). It delivers adequately heated and humidified gas at up to 60 L/min of flow.

Heated humidified oxygen at high flow rates of 30–60 L/min are better tolerated than oxygen by face mask. It facilitates decreased respiratory rate, decreased work of breathing, and better oxygenation in patients.[1] HFNC is best applied in a monitored setting such as the intensive care unit (ICU), step-down ICU, or in the emergency department.[2] This is because patients in need of HFNC are at risk of severe respiratory failure and may require close monitoring for mechanical ventilation.[3]

■ PHYSIOLOGICAL EFFECTS OF HIGH FLOW NASAL CANNULA

Physiological effects of HFNC are:
- Reduction of anatomical dead space
- Positive end-expiratory pressure (PEEP) effect
- Constant fraction of inspired oxygen
- Good humidification (37°C containing 44 mg H_2O/L [100% relative humidity]). Warm humid gas is associated with better conductance and pulmonary compliance compared to dry, cooler gas.
- End-expiratory lung impedance increases with rising flow rate suggesting an increase in end-expiratory lung volume (EELV).

The flow must therefore be set to match the patient's inspiratory demand and/or the severity of the respiratory distress. This is because delivered flow is higher than the patient's spontaneous inspiratory demand and the difference between the delivered flow rate and the patient's inspiratory flow rate is therefore reduced.

The anatomical dead space is decreased via washout of the nasopharyngeal space. Consequently, a larger fraction of the minute ventilation participates in gas exchange.

An improved thoracoabdominal synchrony decreases the work of breathing. Also HFNC mechanically stents the airway thereby attenuating the inspiratory resistance.

The heated and humidified gas provided by HFNC also improves mucociliary function, which facilitates clearance of secretions, preventing atelectasis, and improving the ventilation/perfusion.

PREDICTORS OF HIGH FLOW NASAL CANNULA TREATMENT FAILURE IN PATIENTS WITH ACUTE HYPOXEMIC RESPIRATORY FAILURE

All patients with HFNC must be strictly monitored especially for oxygenation, respiratory rate and pattern, and the need for vasopressors. All these variables have been implicated in HFNC failure. It is important not to delay intubation in patients who fail, as a delay is associated with a high mortality.

Timely intubation is thus critical in patients with acute hypoxemic respiratory failure.[4]

PREDICTORS OF HIGH FLOW NASAL CANNULA SUCCESS

The existence of accurate, early predictors of HFNC success is important. A propensity-score analysis done by Kang et al. associated early intubation (within the first 48 hours) with better ICU survival.[4] In spite of its limitations, the study by Kang et al. raises an important issue regarding delayed intubation which might have worse clinical outcomes in patients with acute respiratory failure.

Therefore, the ability to identify accurate predictors of success on HFNC in patients who are likely to fail is extremely important.

Sztrymf et al.[5] reported that respiratory rate as well as the percentage of patients exhibiting thoracoabdominal asynchrony as early as 30 minutes and 15 minutes after the beginning of HFNC were significantly higher in patients who required endotracheal intubation. Also, the PaO_2/FiO_2 ratios, 1 hour after the start of HFNC, were significantly lower in patients requiring invasive mechanical ventilation.

PATIENT MONITORING

Patient should be observed closely for the first 8 hours to troubleshoot as well as monitor for any deterioration.[6] Monitoring should be for subjective as well as objective signs:
- Subjective: Severity of dyspnea
- Objective: SaO_2 and respiratory rate.

  For assessing the response to HFNC, the following questions need to be asked:
  - Has the patient's tachypnea improved?
  - Is there any improvement in the work of breathing?
  - Is the FiO_2 requirement decreasing ($FiO_2 < 60\%$) while achieving target saturations?

Certain clinical and oxygenation criteria are associated with HFNC failure and need to be constantly monitored. Signs suggestive of an impending respiratory failure and the need for mechanical ventilation are:

- Increasing respiratory rate (RR)
- Progressive hypoxemia
- Thoracoabdominal asynchrony
- $SpO_2:FiO_2$ ratio
- Failure to achieve correct oxygenation ($PaO_2 < 60$ mm Hg despite HFNC flow ≥30 L/min, and FiO_2 of 1.0
- Respiratory acidosis ($PaCO_2 > 50$ mm Hg with pH > 7.25)
- Decreased level of consciousness and inability to clear secretions
- Severe hemodynamic instability (norepinephrine >1 µg/kg/min)
- Cardiac arrest/arrhythmias
- Other criteria suggesting failure are encephalopathy or agitation inability to clear secretions, and inability to tolerate any of the interfaces.

A patient should be promptly intubated if they have failed noninvasive ventilation and there is neither stabilization nor improvement in the clinical condition.

Sztrymf and his colleagues in their study on beneficial effects of HFNC demonstrated that its use was associated with a significant reduction in respiratory rate, heart rate, dyspnea score, supraclavicular retraction thoracoabdominal asynchrony and a significant improvement in SpO_2.

These improvements were evident within the first 15–30 min after applying HFNC and lasted throughout the study period without any unexpected side-effects.[5]

Respiratory Rate Oxygenation Index

Respiratory rate oxygenation index is an easy-to-use index that is a determinant of HFNC success. It predicts the need for mechanical ventilation. It is calculated from the measured respiratory variables assessing respiratory failure, increasing the ability to discriminate between patients who would succeed on HFNC and those who could fail.[7]

Roca and collaborators derived this index to assess the need for mechanical ventilation in a cohort of community-acquired pneumonia patients who were placed on HFNC.[7]

ROX index = $(SpO_2/FiO_2)/RR$

The indicator, named ROX, was found to be superior to the respiratory rate or PaO_2/FiO_2 ratio to predict HFNC success at 12 hours from ICU admission.[7]

A ROX index ≥ 4.88 at 12 hours from the time of ICU admission was associated with a lower risk for mechanical ventilation even after adjusting for confounding variables.[7]

The index can predict the need for mechanical ventilation in patients with pneumonia and in hypoxemic acute respiratory failure but its external validation is still needed before its regular implementation in clinical practice.[7]

Respiratory rate oxygenation index has a positive predictive value of 89.4%. It demonstrated that the best prediction accuracy was 12 hours after HFNC initiation—area under the ROC curve 0.74; $P < 0.002$.[7]

If the index increases at 18 hours after initiation, then patients' chances of succeeding on HFNC are higher.[7]

SpO_2/FiO_2 Ratio

As most of the nonintubated ARF patients are currently managed with noninvasive hemodynamic monitoring, SpO_2/FiO_2 correlates well with PaO_2/FiO_2 ratio.[8,9] It has been demonstrated that patients with ARDS diagnosed by the SpO_2/FiO_2 ratio have very similar characteristics and outcomes compared with those patients diagnosed by PaO_2/FiO_2 ratio.

■ SETTINGS OF HIGH FLOW NASAL CANNULA

Three basic parameters need to be set on HFNC which are also *important from the point of view* of weaning the patient from HFNC.
1. Flow rate
2. FiO_2
3. Temperatures—31°C, 34°C, and 37°C.

Flow Rate

During normal and quiet breathing, the peak inspiratory flow rate is around 30–40 L/min. During heavy workloads, mean flow rates can increase to more than 70 L/min as seen in patients with acute respiratory failure.[10]

The peak inspiratory flow rate of tachypneic patients exceeds the flow rates supplemented by conventional oxygen devices, leading to a dilution of the gas administered and reducing the amount of oxygen that finally reaches the alveoli.

However, the single inspiratory limb of HFNC allows for airflows as high as 50–60 L/min to achieve inspired oxygen fractions (FiO_2) as high as 95–100%. Higher flows allow clinicians to better match the inspiratory demands of patients who are in acute hypoxemic respiratory failure.

If the patient has clinical signs of acute respiratory failure with a PaO_2/FiO_2 of >300, HFNC should be applied with 100% FiO_2 and flow rate of 50–60 L/min.

The proposed initial flow rate differs between studies with some authors suggesting initial lower flow rates 35–40 L/min[11] while others suggest initial maximal flow rates of 60 L/min to rapidly relieve dyspnea and avoid muscle fatigue.[12,13]

It is better to optimize the flow rate first in order to keep the $FiO_2 \leq 60\%$. The flow delivered will try to satisfy the inspiratory demand, minimizing the entrainment of room air and thus ensuring administration of the required FiO_2. Very high flows can increase the tidal volume sometimes causing alveolar overdistension, especially in patients with preexisting lung injury.

Increasing the flow rate is usually preferred to increasing the FiO_2 as an initial strategy to improve peripheral oxygenation, but if this does not happen then increasing the FiO_2 might achieve target SaO_2 levels. Thus high flow rates have shown to result in an improved breathing pattern by increasing tidal volume and decreasing respiratory rate.[14]

Mauri et al. in their study[15] on acute hypoxemic respiratory failure patients showed that by increasing flow rates, there was an improved inspiratory drive and effort, oxygenation, efficiency of minute ventilation, EELV and lung mechanics. The improvement of oxygenation,

EELV and mechanics showed a linear correlation with flow rates with nearly constant improvement at increasing flow. Also optimum flow for each physiologic variable studied did not always correspond to the highest flow rate (i.e. 60 L/min), with considerable variability between patients, indicating that personalized bedside titration of HFNC flow rate (possibly starting from the highest working downward) seemed to be more beneficial.

Similar to conventional oxygen devices, open mouth breathing will mitigate the advantage obtained from using high flow rates to a certain extent.[15]

FiO_2

High flow nasal cannula therapy should be started as early as possible. It seems logical to start with a FiO_2 of 1.0. The FiO_2 (range 0.21–1.0%) is adjusted to target the required SaO_2.

Temperature

Starting the HFNC at lower temperature and gradually increasing it over sometime is a reasonable clinical approach which is better tolerated by most patients as shown by Mauri and his colleagues in their study.[16]

WEANING FROM HIGH FLOW NASAL CANNULA

Patients can tolerate HFNC continuously for prolonged periods. There is no fixed protocol or guidelines to wean the patients from HFNC but it is appropriate that once the patient is progressing well on HFNC, weaning can be initiated by first by decreasing the FiO_2 and then when the $FiO_2 < 0.5$, the flow rate can be reduced. When the $FiO_2 < 0.5$ and the flow rate < 25 L/min.

High flow nasal cannula can be replaced by conventional low-flow oxygen devices. As the use of HFNC is relatively recent there are no standard guidelines in place. However, Ischaki et al. in their review article on HFNC have recommended an algorithm for the use of HFNC in acute hypoxemic respiratory failure.

CONCLUSION

Patients should be carefully monitored for the initial hour after initiation of HFNC.

Those who respond to HFNC generally have some improvement in respiratory parameters with an hour. Those who fail to respond will show signs of persistent respiratory embarrassment such as $SpO_2 < 88–90\%$, respiratory rate > 35 breaths/min, thoracoabdominal asynchrony and accessory respiratory muscle use.

Patients with a failed trial of HFNC should be promptly intubated.

SUMMARY

- HFNC is best applied in a monitored setting such as the ICU, the step-down unit, or the emergency department. It is important not to delay intubation in patients who fail HFNC, as a delay is associated with a high mortality.
- All patients with HFNC must be strictly monitored especially for oxygenation, respiratory rate and pattern, and need for vasopressors. All these variables have been implicated in HFNC failure.

Flowchart 1: Recommended algorithm for high flow nasal cannula use in acute hypoxemic respiratory failure in immunocompetent or immunocompromised patients.

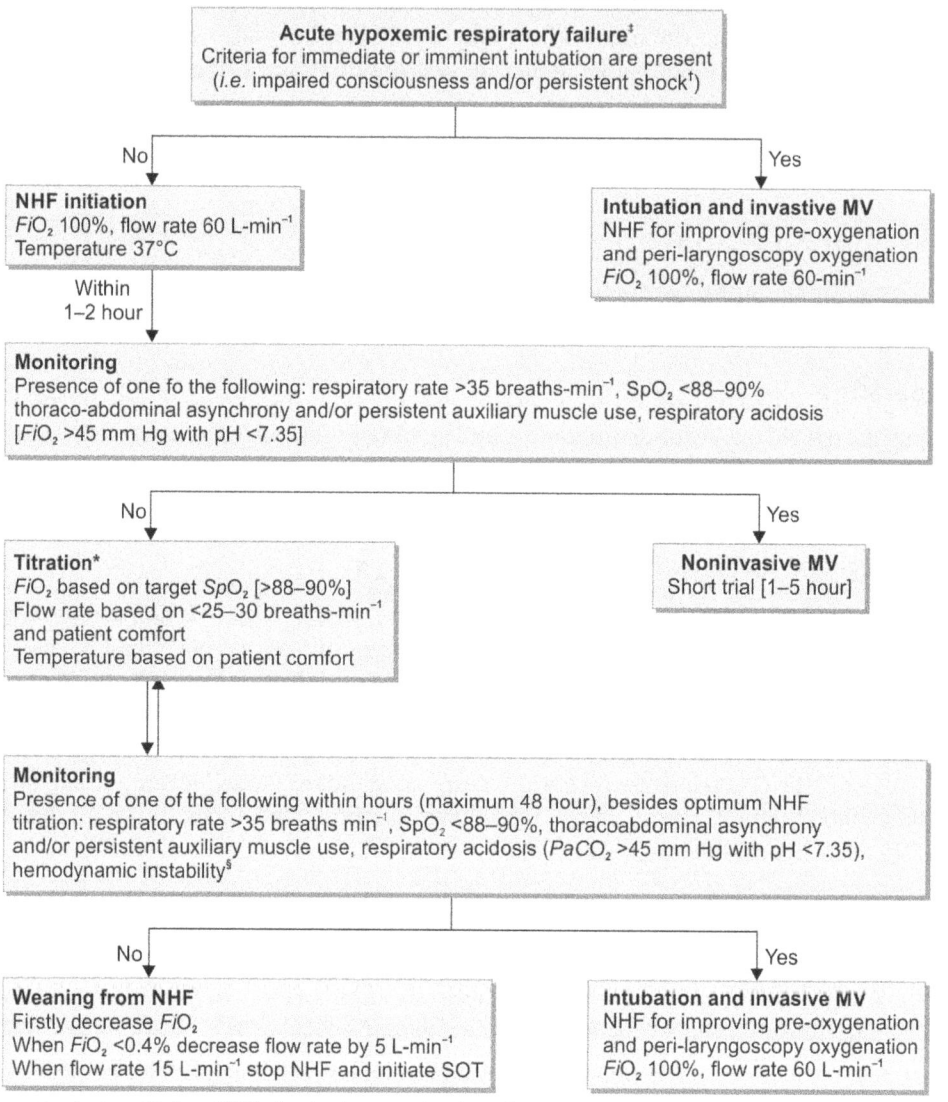

(MV: mechanical ventilation; SOT: standard oxygen treatment)
Note: *Arterial oxygen tension (PaO_2)/inspiratory oxygen fraction (FiO_2) < 300 (patients with arterial carbon dioxide tension [$PaCO_2$] > 45 mm Hg are excluded);[†] systolic arterial blood pressure < 90 mm Hg despite adequate fluid administration; ‡the rationale for change in nasal high flow (NHF) are as follows:
- Flow rate could be adjusted downward by oxygen saturation measured by 5–10 L/min per 1–2 h if none of the negative prognostic factors are present. However, if targets of arterial oxygen saturation measured by pulse oximetry (SpO_2) and respiratory rates are not achieved, while the flow rate is <60 L/min, increase of flow rate by 5–10 L/min is preferred in raising FiO_2
- Increase in FiO_2 causes increase in PaO_2 and SpO_2
- Temperature can be set at 37°C or lower (31–34°C) based on patient's comfort; §hemodynamic instability is defined by heart rate > 140 beats/min or change > 20% from baseline and/or systolic arterial blood pressure > 180 mm Hg, < 90 mm Hg or decrease > 40 mm Hg from baseline.

Source: Adapted from Ischaki E, Pantazopoulos I, Zakynthinos S. Nasal high flow therapy: a novel treatment rather than a more expensive oxygen device. Eur Respiratory Review. 2017:26.

- HFNC oxygen therapy comprises an air/oxygen blender, an active humidifier, a single heated circuit, and a nasal cannula. It delivers adequately heated and humidified gas at up to 60 L/min of flow.
- Physiological benefits of high-flow nasal cannula oxygenation (HFNCO) compared to conventional oxygen therapy are higher and provide a more stable FiO_2.
- The flow must be set to match the patient's inspiratory demand and/or the severity of the respiratory distress. Most of the benefits are from the high flow rates and the heated and humidified gas. The delivery of warm, humidified gas has been associated with better tolerance and comfort improving the mucociliary function and increasing mucus clearance.
- Adult devices provide a flow of 50–60 L/Min. It is important to maximize the flow rates initially and then increase the FiO_2 as per oxygen saturation goal.
- Once the patient is progressing well on HFNC, weaning can be initiated by first decreasing the FiO_2 and when the $FiO_2 < 0.5$, the flow rate can be reduced. When the $FiO_2 < 0.5$ and the flow rate < 25 L/min, HFNC can be replaced by conventional low flow oxygen devices.

REFERENCES

1. Messika J, Ben Ahmed K, Gaudry S, Miguel-Montanes R, Rafat C, Sztrymf B, et al. Use of high-flow nasal cannula oxygen therapy in subjects with ARDS: A 1-year observational study. Respir Care. 2015;60(2):162-9
2. Lenglet H, Sztrymf B, Leroy C, Brun P, Dreyfuss D, Ricard JD. Humidified high flow nasal oxygen during respiratory failure in the emergency department: feasibility and efficacy. Respir Care. 2012;57(11):1873-8.
3. Jones PG, Kamona S, Doran O, Sawtell F, Wilsher M. Randomized controlled trial of humidified high-flow nasal oxygen for acute respiratory distress in the emergency department: The HOT-ER Study. Respir Care. 2016;61(3):291-9.
4. Kang BJ, KohY, Lim CM, Huh JW, Baek S, Han M, et al. Failure of high-flow nasal cannula therapy may delay intubation and increase mortality. Intensive Care Med. 2015;41(4):623-32
5. Sztrymf B, Messika J, Bertrand F, Hurel D, Leon R, Dreyfuss D, et al. Beneficial effects of humidified high flow nasal oxygen in critical care patients: a prospective pilot study. Intensive Care Med. 2011;37(11):1780-6.
6. Soo Hoo GW, Santiago S, Williams AJ. Nasal mechanical ventilation for hypercapnic respiratory failure in chronic obstructive pulmonary disease: determinants of success and failure. Crit Care Med. 1994;22(8):1253-61.
7. Roca O, Messika J, Caralt B, García-de-Acilu M, Sztrymf B, Ricard JD, et al. Predicting success of high-flow nasal cannula in pneumonia patients with hypoxemic respiratory failure: The utility of the ROX index. J Crit Care. 2016;35:200-5.
8. Chen W, Janz DR, Shaver CM, Bernard GR, Bastarache JA, Ware LB. Clinical characteristics and outcomes are similar in ARDS diagnosed by oxygen saturation/FiO_2 ratio compared with PaO_2/FiO_2 ratio. Chest. 2015;148(6):1477-83.
9. Rice TW, Wheeler AP, Bernard GR, Hayden DL, Schoenfeld DA, Ware LB. Comparison of the SpO_2/FiO_2 ratio and the PaO_2/FiO_2 ratio in patients with acute lung injury or ARDS. Chest. 2007;132(2):410-7.
10. Anderson NJ, Cassidy PE, Janssen LL, Dengel DR. Peak inspiratory flows of adults exercising at light, moderate and heavy workloads. J Int Soc Respir Prot. 2006;23:53-63.

11. Spolitini G, Alotaibi M, Blasi F, Hill NS. Heated humidified high flow nasal oxygen in adults: Mechanism of Action and Clinical implications. Chest. 2015;148:253-61.
12. Gotera C, Diaz Lobato S, Pinto T, Winck JC. Clinical evidence of high flow nasal oxygen therapy and humidification in adults. Rev Port Pnuemol. 2013;19(5):217-27.
13. Frat J-P, Thille AW, Mercat A, Girault G, Ragot S, Perbet S, et al. High-flow oxygen through nasal cannula in acute hypoxemic respiratory failure. N Engl J Med. 2015;372(23):2185-9.
14. Corley A, Caruana LR, Barnett AG, Tronstad O, Fraser JF. Oxygen delivery through high-flow nasal cannulae increase end-expiratory lung volume and reduce respiratory rate in post-cardiac surgical patients. Br J Anaesth. 2011;107(6):998-1004
15. Mauri T, Alban L, Turrini C, Cambiaghi B, Carlesso E, Taccone P, et al. Optimum support by high-flow nasal cannula in acute hypoxemic respiratory failure: effects of increasing flow rates. Intensive Care Medicine. 2017;43(10):1453.
16. Mauri T, Galazzi A, Binda F, Masciopinto L, Corcione N, Carlesso E, et al. Impact of flow and temperature on patient comfort during respiratory support by high flow nasal cannula. Critical Care. 2018;22(1):120.

Section 8

Neonatology and Pediatrics

38. Noninvasive Ventilation in Neonates
39. Heated Humidified High Flow Nasal Cannula Therapy in Neonates and Children
40. Home Respiratory Support in Children: What is Possible in India?
41. Noninvasive Ventilation in Acutely Ill Children

Chapter 38

Noninvasive Ventilation in Neonates

Kirti M Naranje, Anita Singh, Niranjan Thomas

INTRODUCTION

Noninvasive ventilation (NIV) is the delivery of mechanical ventilation (MV) to lungs without an endotracheal tube or tracheostomy in the airway. NIV is a gentler form of ventilation. NIV strategy is increasingly being recognized as a primary modality of treatment of respiratory distress in neonates, in order to reduce the side effects of invasive MV and prevent ventilator-induced lung injury (VILI).

Noninvasive ventilation strategy includes continuous positive airway pressure (CPAP), noninvasive positive pressure ventilation (NIPPV), and heated humidified high-flow nasal cannula (HFNC) system.[1] Nasal CPAP is the predominant form of NIV used in neonates. Bilevel CPAP, sigh continuous positive airway pressure (SiPAP), nasal high-frequency ventilation (NHFV), and nasal neurally adjusted ventilator assist (NAVA) are newer modes of NIV which are used infrequently. Heated humidified HFNC will be discussed in a separate chapter.

In this chapter, we discuss the indications, contraindications, practical application, setting up, weaning, and complications of the commonly used NIV modes CPAP and NIPPV.

NASAL CONTINUOUS POSITIVE AIRWAY PRESSURE

Nasal continuous positive airway pressure (NCPAP) is a mode of NIV in which there is application of positive pressure to the airways of a spontaneously breathing baby throughout the respiratory cycle.[2] NCPAP works in preterm neonates with respiratory distress predominantly by the following mechanisms:[3]
- It expands the collapsed alveoli thereby increasing the functional residual capacity
- It splints the airway
- It reduces the work of breathing
- It improves the pattern and regularity of respiration.

Indications

Nasal continuous positive airway pressure is used predominantly in respiratory conditions where there is a tendency of alveoli to collapse or they are filled with fluid.
- *Respiratory distress syndrome (RDS)*: Early use of NCPAP in the delivery room offers both short-term and long-term benefits to premature neonates (<30 weeks) with RDS. It decreases or prevents the need of MV and reduces the incidence of combined outcome of

bronchopulmonary dysplasia (BPD) or death at 36 weeks of corrected gestation. It does not increase the risk of adverse consequences in the long-term.[4-6]
- *Apnea of prematurity (AOP)*: NCPAP reduces the frequency of apnea by rib cage stabilization, improvement in oxygenation, and reduction in supraglottic resistance. It is helpful in reducing the attacks of obstructive apnea by means of splinting the airways.[7]
- *Postextubation*: NCPAP helps in preventing postextubation atelectasis and apnea. It is particularly useful if used at CPAP of 5 cm H_2O and if extubation occurs within the first 14 days of life.[8,9]
- *Delivery room CPAP during resuscitation*: The use of CPAP in the delivery room has been incorporated in the sixth edition of neonatal resuscitation program. In the delivery room, CPAP is given by T-piece resuscitator. This device has positive end-expiratory pressure (PEEP) control knob at the patient end which helps in regulation of delivery of PEEP. Peak inspiratory pressure (PIP) can be controlled by a knob at the equipment side. Delivery room CPAP use reduces the need of surfactant and BPD.
- *Other indications*: NCPAP can be used in term neonates with respiratory distress and saturations less than 90% on oxygen hood. A recent multicenter randomized controlled trial from India supports the use of NCPAP in neonates with meconium aspiration syndrome and respiratory distress.[10] Other uses include transient tachypnea of the newborn, tracheobronchomalacia, chronic lung disease, and bronchiolitis.

Contraindications

Nasal continuous positive airway pressure is contraindicated in congenital diaphragmatic hernia, tracheoesophageal fistula, choanal atresia, cleft palate, newborns with poor respiratory efforts, and those with severe cardiovascular instability.

PRINCIPLE OF CONTINUOUS POSITIVE AIRWAY PRESSURE

In CPAP mode of ventilation, positive pressure is generated in the expiratory limb of the breathing circuit when constant/variable flow is obstructed by constant/variable resistance.[11] Such pressure which is applied to spontaneous respiratory efforts both during inspiration and expiration is CPAP. A schematic diagram for understanding of CPAP function is shown in **Figure 1**.

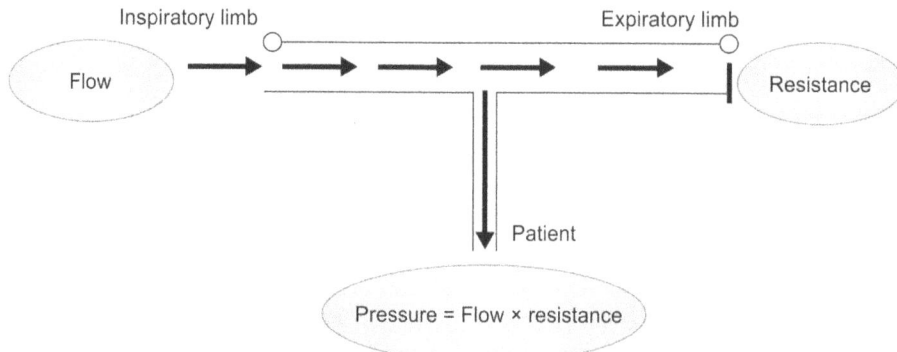

Fig. 1: Principles of continuous positive airway pressure.

Continuous Positive Airway Pressure Types

There are two basic types based on the flow pattern:
1. *Continuous flow devices*: Pressure is generated by changing the resistance. Flow is constant. Examples: Bubble CPAP and Ventilator CPAP.
2. *Variable flow devices*: Pressure is generated by changing the flow. Resistance is constant. Examples: Infant flow driver CPAP, Arabella system, and Viasys.

A comparative table for various types of CPAP is given in **Table 1**. Setting up of NIV involves several aspects for its complete understanding. It includes principles of functioning, types of equipment, components of NIV, type of interfaces, and setting up and initiation of NIV.

Table 1: Comparison of different types of continuous positive airway pressure (CPAP).

Type of CPAP	Ventilator CPAP	Bubble CPAP	Infant flow driver
Mechanism	CPAP is generated by expiratory valve	CPAP is generated by the bubble chamber	CPAP is generated just distal to patient prongs
Flow	Constant	Constant	Variable
CPAP level	Change in pressure is by changing the resistance of the valve	Change in pressure is by changing the length of immersion	Change in pressure is by changing the flow
Advantages	➢ Can be changed to invasive ventilation, if needed	➢ Inexpensive ➢ Bubbling produces better gas exchange ➢ Leaks can be identified as bubbling stops	➢ Reduced work of breathing ➢ Maintains uniform CPAP ➢ Improved lung recruitment
Disadvantages	Expensive	➢ Risk of inadvertent high pressure ➢ No reliable pressure monitor display	➢ Expensive ➢ The physiologic benefits do not translate into improved clinical outcomes

Components of Continuous Positive Airway Pressure

Following are the components of CPAP **(Fig. 2)**:

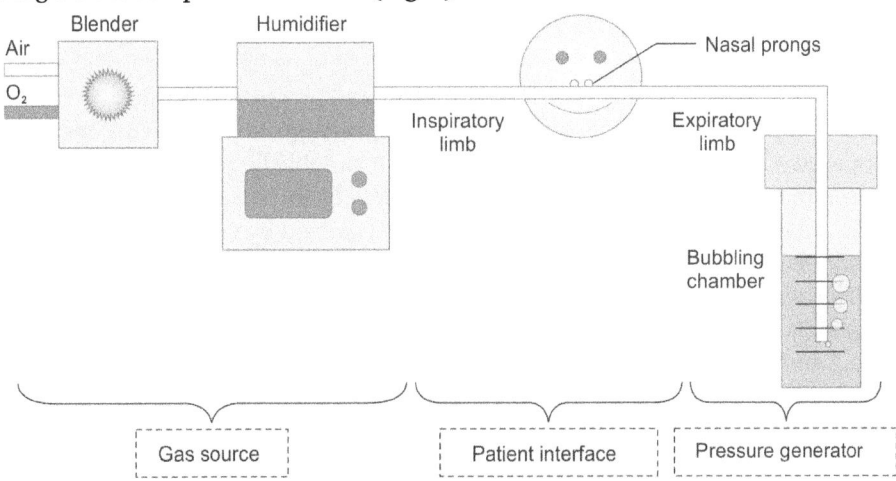

Fig. 2: Components of CPAP delivery system.
(*Source*: Chinnasamy K, Plakkal N, Sivanandan S. CPAP and high flow nasal cannula. In: Bhat BV, Plakkal N (Eds). NICU Protocols of JIPMER. India: Indian Journal of Pediatrics; 2019. pp. 195-205.)

- *Pressure generating device*: Pressure generating mechanism varies according to the type of CPAP.
  - *Continuous flow devices:*
    - Bubble CPAP: Pressure is generated by submerging the expiratory limb into a water chamber and adjusted by altering its depth **(Fig. 3)**. Gas flow is increased until continuous bubbling is achieved. The bubbles in the water chamber have been postulated to provide chest vibrations which may improve gas exchange.

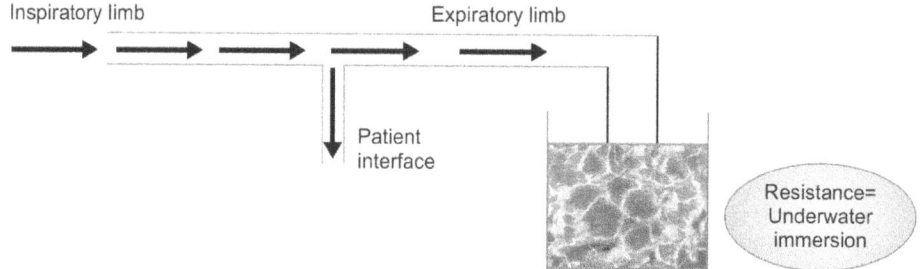

Fig. 3: Depth of underwater immersion regulates continuous positive airway pressure (CPAP) in a bubble CPAP system.

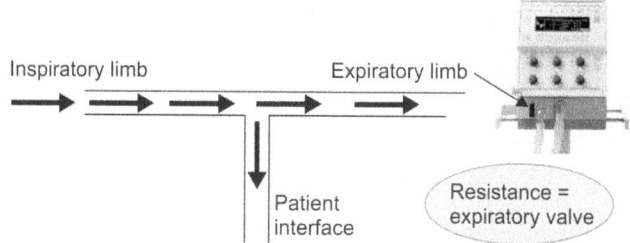

Fig. 4: Expiratory valve regulates continuous positive airway pressure (CPAP) in a ventilator.

    - Ventilator: Pressure is generated at the exhalation valve **(Fig. 4)**. The CPAP level is increased or decreased by varying the ventilator exhalation orifice size. This type of CPAP has an integrated nasal interface and pressure generator.
  - *Variable flow devices*: CPAP level is generated by varying the flow near the nasal interface. Special prongs and flow generator are used for variable flow CPAP. A higher gas flow is used in these devices and pressure is generated by increased resistance as gas leaves the nasal device (Coanda effect). Pressure is changed by varying the flow of gas into the device **(Figs. 5A to C)**. Because of fluidic flip of inspiratory gases during exhalation, the work of breathing is decreased in variable flow system.[12] In physiological studies variable flow CPAP has been shown to achieve consistent CPAP.[13]
- *Heating and humidification*: The inspiratory gases delivered to the baby should be heated and humidified as poor humidification results in mucosal injury, mucociliary dysfunction, and bronchospasm. Servo-controlled humidifiers are preferable.
- *Blended gas source*: For delivery of optimum fractional concentration of inspired oxygen [fraction of inspired oxygen (FiO_2)] to maintain target saturation in the range of 90–95%, a blender is a must. It helps in prevention of free radical oxygen injury, chronic lung disease, and retinopathy of prematurity.

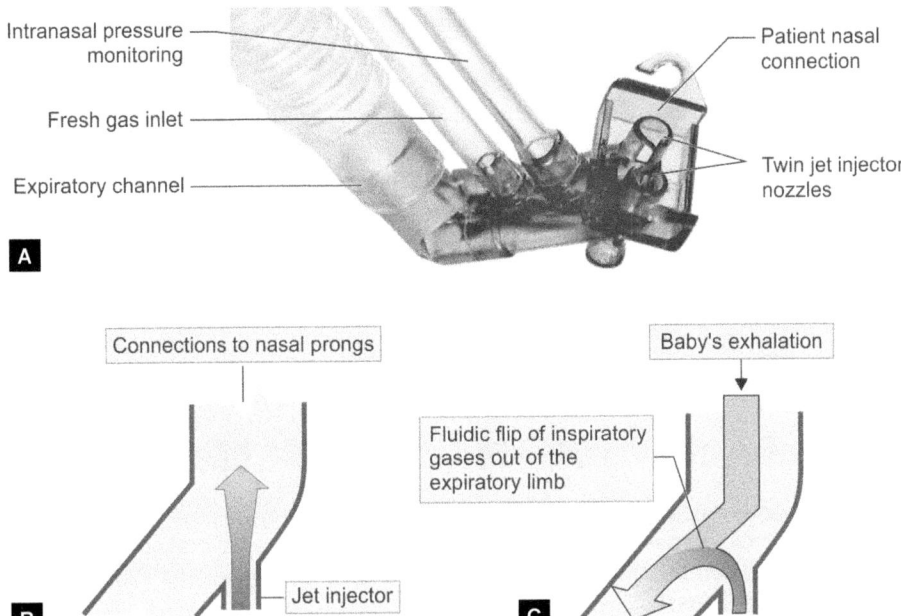

Figs. 5A to C: (A) Photograph of the infant flow driver pressure generator without the nasal prongs; (B and C) Schematic representations of the "fluid flip" of the variable-flow continuous positive airway pressure (CPAP) device; (B) During the child's inspiration, the gas flow is directed towards each nostril due to Bernoulli's effect to maintain a constant pressure; (C) During the child's exhalation, the Coandă effect causes inspiratory flow to "flip" and leave the generator chamber via the expiratory limb. (*Courtesy*: Electro Medical Equipment, Ltd.; Brighton, England.)

- *Patient interface:* The various types of nasal interfaces are:
  - Nasal prongs
  - Nasal mask
  - Nasal cannula
  - Nasopharyngeal prongs

  Amongst all nasal interfaces the short binasal prongs have been shown to be most effective.[14] Various types of nasal interfaces and their fixation have been shown in **Figures 6 and 7**. Nasal interfaces vary in size, configuration, material, and diameter. These factors affect the resistance to flow and may lead to variation in the pressure delivered at the baby's nares or nasopharynx.

- *Nasal prongs:* Nasal prongs are the most commonly used interface for NCPAP. The various types of nasal prongs have been compared by De Paoli et al. for pressure drop for various rates of gas flow.[15] It was observed that there was much variation in pressure drop amongst different devices and least pressure drop occurred with the infant flow system. In a Cochrane review, the same authors have concluded that binasal short prongs are more effective than nasopharyngeal prongs for avoiding reintubation.

- *Nasal mask:* Nasal mask has a configuration similar to the shape of the nose. It is helpful when nares are very small to accommodate nasal prongs. They are also used along with nasal prongs alternatively for an interval to minimize the pressure effects of the prongs on nares.

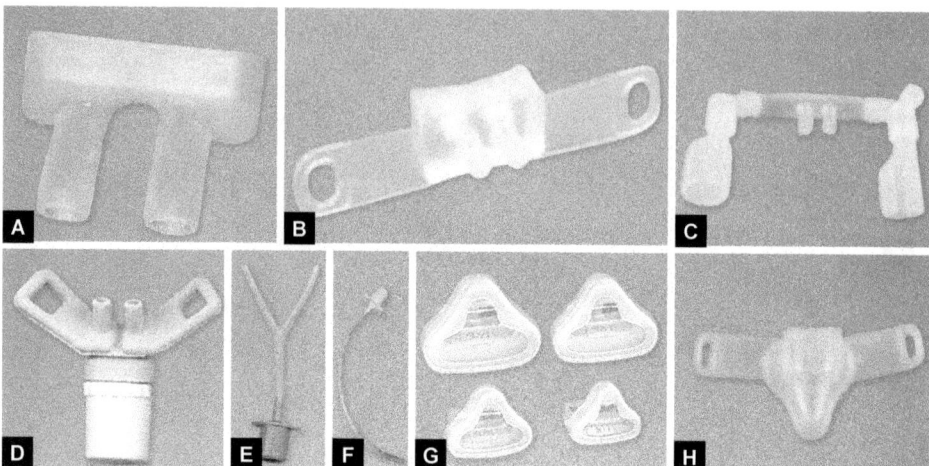

Figs. 6A to H: Various types of nasal interfaces. (A) Fisher and Paykel nasal prongs; (B) Draeger nasal prongs; (C) Hudson nasal prongs; (D) Argyle nasal prongs; (E) Nasopharyngeal prongs; (F) Endotracheal tube can be used as single nasopharyngeal; (G) Fisher and Paykel nasal mask; (G and H) Draeger nasal mask.

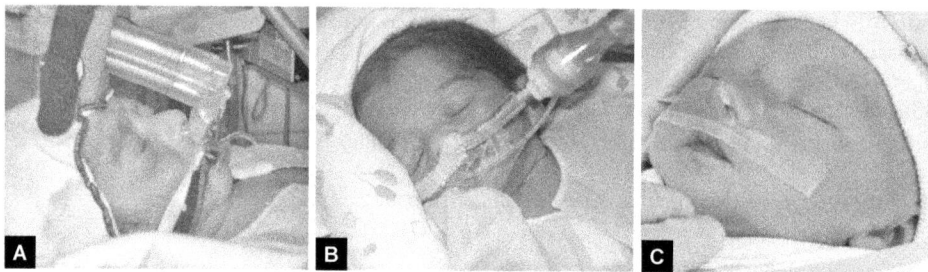

Figs. 7A to C: (A) Secure fixation of nasal prongs; (B) Endotracheal tube being used as a single nasopharyngeal prong; (C) Application of protective dressing (Cannulaide) for decreasing nasal trauma.

- *Nasal cannula*: Nasal cannula is generally used for oxygen delivery. It may provide some distending pressure depending on the flow rate, size of the cannula, degree of leak, and size of the nares. The RAM nasal cannula which was originally designed for oxygen delivery is also found to be a useful NCPAP interface. It bears short binasal prongs on larger caliber tubing than the standard oxygen cannula.
- *Nasopharyngeal prongs*: Long nasal or nasopharyngeal prongs lead to increased resistance and high work of breathing. It could be either single or binasopharyngeal prongs. A cut endotracheal tube from the nares to the nasopharynx may work as a single nasopharyngeal prong **(Fig. 7B)**. Nasopharyngeal prongs are infrequently used.

Other parts of the nasal interface kit include caps, fixing straps, and nasal tubings. A comparative table of the different types of nasal interfaces is given in **Table 2**.

Table 2: Comparison of various continuous positive airway pressure (CPAP) interfaces.

Interface type	Advantages	Disadvantages
Nasal prongs, e.g., Fisher and Paykel, Argyll, Hudson, and Draeger	➤ Lower resistance ➤ Easily available	➤ Nasal trauma ➤ Difficult to fix
Nasopharyngeal prongs, e.g., cut endotracheal tube	➤ Easily available ➤ More secure fixation	➤ More resistance ➤ Easily blocked ➤ Likely to get kinked
Nasal cannula, e.g. RAM's cannula	➤ Easily applicable	➤ Unreliable pressure, fraction of inspired oxygen (FiO_2) ➤ Large leaks around the cannula
Nasal mask	➤ Less nasal trauma	➤ Difficulty in maintaining good seal

How to Set up a Continuous Positive Airway Pressure?

- Identify the baby with respiratory distress and in need of CPAP by respiratory distress scoring (Silverman-Anderson Score ≥3 in preterm babies and ≥5 in term neonates).
- Monitor and record the vitals.
- Connect air and oxygen tubing to pressurized central source or to air compressor and oxygen cylinder. Attach the tubings to blender for controlled FiO_2 delivery. Switch on the humidifier.
- Assemble the sterile CPAP circuit. Disposable circuits are preferable.
- *Inspiratory limb*: Components of inspiratory limb are from flow meter to humidifier and then tubing carrying heated and humidified gas from humidifier to patient end at the nasal interface.
- *Expiratory limb*: In case of bubble CPAP it goes from the patient's nasal interface to the water chamber where depth of its insertion determines the pressure. In case of ventilator CPAP the expiratory limb goes from patient's nasal interface to expiratory valve of the ventilator.
- The most important aspect of CPAP set up is positioning and fixation of nasal interface. The ideal technique of fixation depends on the type of CPAP equipment.
- Identify the right-sized prongs and mask with the help of manufacturer's guide. The nasal prong should fit snugly in the nasal cavity to avoid significant leak. Loose prongs will not deliver CPAP adequately and tight prongs will lead to nasal trauma. A small piece of Tegaderm which covers the philtrum and nasal septum can help in decreasing nasal injury due to CPAP interface. The same purpose can be done by other commercially available protective dressings; e.g. Cannulaide **(Fig. 7C)**. A gap of 2-3 mm should be maintained between the nasal septum and nasal prongs to decrease the chances of trauma to the nasal septum **(Fig. 7A)**. A nasal trauma monitoring chart is given in **Figure 8**.
- Fix the proper sized cap. The cap is chosen on the basis of head circumference and weight. The cap should be placed above the eyebrows, passing over the ears and reaching up to the back of the neck.
- Fix the cap, prongs, and interface with the help of fixing straps and velcro. The set pressure may not be delivered to the baby if the mouth remains persistently open. A chin strap or pacifier may be used to counter this. There is increase of pressure in the nasopharynx by 2-3 cm of H_2O if chin strap is used.
- Connect the ventilator circuit.
- Humidifier should be filled with distilled water.

Section 8: Neonatology and Pediatrics

		\multicolumn{21}{c	}{Score}
Date																						
Shift		AM	PM	Night shift	AM	PM	Night shift	AM	PM	Night shift	AM	PM	Night shift	AM	PM	Night shift	AM	PM	Night shift	AM	PM	Night shift
Internal nare	Left																					
	Right																					
External nare	Left																					
	Right																					
Philtrum																						
Septum																						
Total score																						

Score: 0 = normal, 1 = pink/red, 2 = bleeding/ulcer/scab, 3 = skin tear

Fig. 8: Nasal trauma scoring chart for babies on continuous positive airway pressure (CPAP).

- Connect the circuit to the nasal interface. Check for any leaks.
- Orogastric tube should be in situ which helps in gastric decompression and feeding. CPAP is not a contraindication for enteral feeding and normal feeding protocol should be followed in a baby on NCPAP.
- CPAP delivery in neonates involves giving heated humidified (37°C and 100%) oxygen and air mixture with oxygen concentration range of 21–100% at a flow of 6–8 L/min to achieve a pressure of 4–8 cm of H_2O. The initial setting of CPAP for a neonate depends on the indication for CPAP and will be discussed in the section on clinical application of NIV.

Initial Settings

Presence of good spontaneous breathing is a prerequisite for starting NCPAP. CPAP delivery in neonates involves giving heated humidified (37°C and 100%) oxygen and air mixture with oxygen concentration (FiO_2) range of 21–100% at a flow of 6–8 L/min to achieve pressure of 4–8 cm of H_2O. Initial settings of pressure and FiO_2 in various disease conditions are as follows:
- Neonate with respiratory distress—pressure: 5 cm of H_2O and FiO_2: 30–60%
- Apnea—pressure: 4 cm of H_2O and FiO_2: <25%
- Postextubation—pressure: 5 cm of H_2O and FiO_2: Same as it was on MV.

Adjustment of Continuous Positive Airway Pressure Settings

Adjustment of settings is primarily based on clinical assessment of respiratory distress. Chest X-ray (CXR) and blood gas further helps in titration of CPAP parameters.
- *Pressure*: In case of persistent retractions the CPAP pressure is to be increased in steps of 1 cm H_2O to a maximum of 8 cm H_2O. Pressure is adjusted to minimize chest retractions, visualization of 6–8 posterior ribs on CXR and partial pressure of arterial oxygen (PaO_2) >50 mm Hg.
- *Flow*: Usually kept at 6–8 L/min. In case of bubble CPAP if no or poor bubbling is seen, check for leaks in the circuit and then increase the flow. Too high flows result in wastage of gases, turbulence, and inadvertent high pressure.
- *FiO_2*: In case of oxygen saturation less than 90%, the FiO_2 should be titrated in steps of 5% to maintain target saturations [peripheral capillary oxygen saturation (SpO_2)] of 90–95%. Increase pressure before FiO_2 for better oxygenation.

Weaning from CPAP

- When the disease process is passive, consider weaning from CPAP.
- For apnea, NCPAP may be discontinued after 24–48 hours of apnea free period.
- Gradual decrease of FiO_2 from 30 to 21% (steps of 5%).
- Decrease CPAP to 4 cm H_2O (steps of 1 cm H_2O).
- If CPAP of 4 cm H_2O and FiO_2 <30% and clinically well (no respiratory distress, SpO_2 >90% and normal blood gas), remove CPAP.

Failure of CPAP

Before considering failure, ensure the following:
- Neck position is appropriate and airway is clear
- Nasal prongs or mask are correct size and fit properly
- There is no leak in the circuit
- Humidification is adequate and no condensation is there in the circuit
- Surfactant, if needed, was given and the neonate is not fighting the machine.

Presence of the following failure criteria warrants administration of surfactant and/or MV:
- Increase in oxygen needs with FiO_2 more than 60% on CPAP >8 cm H_2O, associated with increased work of breathing.[16]
- Respiratory acidosis with pH <7.20 with partial pressure of carbon dioxide (PCO_2) >65 mm Hg.
- Recurrent apnea, presence of retractions, and grunting even on maximum permissible settings on CPAP are also indications for MV.

NONINVASIVE POSITIVE PRESSURE VENTILATION

Noninvasive positive pressure ventilation is a bridge between CPAP and invasive ventilation. NIPPV is a form of ventilatory assistance which provides greater level of respiratory support than NCPAP. In neonates, with poor respiratory drive and weak inspiratory efforts, NCPAP may be ineffective and will lead to failure. NIPPV provides positive pressure above CPAP to the neonate's spontaneous efforts which are patient triggered (synchronized) or machine triggered and time cycled. It is given either as synchronized or nonsynchronized NIPPV with conventional ventilators. NIPPV may prevent intubation in a larger percentage of neonates who fail NCPAP.

Indications

- *Respiratory distress*: Early NIPPV appears to be superior to NCPAP alone for decreasing respiratory failure and the need for intubation and endotracheal tube ventilation among preterm infants with respiratory distress syndrome. However, it does not decrease mortality or the incidence of BPD.[17] NIPPV can be used in any neonate with respiratory distress as initial support.
- *Apnea of prematurity*: NIPPV has positive effects on preterm infants with severe and frequent apnea.[18]
- *Postextubation*: Use of NIPPV increases extubation success.[19]
- *NCPAP failure*: A trial of NIPPV can be considered in newborns who do not tolerate NCPAP.

Noninvasive Positive Pressure Ventilation Devices

The devices which can be used to give NIPPV include any conventional ventilators with time cycled pressure limited mode which is capable of providing NCPAP and intermittent mandatory ventilation can deliver NIPPV. With this there would be some alarms about leak and low pressure which can be taken care of by adjustments in ventilatory settings.

The devices for synchronized noninvasive positive pressure ventilation (SNIPPV) are few. SNIPPV can also be delivered with the noninvasive assist/control (N-A/C) and noninvasive pressure support ventilation (N-PSV) modes to assist every spontaneous breath. SNIPPV can be provided by Servo-I ventilator from Maquet Medical System, Sechrist IV-200 SAVI ventilator and nasal flow-synchronized ventilator from Ginevri. SNIPPV has been shown to be better in terms of improved pulmonary mechanics, stability of chest wall, increased tidal and minute volumes, thoracoabdominal motion synchrony, and decreased flow resistance and work of breathing. However, clinical outcomes have not been different for various short-term and long-term neonatal morbidities when NIPPV is compared to SNIPPV.

The method of synchronization involves detection and feedback of patient's inspiratory efforts. The common methods of synchronization are:

- Graseby pressure capsule is a transducer sensor which is placed on the abdomen. It detects abdominal movement as respiratory effort for feedback and synchronization. It is the most commonly used method of synchronization.
- Flow sensors at the patient end on the nasal interface detect patient's inspiratory efforts. It requires frequent sensitivity adjustments for leak compensation around patient's efforts.
- *Neurally adjusted ventilator assist*: It uses electrical activity of diaphragm (EAdi) as inspiratory effort. To detect EAdi, a special sensor is placed in the esophagus, similar to the placement of an orogastric tube.
- *Internal flow sensors*: In some ventilators, flow sensor is inside rather than being at patient's end, but its use in NIV is lacking.

Noninvasive Positive Pressure Ventilation Nasal Interface

Almost all the nasal interfaces which are used to deliver NCPAP can be used for NIPPV. There are no comparative studies to suggest that any one of the nasal interfaces is better than another. In view of the same, the short binasal prongs are recommended, given the ease of use, and decreased susceptibility to blockage secondary to secretions as in case of NCPAP.

Initial Settings

Initial settings for various respiratory conditions are given in **Table 3**.

Adjustment of Noninvasive Positive Pressure Ventilation Settings

- *PIP*: Adjustment of PIP is done based on chest expansion, blood gas parameters (PaO_2 and $PaCO_2$), and target oxygen saturations of 90–95%.
- *PEEP*: PEEP is adjusted according to chest retractions, lung expansion on CXR, and target oxygen saturations of 90–95%.
- FiO_2: Alterations are made to maintain target oxygen saturations of 90–95% and PaO_2 >50–60 mm Hg.
- *Frequency*: It is modified according to central respiratory drive and $PaCO_2$ values.

Table 3: Initial settings in various disease conditions.

Condition	*PIP*	*PEEP*	*FiO2*	*Frequency*	*Time*
Respiratory distress	2–4 cm H_2O above PIP during manual ventilation	5 cm H_2O	40–50%	40/min	0.35–0.45 s
Postextubation	14–16 cm H_2O (based on PIP during invasive MV)	5 cm H_2O	Same as during invasive MV	20–25/min	0.35–0.45 s
Apnea of prematurity	14–15 cm H_2O	4 cm H_2O	21–30%	20–25/min	0.35–0.45 s

(FiO_2: fraction of inspired oxygen; MV: mechanical ventilation; PEEP: positive end-expiratory pressure; PIP: peak inspiratory pressure)

Failure of Noninvasive Positive Pressure Ventilation

Failure of NIPPV is considered when the following criteria are present:

- FiO_2 requirement more than 70% with maximum settings of PIP >22 mm Hg and PEEP >8 cm H_2O.[16]
- Presence of respiratory acidosis with pH <7.25 and $PaCO_2$ >60 mm Hg.
- Recurrent episodes of apnea requiring bag and mask ventilation.

MONITORING AND NURSING CARE

Monitoring in a baby on NIV includes monitoring of the neonate, the CPAP machine, and the nasal interface **(Fig. 9)**.

Patient name:
Medical registration no:
Diagnosis:
NICU day:

Page-1 →	Date and time	HR	Color	RD score	MAP/PI	PEEP	Flow	FiO_2	SPO_2	Apnea	Blood gas	CXR

Page-2 →	Date and time	Humidifier water lavel	Humidifier temperature	Humidifier mode	CPAP *exp. limb depth	Bubbles*	Nasal interface	Nasal trauma	Fixing straps	OG tube	Oral secretions	Circuit leak

*If bubble CPAP is used

Fig. 9: Sample monitoring chart for newborns on NIV. (CPAP: continuous positive airway pressure; CXR: chest X-ray; FiO_2: fraction of inspired oxygen; HR: heart rate; MAP: mean airway pressure; NICU: neonatal intensive care unit; NIV: noninvasive ventilation; OG: orogastric; PEEP: positive end-expiratory pressure; PI: inspiratory pressure; SpO_2: peripheral capillary oxygen saturation)

- Neonate:
  - Vitals: Temperature, heart rate (HR), respiratory rate, capillary filling time (CFT), SpO_2, perfusion index (PI), and blood pressure (BP).
  - Airway: Look for oronasal secretions which can obstruct the airway. If mouth remains persistently open and CPAP delivery is not adequate with persistent distress, chin strap may be considered.
  - Respiratory: An objective scoring system such as Downes or Silverman-Anderson Score **(Tables 4 and 5)** can be used. Watch for apnea and monitor for nasal trauma.

Table 4: Modified Downes score system for term newborn.

Score	0	1	2
Respiratory rate	<60	60–80	>80 or apneic episodes
Central cyanosis	None	None on room air	Present on 40% fraction of inspired oxygen (FiO_2)
Retractions	None	Mild	Moderate to severe
Grunting	None	Audible with stethoscope	Audible without stethoscope
Air entry	Good	Decreased	Barely audible

Mild: 0–3; moderate: 4–6; severe: 7–10
A score of >6 is indicative of impending respiratory failure.

Table 5: Silverman-Anderson scoring system for preterm neonate.

Score	0	1	2
Upper chest retractions	Synchronized	Lag during inspiration	See-saw respiration
Lower chest retractions	None	Just visible	Marked
Xiphoid retractions	None	Just visible	Marked
Nasal flaring	None	Minimal	Marked
Expiratory grunt	None	Audible with stethoscope	Audible with unaided ear

A score of >6 is indicative of impending respiratory failure.

  - Hemodynamic stability.
  - Central nervous system: Activity, irritability, and pain.
  - Monitor for abdominal distension. Orogastric tube may be left open half an hour after feeding and the end of the tube should be above the patient level to decompress the stomach. CPAP belly is a benign phenomenon in which abdomen appears full in a baby on CPAP. It is not an indication to stop feeds.
- Investigations:
  - Chest X-ray: A CXR may be obtained at the time of admission to look for lung pathology and expansion. A lung expansion up to six anterior and eight posterior ribs is normal. Further X-rays should be done in case of acute deterioration.
  - Blood gas analysis: Normal targets for blood gas are as:
    - PaO_2: 60–80 mm Hg
    - SpO_2: 90–95%
    - $PaCO_2$: <50–60 mm Hg

- pH: ≥ 7.25
- Lactate: More than 2 mmol/L
○ *Equipment and interface*:
  - Ensure appropriate size of cap/mask and proper fit.
  - Secure fixation of interface and ensure small gap between the interface and columella.
  - Check for displacement of prongs/blockage of prongs with secretions. If any, then clean and ensure patency of prongs. If there are secretions in nose then, clean the nostrils with saline and suction the secretions.
  - Look for bubbles in case of bubble CPAP. Monitor for depth of insertion of the tube of expiratory limb for CPAP generation.
  - Ensure that the humidifier is working properly and chamber is filled with sterile water. No condensation should be there in circuit.
  - Monitor set and delivered parameters.

COMPLICATIONS OF NONINVASIVE VENTILATION

These are common to both NCPAP and NIPPV.
○ *Nasal effects*: Interface-related nasal erosions, necrosis, and nasal obstruction.
○ *Pulmonary effects*: Pneumothorax and pulmonary interstitial emphysema, especially seen with high pressure settings in NIPPV.
○ *Gastrointestinal effects*: Abdominal distension and perforation.
○ *Cardiovascular effects*: Decreased venous return and cardiac output, hypotension, raised intracranial pressure, and decreased glomerular filtration rate.
○ Rare complications include subcutaneous emphysema of scalp, pneumocephalus, perforated ear drum, local infections, and sepsis.

BILEVEL CONTINUOUS POSITIVE AIRWAY PRESSURE

Devices that cycle between two levels of positive airway pressure at set frequency [bilevel positive airway pressure (BiPAP). These devices generate PIP typically between 9 and 11 cm of H_2O and use longer inspiratory time. Examples of BiPAP devices are the flow-driver "SiPAP" and infant flow driver advance by CareFusion.

This form of respiratory support utilizes two levels of positive pressure in the airway, where the neonate can breathe spontaneously. It increases mean airway pressure without attaining peak values typical of positive pressure ventilation. Its indications for use in neonatology include mild to moderate RDS and as a rescue strategy in babies who do not tolerate intubation, surfactant administration, and extubation to CPAP (INSURE) before MV.[1] Suggested initial settings are as follows:
○ Low level of pressure: 4–6 cm H_2O
○ High level of pressure: 8–20 cm H_2O
○ Time of high level pressure (Ti): 0.7–1 second
○ Rate: 20–40 pre minute
○ FiO_2 adjusted to maintain SpO_2 90–95%.
Monitoring and side effects are same as other methods of NIV.

NEWER METHODS

- *SiPAP*: SiPAP is a second-generation respiratory infant flow device that provides patient triggered, bilevel nasal CPAP for the spontaneously breathing newborn through the delivery of sighs above a baseline CPAP pressure.[20]
- *NHFV*: NHFV uses lower pressure and smaller volumes at a higher frequency and may be more lung protective than are other higher pressure NIV modes. In this mode high frequency breaths are delivered by nasal interface. It uses smaller pressures and tidal volumes at higher frequencies as compared to other forms of NIV. The ventilators which can apply NHFV are Infrasonics Infant Star and Draeger VN500. The nasal interface is either a nasopharyngeal endotracheal tube or binasal prongs.
- *NAVA*: NAVA is a novel form of noninvasive respiratory support which is used in both intubated and nonintubated babies and it uses the electrical activity of the diaphragm to determine the timing and magnitude of inspiratory pressure delivery during spontaneous breathing.[20] To detect EAdi, miniature electrodes are used which are fixed on conventional feeding tube. The EAdi signal is used to trigger and cycle the ventilator. The EAdi signal cannot be acquired in case of apnea, deep sedation, and poor respiratory drive. NIV-NAVA is possible only in neonates with good respiratory effort.

KEY POINTS

- Use of NIV is increasing in neonatology in order to prevent adverse effects associated with invasive ventilation.
- Respiratory distress syndrome, AOP, and postextubation respiratory support are the three main indications for NIV.
- Early use of NCPAP in preterm neonates with RDS decreases the need for MV in short-term and BPD and/or death at 36 weeks corrected gestation.
- NIPPV acts as a bridge between CPAP and invasive ventilation.
- The main indication for use of bilevel CPAP is for mild-to-moderate respiratory distress.
- Close monitoring and good nursing care are required for optimal outcomes.

REFERENCES

1. Courtney SE, Barrington KJ. Continuous positive airway pressure and noninvasive ventilation. Clin Perinatol. 2007;34(1):73-92.
2. Diblasi RM. Nasal continuous positive airway pressure (CPAP) for the respiratory care of the newborn infant. Respir Care. 2009;54(9):1209-35.
3. Maffei G, Gorgoglione S, Vento G. Noninvasive ventilation: systemic approach and new perspectives for preterm infants. J Clin Neonatol. 2017; 6:135-43.
4. Morley CJ, Davis PG, Doyle LW, Brion LP, Hascoet JM, Carlin JB. COIN Trial Investigators. Nasal CPAP or intubation at birth for very preterm infants. N Engl J Med. 2008;358:700-8.
5. SUPPORT Study Group of the Eunice Kennedy Shriver NICHD Neonatal Research Network, Finer NN, Carlo WA, Walsh MC, Rich W, Gantz MG, et al. Early CPAP versus surfactant in extremely preterm infants. N Engl J Med. 2010;362:1970-9.
6. Subramaniam P, Ho JJ, Davis PG. Prophylactic nasal continuous positive airway pressure for preventing morbidity and mortality in very preterm infants. Cochrane Database Syst Rev. 2016;(11):CD001243.
7. Martin RJ, Abu-Shaweesh JM. Control of breathing and neonatal apnea. Biol Neonate. 2005;87:288-95.
8. Davis PG, Henderson-Smart DJ. Nasal continuous positive airways pressure immediately after extubation for preventing morbidity in preterm infants. Cochrane Database Syst Rev. 2003;2:CD000143.

9. Sweet DG, Carnielli V, Greisen G, Hallman M, Ozek E, Plavka R, et al. European consensus guidelines on the management of neonatal respiratory distress syndrome in preterm infants—2013 update. Neonatology. 2013;103:353-68.
10. Pandita A, Murki S, Oleti TP, Tandur B, Kiran S, Narkhede S, et al. Effect of Nasal Continuous Positive Airway Pressure on Infants with Meconium Aspiration Syndrome: A Randomized Clinical Trial. JAMA Pediatr. 2018;172(2):161-65.
11. Gupta S, and Donn SM. Continuous positive airway pressure: physiology and comparison of devices. Semin Fetal Neonatal Med. 2016;21:204-11.
12. Pandit PB, Courtney SE, Pyon KH, et al. Work of breathing during constant- and variable-flow nasal continuous positive airway pressure in preterm neonates. Pediatrics. 2001;108:682-85.
13. Moa G, Nilsson K, Zetterström H, Jonsson LO. A new device for administration of nasal continuous positive airway pressure in the newborn: an experimental study. Crit Care Med. 1988;16:1238-42.
14. Courtney SE, Pyon KH, Saslow JG, et al. Lung recruitment and breathing pattern during variable versus continuous flow nasal continuous positive airway pressure in premature infants: an evaluation of three devices. Pediatrics. 2001;107:304-08.
15. De Paoli AG, Davis PG, Faber B, et al. Devices and pressure sources for administration of nasal continuous positive airway pressure in preterm neonates. Cochrane Database Syst Rev. 2008;23(1):CD002977.
16. Kallem VR, Murki S. Noninvasive Ventilation: CPAP, HHHFNC and NIPPV. In Bhat R, Kumar P, Vidyasagar D, (eds). The Handbook of Neonatology. India: Indian Journal of Pediatrics. 2018;313-23.
17. Lemyre B, Laughon M, Bose C, Davis PG. Early nasal intermittent positive pressure ventilation (NIPPV) versus early nasal continuous positive airway pressure (NCPAP) for preterm infants. Cochrane Database Syst Rev. 2016;12:CD005384.
18. Lemyre B, Davis PG, de Paoli AG. Nasal intermittent positive pressure ventilation (NIPPV) versus nasal continuous positive airway pressure (NCPAP) for apnea of prematurity. Cochrane Database Syst Rev. 2002;(1):CD002272.
19. Lemyre B, Davis PG, De Paoli AG, Kirpalani H. Nasal intermittent positive pressure ventilation (NIPPV) versus nasal continuous positive airway pressure (NCPAP) for preterm neonates after extubation. Cochrane Database Syst Rev. 2017;2:CD003212.
20. DiBlasi RM. Neonatal noninvasive ventilation techniques: do we really need to intubate? Respir Care. 2011;56(9):1273-94.

Chapter 39

Heated Humidified High Flow Nasal Cannula Therapy in Neonates and Children

Rajeev Kumar Thapar, Safal Muhammed MK

▍INTRODUCTION

Heated humidified high flow nasal cannula (HFNC) oxygen therapy was described as a mode of respiratory therapy in premature neonates as early as 1991;[1] however, in recent years, it has gained recognition as the first-line respiratory support in all age groups, for various indications and also, in different settings. HFNC is a technique for providing noninvasive ventilation by delivering high-flow rates using specific devices.

Over the years, a lot of experience in using HFNC has accumulated in respiratory distress syndrome, apnea of prematurity, anticipated/impending respiratory failure, and management of babies immediately after extubation and in various clinical settings such as emergency departments, wards, intensive care units (ICUs), and labor rooms.[2]

Conventionally, nasal cannulae were used for oxygen therapy. However, with the understanding that an appropriate flow rate of gas (air, oxygen, or its mixture) with a snug or a loose fit of the cannula can generate positive pressure; high-flow nasal cannula is being increasingly recognized as an effective means for providing noninvasive ventilation.[1] There is currently no single, simple definition of "high flow" but it is generally agreed that a system that delivers an oxygen-air mixture that meets or exceeds the patient's spontaneous inspiratory demand is a high-flow system. Gas flow rates exceeding 1–2 liters/min (LPM) in neonates were considered high flow but recently flows up to 8 LPM in toddlers and up to 60 LPM have been used in adults.

Based on physiological studies by Hough et al., flow rates more than 1.7 L/kg/min (rounded to 2 L/kg/min) were recommended.[3] There is no recommendation on the upper flow limits but in various studies of infants with bronchiolitis, flow rates of 2 L/kg/min were found to be well tolerated.[4] These high-flow rates need heating and humidification. Devices that can effectively heat and humidify gas at very high-flow rates are considered HFNCs. The advantages of heating and humidification are in preventing drying of nasal passages, mucosal injury, and impaired secretion clearance, which is seen with dry, cold air at high flow rates.

Evidence that nasal cannula can provide continuous positive airway pressure (CPAP) has been available for some time now. Since the pressure delivered cannot be titrated reliably, nasal cannula was not conventionally considered as a mode for providing nasal CPAP in infants. Recent studies, however, have demonstrated that HFNC was as efficacious and safe as conventional CPAP and also delivered comparable distending pressures.[5]

MECHANISMS OF ACTION

Nasal CPAP (NCPAP) acts by providing a continuous distending pressure to the airways and improving the functional residual capacity (FRC). The cardinal difference between nasal CPAP and HFNC is that the pressure delivered by the latter is unpredictable and variable whereas nasal CPAP devices deliver constant distending pressures.[6] Hence nasal CPAP devices require snugly fitting nasal cannula with minimal leakage. HFNC, on the other hand, requires smaller caliber cannula to ensure that a certain amount of air leak always exists. This leak is a safety measure to minimize the risk of delivering excessively high distending pressure, which can cause barotrauma and pneumothorax.

HFNC supports respiration through multiple mechanisms:[3]

- Reduces the dead space by flushing the upper airways of CO_2, thus improving the gas exchange at the alveolar level.
- Provides constant distending pressure which helps in alveolar recruitment; however, the distending pressure delivered depends upon the flow rate and the leak around the nasal cannula.
- HFNC provides a sufficiently high inspiratory flow rate which helps in splinting airways, reducing the patient's inspiratory work of breathing.
- By providing a flow rate which is greater than the minute ventilation of the patient, HFNC minimizes the inspiration of room air. The upper airways are filled with the higher concentration of O_2 as per the set fraction of inspired oxygen (FiO_2). These two factors help to ensure that HFNC devices deliver the FiO_2 set by the treating clinician.
- Humidification minimizes the effects of drying and cooling of the inspired air, which improves the aerodynamics and minimizes injury to the respiratory epithelium. It also minimizes injury to the nasal alae and septum which may be seen in infants who receive nasal CPAP for a long time. Humidification and warming of the gases in the upper airway require energy; this is conserved in HFNC.
- The nasopharynx normally offers resistance to the inspiratory gas flow. Due to the high flow of gases with HFNC, this resistance is decreased.

Patients tend to tolerate HFNC much better than conventional noninvasive ventilation using face mask. It is easier for them to expectorate secretions. Patients can continue to receive enteral feeds (if the primary pathology permits), express themselves verbally and actively participate in physical therapy. Avoiding the application of face mask and sedation augments the comfort level of the patients and hastens recovery.

LIMITATIONS

High flow nasal cannula is not useful in diseases in which delivery of a constant CPAP is mandatory. Examples of conditions where HFNC is not beneficial include bronchomalacia, neuromuscular disorders, clinically significant lung collapse, and severe hypoxemia.

It must be reiterated to all the support staff and paramedics involved in patient care that HFNC is not just a "simple nasal cannula." On the contrary, HFNC provides a high level of respiratory support which is almost equivalent to nasal CPAP. Any patient on HFNC not demonstrating significant improvement in respiratory distress or work of breathing must be immediately assessed to identify requirement of more aggressive modes of respiratory support. Thus training of the support staff is necessary to prevent underdiagnosis of clinical deterioration of a patient on HFNC.

The side effects of HFNC include gas trapping, air leak, and nasal mucosal injury. The latter two occur at much lower rates as compared to NCPAP.

INDICATIONS OF HIGH FLOW NASAL CANNULA

HFNC in Neonates[6,7]

- Mild/moderate respiratory distress; as an alternative to NCPAP
- Requiring > 1 L/min of oxygen therapy
- Postextubation scenario
- Nasal trauma from NCPAP
- Apnea of prematurity[8]
- Chronic lung disease (CLD)

The bulk of the literature supporting the use of HFNC in neonates is for its use as postextubation support; as compared to nasal CPAP, it causes less nasal trauma and is also associated with less pneumothorax.[9] Further evidence is required comparing HFNC with other forms of noninvasive respiratory support immediately after birth as the primary mode of ventilation.[10,11]

HFNC in Infants and Older Children

Currently, there is ample evidence available that indicates that HFNC therapy is feasible, effective, safe, and well tolerated as a form of respiratory support in infants with bronchiolitis.[4,12-14] Studies have demonstrated reduced work of breathing and improved gas exchange when HFNC is used in infants with bronchiolitis. It is indicated for hypoxemic infants who do not respond to standard subnasal oxygen therapy. However, in children with increased work of breathing, nasal CPAP has been shown to be better.[13] HFNC has also been shown to be safe, with very low incidence of air leaks.[14] Over the last decade, HFNC is not only being used in the pediatric intensive care units (PICUs), but also in other areas such as pediatric emergency department and general pediatric wards. In fact, it might be possible to decrease ICU admissions due to bronchiolitis with the administration of HFNC outside the ICU.[14]

High flow nasal cannula was found to be safe and effective in improving hypoxemia after extubation in infants after elective cardiac surgery in a single center prospective trial.[15] The use of HFNC for this indication requires further validation in larger studies.

High flow nasal cannula has been evaluated in acute exacerbations of bronchial asthma, another common lower airway obstructive disease of childhood. In a Spanish pilot trial published in 2018, children with moderate-to-severe asthma exacerbations responded better to HFNC as compared to conventional oxygen therapy in the first 2 hours after therapy was started in the emergency department.[16] Other studies in children with acute exacerbations of asthma presenting to the emergency department or in the PICU have shown it to be superior to standard oxygen therapy but not superior to noninvasive ventilation [CPAP or (bilevel positive airway pressure (BIPAP) therapy].

Other indications for HFNC in older children include pneumonia, cardiac illnesses, and postextubation.[17] Studies have shown decrease in PICU admissions and intubations in the years after introduction of HFNC in supporting children with a variety of respiratory, cardiac, and neurological illnesses.[9,14,18] However, evidence-based literature is scarce and there is a need to formulate protocols for initiation, escalation, and weaning of HFNC.

ADMINISTRATION OF HIGH FLOW NASAL CANNULA

High flow nasal cannula devices allow the clinician to set the flow rate and FiO_2. While FiO_2 is determined by the primary pathology and its severity, the flow rate is often limited by the patient characteristics **(Fig. 1)**.

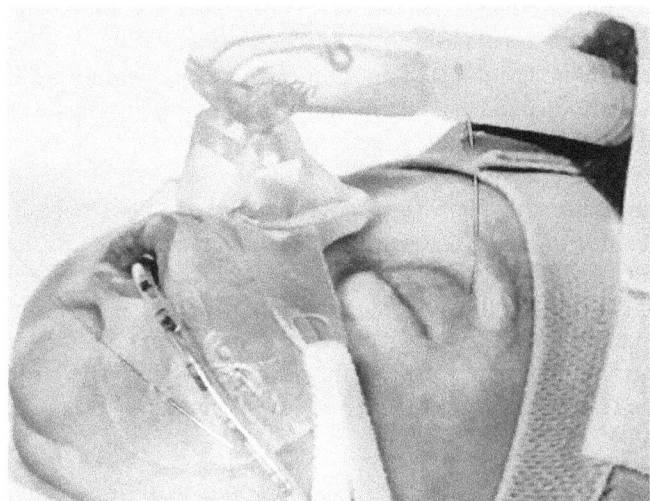

Fig. 1: A newborn receiving high flow nasal cannula therapy.

Initiation, escalation, and weaning protocols vary widely. Conventionally, the flow rate used at initiation of HFNC was limited to 2 L/min in term and preterm neonates. The suggested formula "0.92 + 0.68 w" (w is the weight of the patient in kg) can give the initial flow rate at which HFNC therapy may be started.[8] However, literature review has revealed many protocols which have used higher flow rates safely and successfully.[19] Most protocols use 2 L/kg/min for the first 10 kg body weight and an additional 0.5 L/kg/min for each kg above 10 kg. Each unit can standardize their own protocol for setting the initial and subsequent settings for flow rate based on patient characteristics.

The FiO_2 is set to achieve oxygen saturation greater than 92% and can vary depending on the primary pathology of the patient. The humidifier temperature is set to 34–37°C and adjusted to limit condensation in the tubing. Nasal cannula size is usually half the nostril diameter. It might be useful to reduce mouth leaks with a pacifier in smaller infants **(Figs. 2A to C)**.

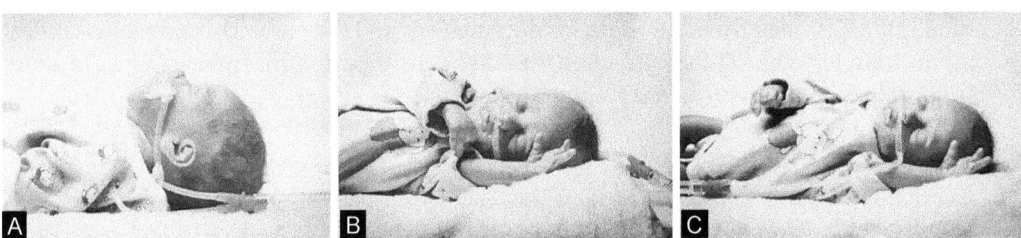

Figs. 2A to C: High flow nasal cannula (HFNC) delivery. Note the relative comfort of the newborn on HFNC vis-à-vis continuous positive airway pressure in terms of ease of handling and better mobility.

Once HFNC therapy is started, meticulous monitoring is required to identify the response to the therapy. Failure of therapy must be identified early to immediately step up the respiratory support by identifying worsening tachypnea, increased FiO_2 requirement, thoracoabdominal dyssynchrony, altered mental status, and respiratory acidosis. Early predictors of HFNC failure include higher venous PCO_2 (>50 mm Hg), lower pH (<7.30), and degree of tachypnea at the onset, failure of FiO_2 requirement to fall below 0.5 during the first 2 hours of therapy.[20] Failure of HFNC requires introduction of nasal CPAP or invasive ventilation.

Clinical improvement is indicated by reduced work of breathing, improving oxygen saturation, improved thoracoabdominal synchrony, and improved overall comfort level of the patient and normal blood gas analysis. Responders showed a decrease in respiratory rate and heart rate within 90 minutes of the start of HFNC therapy.

Weaning practices from high flow vary between different units. Generally, there is no need for a prolonged weaning process. As the primary pathology resolves, FiO_2 requirement comes down and the set FiO_2 is gradually reduced initially. Once FiO_2 is brought down to an acceptable range (usually 0.4), weaning of the flow rate may be started. Once the primary pathology has resolved and the patient is stable with FiO_2 of 0.21 and flow rate 1 L/min, the patient can be taken off HFNC.[11] Another approach to weaning is by giving "holidays" from HFNC to assess the need for further respiratory support and once these "holidays" are uneventful, the patient can be taken off HFNC.

CONCLUSION

High flow nasal cannula is a safe and effective mode of noninvasive ventilation, which is comparable to conventional CPAP. It has been used successfully in many conditions such as post-extubation respiratory support and mild-moderate respiratory distress syndrome in preterm neonates and bronchiolitis in children. Though it is not as effective as nasal CPAP in all clinical scenarios, HFNC has some advantages over nasal CPAP such as reduced nasal trauma, easier enteral feeding, etc. As more evidence is gathered, HFNC is likely to become a primary mode of respiratory support in several respiratory diseases, both in neonates and older children.

KEY POINTS

- HFNC is a mode of noninvasive ventilation, which can basically provide oxygen at a high flow and generate a certain amount of CPAP.
- There are many conditions in which HFNC can be used. However, maximum evidence is available for its use for postextubation respiratory support and mild-to-moderate respiratory distress syndrome in neonates and bronchiolitis in older infants.
- While HFNC is "user friendly" (both for the caregiver and the patient), meticulous clinical monitoring is essential for patients with early consideration for increasing respiratory support for patients who do not respond or worsen.

REFERENCES

1. Locke RG, Wolfson MR, Shaffer TH, Rubenstein SD, Greenspan JS. Inadvertent administration of positive end-distending pressure during nasal cannula flow. Pediatrics. 1993;91:135-8.
2. Shoemaker MT, Pierce MR, Yoder BA, Di Geronimo RJ. High flow nasal cannula versus nasal CPAP for neonatal respiratory disease: a retrospective study. J Perinatol. 2007;27:85-91.

3. Hough JL, Pham TM, Schibler A. Physiologic effect of high-flow nasal cannula in infants with bronchiolitis. Pediatr Crit Care Med. 2014;15: e214-9.
4. McKiernan C, Chua LC, Visintainer PF, Allen H. High flow nasal cannulae therapy in infants with bronchiolitis. J Pediatr. 2010;156:634-8.
5. Spence KL, Murphy D, Kilan C, McGonigle R, Kilani RA. High-flow nasal cannula as a device to provide continuous positive pressure in infants. J Perinatol. 2007;27:772-5.
6. Yoder BA, Stoddard RA, Li M, King J, Dirnberger DR, Abbasi S. Heated, humidified high-flow nasal cannula versus nasal CPAP for respiratory support in neonates. Pediatrics. 2013;131:e1482-90.
7. Milési C, Boubal M, Jacquot A, Baleine J, Durand S, Odena MP, et al. High-flow nasal cannula: recommendations for daily practice in pediatrics. Ann Intensive Care. 2014;4:29.
8. Sreenan C, Lemke RP, Hudson-Mason A, Osiovich H. High-flow nasal cannulae in the management of apnea of prematurity: a comparison with conventional nasal continuous positive airway pressure. Pediatrics. 2001;107:1081-3.
9. Schibler A, Pham TM, Dunster KR, Foster K, Barlow A, Gibbons K, et al. Reduced intubation rates for infants after introduction of high-flow nasal prong oxygen delivery. Intensive Care Med. 2011;37:847-52.
10. Wilkinson D, Andersen C, O'Donnell CP, De Paoli AG, Manley BJ. High flow nasal cannula for respiratory support in preterm infants. Cochrane Database Syst Rev. 2016;2:CD006405.
11. Hegde D, Mondkar J, Panchal H, Manerkar S, Jasani B, Kabra N. Heated humidified high flow nasal cannula *versus* nasal continuous positive airway pressure as primary mode of respiratory support for respiratory distress in preterm infants. Indian Pediatr. 2016;53:129-33.
12. Lin J, Zhang Y, Xiong L, Liu S, Gong C, Dai J. High flow nasal cannula therapy for children with bronchiolitis: a systematic review and meta-analysis. Arch Dis Child. 2019;104:564–76.
13. Milési C, Essouri S, Pouyau R, Liet JM, Afanetti M, Portefaix A, et al. High flow nasal cannula (HFNC) versus nasal continuous positive airway pressure (nCPAP) for the initial respiratory management of acute viral bronchiolitis in young infants: a multicenter randomized controlled trial (TRAMONTANE study). Intensive Care Med. 2017;43:209-16.
14. Daverio M, Da Dalt L, Panozzo M, Frigo AC, Bressan S. A two-tiered high-flow nasal cannula approach to bronchiolitis was associated with low admission rate to intensive care and no adverse outcomes. Acta Paediatr. 2019;108:2056-62.
15. Testa G, Iodice F, Ricci Z, Vitale V, De Razza F, Haiberger R, et al. Comparative evaluation of high-flow nasal cannula and conventional oxygen therapy in paediatric cardiac surgical patients: a randomized controlled trial. Interact Cardiovasc Thorac Surg. 2014;19 :456-61
16. Ballestero Y, De Pedro J, Portillo N, Martinez-Mugica O, Arana-Arri E, Benito J. Pilot clinical trial of high-flow oxygen therapy in children with asthma in the emergency service. J Pediatr. 2018;194: 204-10.
17. Coletti KD, Bagdure DN, Walker LK, Remy KE, Custer JW. High-flow nasal cannula utilization in pediatric critical care. Respir Care. 2017;62:1023-9.
18. Kawaguchi A, Yasui Y, de Caen A, Garros D. The clinical impact of heated humidified high-flow nasal cannula on pediatric respiratory distress. Pediatr Crit Care Med. 2017;18:112-9.
19. Kotecha SJ, Adappa R, Gupta N, Watkins WJ, Kotecha S, Chakraborty M. Safety and efficacy of high-flow nasal cannula therapy in preterm infants: A meta-analysis. Pediatrics. 2015;136:542-53.
20. Kelly GS, Simon HK, Sturm JJ. High-flow nasal cannula use in children with respiratory distress in the emergency department: predicting the need for subsequent intubation. Pediatr Emerg Care. 2013;29:888-92.

Chapter 40

Home Respiratory Support in Children: What is Possible in India?

Kana Ram Jat, Nitin Dhochak

INTRODUCTION

With evolution of health care and better survival of children with chronic respiratory diseases, chronic respiratory support is becoming increasingly important. Patients who require mechanical ventilator support for at least 4 hours a day for a month or longer are classified to have chronic respiratory failure. Long-term respiratory support in children with irreversible or slowly progressive illnesses can lead to unnecessary burden on health care. This can also seriously affect family members, who have significant economic and emotional stress due to prolonged hospital stay. Children with chronic lung diseases requiring long-term respiratory support also do not prefer repeated prolonged hospitalization. These children dislike intensive care units (ICUs) due to excessive light and noise, lack of mobilization, controlled and crowded environment of ICUs. Chronic hypoxia may lead to pulmonary hypertension and adversely affects neurodevelopment, cognition, sleep, and growth. For these reasons, appropriate home respiratory support is an essential part of modern medicine.

Respiratory support can be in the form of invasive ventilation, noninvasive ventilation (NIV) or oxygen supplementation. The aim of home respiratory support is to improve longevity as well as quality of life in children with chronic respiratory diseases. American Thoracic Society (ATS) has issued guidelines for home ventilation and home oxygen support for children recently.[1,2] In view of lack of good quality evidence, most of the recommendations are based on low quality evidence or consensus. Also, these guidelines are based on settings in developed countries and difficulties faced in developing countries like India need special considerations. There is limited literature related to home respiratory support from India. A study from India in adults with chronic obstructive pulmonary disease (COPD) requiring recurrent hospitalizations demonstrated that the use of noninvasive ventilation at home was associated with decrease in mortality, hospitalization, ICU admission, and ventilator requirement.[3] There is another single case report of home mechanical ventilation for COPD from India.[4] There is hardly any such study in children.

In this chapter, we aim to describe the indications, methods, and impact of home respiratory support in these children. We also address the problems encountered in home respiratory support in India and developing countries.

HISTORY, BURDEN, AND INDICATIONS OF HOME RESPIRATORY SUPPORT

The poliomyelitis epidemic in the 1930s to 1940s heralded the beginning of large-scale need for prolonged respiratory support. The machines in those days applied negative pressure around patients' bodies, but over time it has changed to air/oxygen being pushed actively into the respiratory tract by an interface around the nose and mouth. Modern day noninvasive ventilators have similar functioning and are as accurate as the invasive ventilators. Historically, the "Katie Beckett waiver" allowed coverage of home ventilation under Medicaid in USA, easing the financial difficulties in starting and maintaining ventilation at home.[5] As per the EuroVent survey, the prevalence of chronic ventilation support in European countries is estimated to be around 6.6 per 100,000 individuals.[6] Among children, surveys from England and Italy estimated that 6.7 and 4.2 per 100,000 children require home ventilation.[7,8] Temporal trends suggest significant increase in rates of home ventilation support.[7] Data on similar estimations from India are lacking.

Common conditions requiring home ventilation or home respiratory support can be classified as per type of defect. These conditions are summarized in **Table 1**. Those that cause severe chronic hypoxia may be treated with oxygen at home while conditions needing prolonged ventilation will need noninvasive or invasive ventilatory support at home. American Thoracic Society recommendation panel defines hypoxia as follows: in children below 1 year of age, $SpO_2 \leq 90\%$ lasting for 5% of the recording time, if recording continuously *or* $SpO_2 \leq 90\%$ on three occasions if recording intermittently. In children 1 year of age and above hypoxia is defined as $SpO_2 \leq 93\%$ lasting for 5% of the recording time *or* three measurements of $SpO_2 \leq 93\%$, if recording intermittently.[1] Hypoxia for 2 weeks or more is considered as chronic hypoxia in children. Pulse oximetry is sufficient to define hypoxia and PaO_2 is not recommended.

Table 1: Common conditions requiring home ventilation or home respiratory support in children.

Mechanism of respiratory insufficiency	Diseases
Inadequate central inspiratory drive	➤ Congenital hypoventilation syndrome ➤ ROHHAD (rapid-onset obesity with hypothalamic dysregulation, hypoventilation, and autonomic dysregulation) ➤ Brain injury (traumatic) ➤ Hypoxic ischemic encephalopathy sequelae ➤ Encephalitis sequelae ➤ Metabolic encephalopathies
Inadequate respiratory pump	➤ Neuromuscular disorders (Duchene muscular dystrophy, myasthenia gravis, spinomuscular atrophy, Juvenile dermatomyositis) ➤ Diaphragmatic palsy ➤ Spinal cord injury ➤ Guillain-Barré syndrome ➤ Chest wall defects (Kyphosis, scoliosis, pectus excavatum) ➤ Krait poisoning
Parenchymal and vascular problems defects	➤ Bronchopulmonary dysplasia ➤ Cystic fibrosis ➤ Interstitial lung disease (ILD) ➤ Bronchiectasis ➤ Congenital heart diseases
Airway defects	➤ Airway malacia (tracheomalacia, bronchomalacia) ➤ Obstructive sleep apnea ➤ Craniofacial defect

Centers for Medicare and Medicare Services, USA, funds home oxygen if PaO_2 is less than 55 mm Hg, SpO_2 is less than 88%, or PaO_2 is between 55 and 59 mm Hg and SpO_2 89% associated with cor pulmonale, hematocrit more than 55% or pedal edema.[1]

Neuromuscular disorders were the most common conditions requiring NIV at home. Frequency of various disease conditions in three pediatric studies requiring home NIV is described in **Table 2**.

Table 2: Frequency of conditions requiring home ventilation in children.

Study	Neuromuscular defect	Respiratory drive	Airway lesion	Parenchymal defects
Amirnovin et al. 2018[9] (n=164)	53%	—	2%	29%
Goodwin et al. 2011[7] (n=63)	49%	15%	33%	3%
Racca et al. 2011.[8] (n=56)	50%	30%	—	—

Timing of starting mechanical ventilation is commonly following an acute episode of pneumonia/respiratory tract infection where there is difficulty in weaning due to any of the above reasons. Sometimes physical manifestations of respiratory insufficiency in chronic respiratory failure like failure to gain weight, daytime sleepiness, attention deficit, etc. become indications to start home ventilatory support. Polysomnography is an important tool to identify patients suitable for home based respiratory support as well as help in monitoring the therapy. Nocturnal or daytime CO_2 retention is an important indication of starting ventilation.

INTERFACE FOR RESPIRATORY SUPPORT

Ventilatory support in children with chronic respiratory failure can be provided by tracheostomy or a noninvasive interface.

Tracheostomy

Ventilation via tracheostomy is preferred when the child is previous mechanically ventilated with failed weaning, has severe central hypoventilation, craniofacial anomalies or the child is not able to maintain patency of upper airway or clear secretions. Neuromuscular weakness can present as difficulty in weaning and also, over time, it can progress to bulbar weakness associated with poor handling of secretions. Ventilation can be done using an invasive two limb ventilator or a single limb vented circuit.

Tracheostomy adds to the difficulty in caring for the child at home. The child's relatives need to be trained to perform suctioning, and, if necessary, to change the tracheostomy tube in case of obstruction or displacement. Tracheostomy predisposes to increased risk of infections; so, care should be taken to maintain hygiene while managing the tracheostomy tube. Frequency of routine tube change is once weekly, though this recommendation is based on consensus rather than evidence.

Noninvasive Ventilation

Noninvasive ventilation interfaces are increasingly being used in home ventilation support, even in patients with congenital hypoventilation syndromes. The available interfaces include nasal, oronasal and full-face mask, nasal prongs, oral airway, oropharyngeal airway, etc.

Commonly encountered complications are related to pressure and friction effects of face masks leading to maceration and pressure ulceration of skin. This can be decreased by using two interchangeable interfaces during the daytime. Prolonged use in growing children is associated with midfacial growth limitation and deformities. Leakage around the mask is another significant problem. Custom made masks provide less leak and NIV machines can compensate for leaks. Pressure targeted ventilation strategy should be used if significant leak is present as measurement of volume is fallacious in such a case. Care providers are trained to apply the different airway devices.

For both tracheostomy ventilation and NIV, parents or care givers should be trained during hospital admission to operate the ventilator/bilevel positive airway pressure (BIPAP) devices. Change of settings according to changing disease conditions should be taught. All care givers should be trained for basic life support, and bag and mask/tube ventilation. This training needs to be imparted while the patient is admitted in the hospital and the patient should be discharged only after the care providers are confident of managing the ventilation at home.

EQUIPMENT FOR RESPIRATORY SUPPORT

Ventilators

Ventilators for home ventilation are portable ventilators with inbuilt turbines which provide the necessary flow. Earlier portable ventilators had limited leak compensation, ventilator modes and synchrony. But newer generation ventilators are more efficacious at leak compensation and provide multiple operating modes similar to hospital ventilators. These also provide baseline flow which improves the synchrony and provides flow for spontaneous breath in excess of set rate. These can utilize single limb (inspiratory) or double limb circuits (inspiratory and expiratory). Double limb circuits prevent rebreathing and control of breath delivery is better. These can be utilized with tracheostomy tube or NIV interfaces. All these ventilators have battery backup of 1-3 hours and additional batteries should be kept for enhanced mobility/travel, etc. Most guidelines recommend keeping spare ventilator and batteries to take care of accidental malfunction. Usual cost of ventilator in the Indian market ranges from 200,000 to 500,000 INR. These can be acquired on a rental basis too. An indigenously made ventilator "AgVa" provides a low cost solution (costing less than INR 100,000) with ease of operation using smartphone as controller. Long-term data is still not available on the use of this new ventilator.[10]

Commonly operated modes in home ventilation are pressure controlled and volume controlled. In settings of high leakage (loose NIV interface or leakage around tracheostomy tube), pressure control is utilized to provide appropriate flow to maintain inspiratory pressures throughout the inspiratory phase. Ventilator settings are set according to patient needs. Patients with parenchymal defect or recurrent collapses are operated at higher peak expiratory pressure (PEEP) to keep the alveoli open. Peak inspiratory pressure (PIP) is adjusted to provide adequate chest rise after initial setting of 10-12 cm of water above PEEP. Number of supported breaths is decided by the set rate where excessive breaths are allowed but do not receive complete PIP; whereas in assist control modes, all breaths above set rate are supported by similar PIP. Dual limb circuits provide finer control of breaths with efficient analysis of breath and synchrony while single limb circuits are less bulky and provide better mobility. Fraction of inspired oxygen (FiO_2) is determined by flow of oxygen and site of oxygen delivery (more FiO_2 where oxygen is directly delivered near the mask than more proximal delivery.[11]

Bilevel or Continuous Positive Airway Pressure Machines

Bilevel or continuous positive airway pressure machines (BIPAP or CPAP) machines are cheaper and smaller than ventilators. These utilize single limb circuits and exhalation ports are present in the NIV mask/tracheostomy interface. Blowers provide the necessary flow to generate inspiratory (IPAP) and expiratory positive airway pressure (EPAP). Conventionally, BIPAP machines provide larger flow and better leak compensation than ventilators for NIV but newer generation of ventilators also provide leak compensation. BIPAP machines operate at a fixed rate (timed), spontaneous and hybrid (spontaneous/timed) mode. Initial settings are EPAP 4-6 cm of water and IPAP 8-10 cm of water above EPAP. For a given oxygen flow, CPAP mode delivers higher FiO_2 than BIPAP.[11] These machines cost around INR 20,000–50,000 in the Indian market. Smaller size makes these machines favorable for transport.

Duration of daily therapy for both ventilator and BIPAP machines depends on underlying respiratory condition. Most of the patients with neuromuscular weakness and hypoventilation require mechanical support only during part of the day and nighttime. Night-time NIV improves the respiratory condition with unloading/resting of respiratory muscles during sleep, resets the CO_2 sensitivity of respiratory centers, and improves daytime sleepiness/tiredness. Therapy is titrated as per clinical requirement. Polysomnography can assist in titration of setting especially in sleep disordered breathing. During of therapy and pressures might need to be increased during acute infections.

Oxygen Source

Oxygen is an essential part of home respiratory support. It is needed for patients with home ventilation with parenchymal involvement, during infections, excessive secretions, lung collapse or during suctioning. Oxygen supplementation even without positive pressure ventilation is recommended in patients with chronic lung diseases including cystic fibrosis, bronchopulmonary dysplasia, sickle cell disease, pulmonary hypertension, interstitial lung diseases, etc. For sleep disordered breathing, it can be used in patients not tolerating positive airway pressure therapy or awaiting surgery.[2]

Common oxygen sources for home use are oxygen cylinders and oxygen concentrators. Oxygen cylinders contain compressed oxygen. Capacity of oxygen cylinders varies from 40 liters to 7,000 liters. Home use cylinders have capacity up to 500-600 liters. Oxygen cylinders can be availed on rent for short-term use and these can be refilled from nearby oxygen supplier (refill cost varies from INR 100–300). If oxygen requirement is low and it is expected to be required for a few months, oxygen cylinder may be considered. Oxygen concentrators are large devices which concentrate oxygen form air by adsorbing nitrogen in zeolite minerals. These can provide output at 5 liters/minute delivering around 90% oxygen. Some machines can reach flows up to 10 liters/minute. But these machines need continuous power supply. Patients using oxygen concentrators need back up cylinders for power failure and transport of patients. Cost of machines with supply of 5 liters/minute capacity is around INR 40,000 to 50,000. Pulse oxygen delivery system (oxygen conserver device) provides oxygen only during inspiration, not during expiration, thus avoiding wastage of oxygen. It is used in adults, but not recommended in children because of high respiratory rate and low inspiratory volume; however, it may be considered in adolescents.

Humidification is recommended if oxygen flow is greater than 1 L/min and it can be achieved by bubbling or humidification device.

ANCILLARY THERAPIES

Tracheostomy Care

Tracheostomy care includes effective suctioning, change of tracheostomy, and trouble shooting. Caregivers should establish communication with ear nose throat (ENT) specialist near the patient's home to change the tracheostomy tube. Frequency of tracheostomy tube change is based on consensus and most centers change tracheostomy tube once a week. Caretakers can also be trained for tube change once the stoma is old for emergency dislodgement but as a routine tracheostomy should be changed by trained ENT surgeon. Children managed on tracheostomy need heating humidification of gases as the natural humidification of gases by nose and upper airway is bypassed in these patients (temperature target 29-35°C and humidification target 28-35 mg of water/L). Heat and moisture exchanger devices should be used for humidification in tracheostomized patients.

Suctioning should be taught to at least two caretakers for home-based support. Tracheostomy suctioning is need based rather than time based. There is only one study of sterile versus clean suctioning which did not find any difference in infections rates between these groups. Most centers recommend use of either clean or sterile technique as feasible.[12] Suction pressure is set at 80-100 cm for smaller children and 100-120 mm Hg for adolescent and adults. Portable suction devices can be electricity operated or pedal/foot operated. In developing countries like India where power supply is not constant, pedal/foot operated suction machine is very useful and cost effective (costs about 800-1,500 INR/unit). Also, it offers better mobility with ease of carrying out of home.

With improvement in underlying condition, tapering off of tracheostomy tube is planned. Small sized tracheostomy tube is placed to facilitate breathing and speech around the tracheostomy tube. Before planning decannulation, opening of tracheostomy tube is blocked to check for sufficiency of child's reserve to maintain respiration by breathing through the natural airway. Some centers routinely do bronchoscopy to look for granulation around the tracheostomy site before decannulation, but this is not routinely recommended.

Airway Clearance

Most children on chronic ventilation have difficulty in clearance of secretions due to either poor cough (neuromuscular weakness and post-brain injury sequalae) or thick viscid secretions (cystic fibrosis). Amount of secretions increases during infections which can block airways and lead to significant respiratory impairment in these children. Airway clearance techniques should be taught to caretakers which includes postural drainage and chest percussion. In patients with poor cough, mechanical insufflator – exsufflator (cough assist device) should be used for airway clearance. There is insufficient data for or against the use of cough assist devices but in view of short-term benefits and improvements of quality of life, most clinical guidelines recommend its use in patients with neuromuscular weakness.[13] Airway clearance should be done more intensively and frequently during infections. Disease specific therapies (deoxyribonucleotidase or hypertonic saline therapy for cystic fibrosis) should be administered.

Monitoring

Purpose of monitoring includes early identification of adverse events like ventilator dysfunction, adequacy of respiratory support while ensuring minimal disturbance in sleep especially during night-time. Ventilator alarms and monitor alarms should be set loud enough to be detected early. ATS guidelines recommend regular checkup of ventilator devices as recommended by manufacturer.[2] There is debate on how many vital parameters should be monitored. Most clinical guidelines recommend using pulse oximeter for nocturnal monitoring of patients. Cardiopulmonary monitoring usually results in false alarms and frequent sleep interruption of both patient and caregivers; hence it is not routinely indicated in all patients. Percutaneous CO_2 monitoring provides measurement of night-time CO_2 changes and effectiveness of ventilation.[14] These are important in titration of IPAP and EPAP of patients on NIV. ATS guidelines recommend routine pulse oximeter monitoring in these patients.[2]

Oxygen therapy may blunt respiratory drive leading to hypoventilation resulting in CO_2 retention. The child should be monitored for symptoms of CO_2 narcosis and blood CO_2 should be checked during health care facility visit.[15] Parents should be educated about safety at home. They should avoid smoking or keeping inflammable items near oxygen source.

■ TRAINING OF CARE PROVIDERS AND TITRATION OF THERAPY

Initiation of NIV should be preferably done in the hospital, as an inpatient. At least two caregivers who are willing and motivated for long-term care of the child, should be educated and trained to take care of the child, modify ventilator settings, trouble shoot common problems and basic life support. A written plan should be provided for common problems including ventilator alarms, increased secretions, acute infections, etc. Preferably, there should be a tie up with nearby health care center where treatment can be provided if any complication arises. All caregivers should have self-inflating bag and mask, preloaded adrenaline syringe, and spare tracheostomy tubes for resuscitation, if need arises. Long term follow up data in children with chronic ventilation suggests that home respiratory support can be managed by training parents and lay caregivers, and it is not necessary to have a specialized nurse.[16]

Initial optimization of setting for the device for the patient needs to be done in the hospital. For BIPAP devices, EPAP is targeted for optimal recruitment and prevention of collapse. IPAP is titrated to chest expansion and nocturnal CO_2. Synchronization of efforts in spontaneous mode requires patient efforts, which may be problematic in patients with severe neuromuscular weakness where the strength of efforts is inadequate to trigger breaths. Such patients might benefit from timed or spontaneous/timed mode. PIP and PEEP in ventilators are usually set like IPAP and EPAP for BIPAP devices while additional settings like trigger, inspiratory time, pressure support also need to be set. Simple algorithms should be provided for titration of settings. If there is persistent problem despite simple measures, urgent contact with health care should be sought.

WEANING OF HOME RESPIRATORY SUPPORT

As per ATS guidelines child should to considered for weaning from home respiratory support if following conditions are fulfilled: (1) child is relatively stable without current or recent acute problem, (2) child has age and disease appropriate growth and development parameters, (3) acceptable low ventilatory support requirement and improvement in condition that required home respiratory support, (4) respiratory rate and efforts are as expected for underlying disease, (5) acceptable oxygen saturation (not fulfilling definition of hypoxia as earlier), and (6) echocardiography to document absent or improving pulmonary hypertension (in selected patients).[1] Weaning of home respiratory support is done gradually. There are two common approaches—(1) gradually decreasing pressures and set rate; and (2) gradually increasing periods off the ventilator. Patients recovering from acute neuromuscular insult (Guillain-Barre syndrome), and post-brain injury sequelae (encephalitis, traumatic brain injury) usually tolerate off ventilator times during daytime which is gradually increased. Children recovering from acute illness like superimposed infection with increased NIV requirement can be initially weaned by decreasing IPAP and later, gradually increasing ventilator free time. Diaphragmatic pacing can be done in patients with congenital hypoventilation by implanted devices; such children are usually tapered off ventilatory support during daytime. A few patients who have progressive diseases like muscular dystrophies might be weaned initially after starting NIV due to improvement in lung micro-atelectasis and fatigue but gradually these children require hiking of support due to progressive illness. Discontinuation from home oxygen therapy may be considered once a child is stable at oxygen flow less than 0.1 L/min in children below 1 year of age and less than 0.25-0.5 L/min in children above 1 year of age.[1]

FOLLOW-UP AND OUTCOME

It is preferred that children on home ventilator support should have 24 hour hotline for rapid addressal of the complications arising at home while seeking health care support. In a study of 1,199 adult and pediatric patients with chronic home ventilation, 528 daytime and 14 night-time calls were received per month; indicating that there is need for ready assistance to these patients.[17] Regular follow-up should be done in children who are mobile enough to visit clinics or home visits should be scheduled. On each visit, apart from underlying condition, review should be made of respiratory function, growth, and nutrition, and revision of the ventilator titration/weaning plan should be done. Alteration of daytime wakefulness, mood, and growth can be indicators of insufficiency of ventilator support.

Long-term outcome of children on chronic home respiratory support depends on whether the underlying condition is progressive (muscular dystrophies, SMA) or gradually reversible (BPD, Guillain-Barré syndrome). Long term-NIV support in children with DMD is associated with slower decline in pulmonary functions, avoids tracheostomy, and is well tolerated.[18,19]

In India, there is limited evidence regarding the use of home respiratory therapy in children. It is underutilized and the main reason may be financial (unable to afford the devices) and ignorance. There is a lot of scope to introduce and promote home respiratory therapy in India.

Recommendations for home oxygen support are summarised in Box 1.

Box 1: Recommendations: Home respiratory support in children.

Recommendations	Grading of Recommendation	Level of evidence
Home oxygen therapy		
Home oxygen therapy should be prescribed in children with cystic fibrosis having severe chronic hypoxia (SpO_2 < 90%).	Strong	Very low quality (Level IV)
Home oxygen therapy should be prescribed in children with bronchopulmonary dysplasia (BPD) having chronic hypoxia (SpO_2 <93%).	Strong	Very low quality (Level IV)
Home oxygen therapy should be prescribed in children with obstructive sleep apnea having severe hypoxia (SpO_2 < 90%) during sleep and not tolerating/not using positive airway pressure.	Conditional	Very low quality (Level IV)
Home oxygen therapy should be prescribed in children with pulmonary artery hypertension secondary to chronic respiratory disease with chronic hypoxia (SpO_2 <93%).	Strong	Very low quality (Level IV)
Home oxygen therapy should be prescribed in children with interstitial lung disease having chronic hypoxia (SpO_2 < 90%).	Strong	Very low quality (Level IV)
Home ventilation		
For children needing home ventilation, standardized objective discharge criteria should be used to assess medical stability and home situation.	Conditional	Very low quality (Level IV)
There should be one trained awake and attentive caregiver at home round the clock for children requiring home ventilation.	Strong	Very low quality (Level IV)
There should be two trained family care providers for children requiring home ventilation.	Conditional	Very low quality (Level IV)
There should be ongoing education and training to professional and family caregivers for children requiring home ventilation.	Conditional	Very low quality (Level IV)
Equipment for resuscitation, monitoring equipment like pulse oximeter, and suctioning equipment, etc. should be available at home for children requiring home ventilation.	Conditional	Very low quality (Level IV)

KEY POINTS

1. There is increasing need of home respiratory support because of better survival of children with chronic respiratory diseases.
2. In children with chronic respiratory illnesses, parents/caregivers should be motivated to take on the challenge of home respiratory support, provided finances permit it. Good clear communication to this effect would guide the parents to start home respiratory support.
3. Invasive ventilation with portable ventilation, NIV, BIPAP/CPAP, or just oxygen may be used at home depending on the underlying disease.
4. Constant support through phone calls and regular monitoring of children on home respiratory support is crucial for its success.
5. There is a need to promote the use of home respiratory support in children in India.

REFERENCES

1. Hayes D, Wilson KC, Krivchenia K, Hawkins SMM, Balfour-Lynn IM, Gozal D, et al. Home Oxygen Therapy for Children. An Official American Thoracic Society Clinical Practice Guideline. Am J Respir Crit Care Med. 2019;199(3):e5-23.
2. Sterni LM, Collaco JM, Baker CD, Carroll JL, Sharma GD, Brozek JL, et al. An Official American Thoracic Society Clinical Practice Guideline: Pediatric Chronic Home Invasive Ventilation. Am J Respir Crit Care Med. 2016;193(8):e16-35.
3. Suraj KP, Jyothi E, Rakhi R. Role of Domiciliary Noninvasive Ventilation in Chronic Obstructive Pulmonary Disease Patients Requiring Repeated Admissions with Acute Type II Respiratory Failure: A Prospective Cohort Study. Indian J Crit Care Med. 2018;22(6):397-401.
4. Guleria R, Batra YK, Sharma BK, Jindal SK. Domiciliary mechanical ventilation in a patient with severe chronic obstructive lung disease and respiratory failure. Indian J Chest Dis Allied Sci. 1992;34(3):149-52.
5. King AC. Long-term home mechanical ventilation in the United States. Respir Care. 2012;57(6):921-32.
6. Lloyd-Owen SJ, Donaldson GC, Ambrosino N, Escarabill J, Farre R, Fauroux B, et al. Patterns of home mechanical ventilation use in Europe: results from the Eurovent survey. Eur Respir J. 2005;25(6):1025-31.
7. Goodwin S, Smith H, Langton Hewer S, Fleming P, Henderson AJ, Hilliard T, et al. Increasing prevalence of domiciliary ventilation: changes in service demand and provision in the South West of the UK. Eur J Pediatr. 2011;170(9):1187-92.
8. Racca F, Berta G, Sequi M, Bignamini E, Capello E, Cutrera R, et al. Long-term home ventilation of children in Italy: a national survey. Pediatr Pulmonol. 2011;46(6):566-72.
9. Amirnovin R, Aghamohammadi S, Riley C, Woo MS, Del Castillo S. Analysis of a Pediatric Home Mechanical Ventilator Population. Respir Care. 2018;63(5):558-64.
10. Speciality Medical Dialogues. AIIMS team develops smallest ventilator costing only ₹35,000! [online]. Available from https://speciality.medicaldialogues.in/aiims-team-develops-smallest-ventilator-costing-only-rs-35000/. [Last Accessed December, 2019].
11. Samolski D, Antón A, Güell R, Sanz F, Giner J, Casan P. Inspired oxygen fraction achieved with a portable ventilator: determinant factors. Respir Med. 2006;100(9):1608-13.
12. Harris RB, Hyman RB. Clean vs. sterile tracheotomy care and level of pulmonary infection. Nurs Res. 1984;33(2):80-5.
13. Auger C, Hernando V, Galmiche H. Use of Mechanical Insufflation-Exsufflation Devices for Airway Clearance in Subjects with Neuromuscular Disease. Respir Care. 2017;62(2):236-45.
14. Janssens JP, Borel JC, Pépin JL. Nocturnal monitoring of home non-invasive ventilation: the contribution of simple tools such as pulse oximetry, capnography, built-in ventilator software and autonomic markers of sleep fragmentation. Thorax. 2011;66(5):438-45.
15. Balfour-Lynn IM, Field DJ, Gringras P, Hicks B, Jardine E, Jones RC, et al. BTS guidelines for home oxygen in children. Thorax. 2009;64(Suppl 2):ii1-26.
16. Tibballs J, Henning R, Robertson CF, Massie J, Hochmann M, Carter B, et al. A home respiratory support programme for children by parents and layperson carers. J Paediatr Child Health. 2010;46(1-2):57-62.
17. Chatwin M, Heather S, Hanak A, Polkey MI, Simonds AK. Analysis of home support and ventilator malfunction in 1,211 ventilator-dependent patients. Eur Respir J. 2010;35(2):310-6.
18. Brasil Santos D, Vaugier I, Boussaïd G, Orlikowski D, Prigent H, Lofaso F. Impact of Noninvasive Ventilation on Lung Volumes and Maximum Respiratory Pressures in Duchenne Muscular Dystrophy. Respir Care. 2016;61(11):1530-5.
19. McKim DA, Griller N, LeBlanc C, Woolnough A, King J. Twenty-four hour noninvasive ventilation in Duchenne muscular dystrophy: a safe alternative to tracheostomy. Can Respir J. 2013;20(1):e5-9.

Chapter 41

Noninvasive Ventilation in Acutely Ill Children

Samriti Gupta, Jhuma Sankar

BACKGROUND

Noninvasive ventilation (NIV) is increasingly being used in pediatric emergency and critical care units as a form of respiratory support in various conditions requiring respiratory support. Non-invasive ventilation refers to the delivery of assisted ventilation without the use of advanced airways such as endotracheal tube (ET) or a tracheostomy tube. It can be through positive or negative pressure devices and, may be continuous or intermittent. The advantage in using noninvasive over invasive ventilation in the acute setting is that tracheal intubation can be avoided and thus prevents nosocomial infection and also requires lesser use of sedation. Typically non-invasive ventilation involves biphasic positive airway pressure and continuous positive end expiratory pressure. Heated humidified high flow nasal cannula (HHHFNC) has recently gained importance as a form of noninvasive respiratory support because of its ease of use, tolerability, and safety. Evidence is upcoming on the safety of use of NIV in children. However, several challenges with NIV remain including tolerability of the interfaces, risk of aspiration and NIV failure. Patients need to be closely monitored for early detection of NIV failure.

INTRODUCTION

Non-invasive respiratory support in children has gained popularity in recent years because of its less invasive nature, better tolerability and improved outcomes in several acute and chronic respiratory disorders. It includes continuous positive end expiratory pressure (PEEP), noninvasive ventilation (NIV) or biphasic positive airway pressure (BiPAP) and more recently heated, humidified, high flow nasal cannula (HHHFNC).[1] Much of the evidence regarding use of noninvasive respiratory support comes from neonatal and adult population but there is growing evidence of its utilization in pediatric population in last decade.[2] However, there are several unique challenges associated with the application, management, and safety of noninvasive respiratory support in pediatric population. The advantages associated with NIV and other modalities are decreased need for invasive artificial airway, reduced need for sedation and hence better tolerability, reduced risk of ventilator associated pneumonia, improved tolerance to enteral feeding and ability to ambulate.[1-3]

PHYSIOLOGIC PRINCIPLES

Noninvasive ventilation in acute pediatric settings is mainly used in conditions associated with acute respiratory distress and acute respiratory failure. The main objective is to reduce the work of breathing, and improve oxygenation and ventilation and thus prevent invasive mechanical ventilation.

There are three types of noninvasive positive pressure ventilation: (1) CPAP, (2) BiPAP and (3) negative pressure ventilation.[1-3] The latter is rarely used now-a-days. HHHFNC has emerged as an important tool in acute care settings especially in pediatric settings although it is not a traditional form of NIV.[1,4]

Continuous Positive Airway Pressure

It refers to the administration of continuous positive airway pressure during all phases of the respiratory cycle of a spontaneously breathing patient. The mechanisms of action of CPAP described include recruitment of collapsed alveoli, restoration of functional residual capacity and hence improvement in tidal volume. It reduces the work of breathing by unloading of respiratory muscles and improvement in airflow. Also, it helps in stenting of upper airways and is helpful in obstructive disorders of the upper airways. CPAP is most helpful in disorders associated with hypoxemic respiratory failure.[1,3]

Bilevel Positive Airway Pressure

It refers to the application of two pressure levels (inspiratory-IPAP and expiratory-EPAP) designed to enhance ventilation by creating pressure gradients that facilitate the movement of air in and out of the lungs in spontaneously breathing patients. The tidal volume generated depends upon the degree of difference between IPAP and EPAP. It is suitable in both hypoxemic and hypercapnic respiratory failure.[1,3]

High Flow Nasal Cannula

The HHHFNC involves providing heated, humidified oxygen at high flows up to 2 L/kg/min which helps in reducing the dead space in upper airways and also provides some degree of positive end expiratory pressure. HHHFNC causes carbon dioxide (CO_2) washout from the anatomical dead space in the nasopharynx and improves oxygenation. It also provides some degree of CPAP which is variable at different flows. It has been reported that a flow rate of 6L/min may produce a CPAP of 4-5 cm H_2O. Other benefits of HHHFNC include reduced airway resistance, some degree of bronchodilation, improved mucociliary clearance and reduced inflammation.[1,4]

INDICATIONS AND CONTRAINDICATIONS OF NONINVASIVE VENTILATION

Indications of NIV in acute settings are any child with respiratory distress or respiratory failure who is not having severe acute respiratory distress syndrome (ARDS) or urgent need for endotracheal intubation (ETI) and invasive mechanical ventilation (IMV). The conditions include asthma, bronchiolitis, pneumonia, mild to moderate ARDS, immunocompromised children, acute pulmonary edema, and weaning from mechanical ventilation.

The absolute contraindications to NIV include reduced level of consciousness with inability to protect airways, lack of spontaneous respiration and the inability to achieve a good fit with interface.[1-3]

Interfaces

Various interfaces are available for application of NIV. These include nasal prongs, nasal pillows, nasal masks, oronasal masks, total face masks, and nasopharyngeal prongs. The choice of interface depends upon patient's age, tolerability, and acceptance of degree of leak. In small infants, the interfaces of choice are nasal prongs, nasal pillows, and nasal masks. However, these are associated with significant amount of leaks, which may be overcome to some extent with the use of a chin strap. Oronasal masks work well in older children and adolescents in terms of tolerability and reduced system leaks. For those who do not tolerate oronasal masks, nasal masks, and nasal pillows are alternate options. Whole face masks are tolerated better by small infants but not older children.[1,3,5]

Delivery Devices

In acute settings, NIV can be delivered with any ICU ventilator in all ages. The standalone devices to deliver CPAP are available for infants weighing 5–7 kg and pediatric patients more than 20 or 30 kg. Several portable BiPAP machines are available which can also be used in acute settings apart from home care.[1,3]

INITIATION AND MANAGEMENT OF NONINVASIVE VENTILATION

Continuous Positive Airway Pressure

It helps in recruitment of alveoli and keeping the alveoli open by restoring functional residual capacity and hence reduces the work of breathing and improves oxygenation. However, CPAP does not lead to significant increase in tidal volumes and has less effect on CO_2 elimination.

The level of CPAP required depends upon the indication and disease severity. To initiate, 5–8 cm of H_2O of CPAP generally suffice in most of the cases. CPAP level upto 10–12 cm of H_2O may be needed in disorders associated with reduced lung compliance. The general guideline of CPAP use is to increase pressure level gradually to achieve the target oxygen saturation at FiO_2 of 50–60% depending upon the underlying disease process and pulmonary mechanics. Response to CPAP can be measured clinically by achieving reduction in respiratory rates and chest retractions as well as improvement in oxygen saturations leading to overall decreased work of breathing with adequate CPAP levels.

Weaning from CPAP should be initiated when the underlying disease process has started resolving which can be determined clinically and by certain diagnostic parameters like blood gas analysis. FiO_2 should be decreased to minimal acceptable levels typically <40% before decreasing CPAP levels. Discontinuation of CPAP can be done when CPAP levels are <5 cm of H_2O and FiO_2 requirement is <30% while maintaining the predetermined oxygen saturation targets. Weaning can be done directly to standard nasal prongs or to HHHFNC which can further be tapered off.[1-3]

Noninvasive Ventilation/Biphasic Positive Airway Pressure

Initial settings for BiPAP will be patient and disease specific.

Interface

Interface should be chosen wisely and correctly according to patient's age, tolerance, degree of leak and triggering capacity of patient.

Mode

There are three modes of ventilation in NIV which is present in most of the delivery devices—spontaneous, timed and spontaneous/timed mode. These modes are chosen based upon the respiratory drive of the patients and their triggering capacity. Spontaneous mode allows the patient to trigger the breaths and provides pressure support during inspiration without backup rates. Timed mode provides IPAP at a set frequency while allowing patient to trigger breaths in between. However, this mode may lead to asynchrony as machine triggered breaths may get superimposed on patient triggered breaths. Spontaneous/timed mode has an advantage of being a patient triggered mode with backup rates and hence provides patient comfort and safety. Other modes include pressure controlled and volume controlled modes of ventilation as in invasive mechanical ventilation.

Frequency and Inspiratory Time

For timed and spontaneous/timed, a mandatory breathing frequency needs to be selected according to patient's age and requirement of amount of support by the patient. Inspiratory time indicates the time taken for inspiratory phase of respiration and is set according to the age of the patient and disease status. Very long inspiratory times lead to patient asynchrony in case of active expiration.

Expiratory Positive Airway Pressure

The EPAP indicates the PEEP in BiPAP and helps in alveolar recruitment and reduces the alveolar collapse. It should be initiated at 4–5 cm of H_2O and depending upon oxygenation and underlying lung condition, can be increased to 7–8 cm of H_2O in infants and 10–12 cm of H_2O in pediatric patients.

Inspiratory Positive Airway Pressure

It is the positive pressure applied to airways and the difference between IPAP and EPAP is directly proportional to the volume delivered to the patient. It helps in improvement of both oxygenation and ventilation. It should be started at 6–8 cm H_2O and then gradually increased upto 18–20 cm H_2O depending upon the disease status and patient tolerance.

Trigger Sensitivity

The most common trigger variables used are flow and pressure triggers. Flow trigger is more commonly used as it has been shown to reduce the work of breathing. Trigger sensitivity should be set such that the patient should be able to initiate a breath easily without auto-triggering.

Presence of larger leaks in NIV may affect triggering by the patient. This may be reduced by achieving an effective seal between patient interface and the oronasal opening and by use of a device having option of leak compensation.

Other settings include rise time which refers to the time needed to reach the preset pressure during pressure controlled ventilation and depends upon the patient comfort and type of respiratory disorder.

FiO_2 can be regulated when BiPAP is provided by ICU ventilators. In portable BiPAP machines, oxygen supplementation is attached to the device by wall oxygen or if possible by blenders which may help to adjust FiO_2.

Once the patient's underlying condition has started improving and the patient is comfortable, weaning from BiPAP can be initiated. However, leaks in the system have significant effects on maintenance and weaning from BiPAP. One approach is to gradually decrease IPAP and EPAP settings by 1–2 cm of H_2O to the minimal required pressures and then switch the patient to supplemental oxygen. This helps in gradual decrease in the work of breathing. Another approach of reducing mandatory frequency in the presence of leaks results in increased work of breathing as the spontaneous breaths are not supported in the presence of large system leaks.[1-3]

High Flow Nasal Cannula

High-flow nasal cannula, though not a traditional form of NIV, has gained popularity in recent years as noninvasive respiratory support. It has been seen in previous studies that when supplemental oxygen given by nasal prongs is humidified and heated, larger flows can be supplied to the patient without much nasal irritation and discomfort. The flow rates in HHHFNC are typically 2 L/kg/min with maximum upto 60 L/min in adults, However, in neonates, flows beyond 2 L/min are high flows.[1,4]

MEASUREMENT AND MONITORING

Meticulous monitoring is required when NIV is initiated to identify patients who may require invasive mechanical ventilation early. The first hour after initiation of NIV is very crucial for monitoring. Child should be kept nil per orally and continuous cardiorespiratory monitoring should be started. Pulse oximetry and if possible transcutaneous CO_2 monitoring should be done continuously to ensure adequate oxygenation and ventilation respectively. Clinical indicators of respiratory distress, i.e. heart rate (HR), respiratory rate (RR), work of breathing, clinical lung examination and level of consciousness should be regularly monitored and documented. Arterial blood gas analysis is desirable at baseline, 30 minutes and 1 hour after NIV initiation; however, it should be kept in mind that any painful stimulus is known to aggravate respiratory distress. System leaks, patient tolerance and asynchrony should also be monitored.[1,3]

Determination of volume delivery in NIV is inaccurate because of leaks in the system, size of interface and residual volume within the interface. Hence, it can be indirectly indicated by clinical indicators and blood gas analysis.[1]

NONINVASIVE VENTILATION FAILURE/SUCCESS

The goal of NIV is to improve the work of breathing and prevent ETI and invasive mechanical ventilation. However, a few patients may not be able to meet this goal. The success and failure of NIV depends upon several factors like underlying disease status, severity of respiratory failure, comorbidities and timing of NIV initiation. Several studies have tried to determine the predictors of NIV success and failure. The most important predictor of NIV success is improvement in clinical status, work of breathing, pH and PCO_2 within 1 hour after NIV initiation indicating the importance of meticulous monitoring in the first few hours after starting NIV. The predictors of NIV failure include moderate to severe ARDS, higher PRISM or PELOD scores, no improvement in RR, PCO_2 and work of breathing as well as significant hypoxemia within first hour after NIV initiation.[6-8]

Predictors of HHHFNC failure in bronchiolitis include increased PCO_2, failure to reduce RR or normalize HR, and failure to decrease FiO_2 less than 0.5 in the first 1–2 hours.[9]

COMPLICATIONS

Complications associated with NIV are seen most often in the most fragile patients; they include gastric distention, aspiration, pneumothorax, and pressure ulcerations. Complications reported by the use of HHHFNC oxygen therapy are rare and similar to those reported with CPAP and BiPAP, including gastric insufflation, eye irritation, inability to continuously monitor capnography, air leak (e.g. pneumothorax, pneumomediastinum), and failure to recognize treatment failure that delays ETI. Compared with NIV, HHHFNC has improved patient comfort and fewer skin injuries.[1,3]

USE OF NIV IN ACUTE CARE SETTING IN PEDIATRICS: EVIDENCE AND OUTCOMES

There has been a trend toward increasing use of NIV in acute care settings in children in the last two decades and research is still active in this area. The first randomized controlled trial (RCT) of NIV plus standard therapy versus standard therapy alone in acute respiratory failure in children was published in 2008 and showed improvement in HR, RR, PaO_2/FiO_2 ratio and lower rates of endotracheal intubation in NIV group.[10] Similar findings were observed in other studies also.[8,11] There is a significant increase in the use of NIV in children from 11.9 to 21.6% in 2006 and 2012, respectively in an Italian study.[12] Also, the success rates of NIV have been reported as 64–84% in preventing invasive mechanical ventilation in children in various causes of acute respiratory failure.[6,8,11]

Acute Respiratory Distress Syndrome

Noninvasive ventilation in ARDS has shown high failure rates especially in moderate to severe ARDS between 50 and 78%.[8,12] This high failure rate has led to the recommendation by the pediatric acute lung injury consensus conference (PALICC) group in 2015 that NIV, preferably BiPAP, may be considered in children at risk of ARDS or with mild ARDS as initial mode of treatment. However, this can be considered only if they are meticulously monitored by highly trained staff. Full face or oronasal mask is preferred in this setting. ETI and IMV should be considered as treatment of choice in children with moderate to severe ARDS as well as in case of NIV failure in mild ARDS. Also, they recommend the use of sedation to improve patient ventilator synchrony. The use of HHHFNC in ARDS has not been well studied and no recommendations could be made regarding its use by PALICC group.[13]

Asthma

In two pediatric RCTs comparing BiPAP with standard care in asthma including one pilot study, BiPAP showed significant improvement in clinical parameters and asthma scores without increase in adverse effects.[14,15] In asthma, NIV helps in reducing the work of breathing, eliminates auto PEEP, stents small airways, decreases resistance to airflow and improves the delivery of aerosolized bronchodilators. The other observational studies have also shown good tolerance and improved clinical parameters without increase in complications.[16,17] Data is still inconclusive regarding the ability of NIV to prevent ETI and IMV according to recent systematic reviews.[18] Hence, more evidence is still required.

The HHHFNC has also shown promising results in status asthmaticus with clinical improvement and in certain studies, reduction in incidence of IMV.[19] However, larger studies are needed to recommend its use in asthma.

Bronchiolitis

Bronchiolitis is one of the major causes of respiratory distress in infants and young children requiring hospitalization. There are several studies on the use of CPAP and HHHFNC in severe bronchiolitis in infants showing improved RR and work of breathing with both CPAP and HHHFNC and hence an increasing trend toward their use. However, a recent Cochrane review has reported that the evidence for the use of either CPAP or HHHFNC in bronchiolitis is insufficient.[20,21] A retrospective study in 2012 showed a 2.8% increase in NIV per year and decrease in ETI by 1.9% per year with a success rate of 83.2%.

Noninvasive ventilation failure was associated with the presence of comorbid conditions like prematurity, congenital heart disease, chronic lung disease, immunodeficiency and neuromuscular disease.[22] Two small RCTs have shown benefit of CPAP over supplemental oxygen therapy in terms of decrease in respiratory distress score, work of breathing and need for oxygen in severe RSV bronchiolitis. Also, the hospital stay and cost of care was decreased with the use of CPAP without any adverse events.[23,24]

HHHFNC is a reasonable initial therapy to start with in infants with bronchiolitis although it has not been shown to be superior to CPAP in a recent Cochrane review.[21] However, in infants with severe bronchiolitis, HHHFNC should be initiated with careful monitoring as it is safe and has better tolerability than CPAP.

Pneumonia

Noninvasive ventilation in pneumonia similar to ARDS requires careful consideration. A small RCT comparing Noninvasive ventilation with standard oxygen therapy in respiratory failure due to pneumonia in children demonstrated reduction in rates of ETI with NIV up to 72%.[10] Several other trials have also shown benefits of NIV in improving symptoms and laboratory parameters as well as prevention of ETI without any complications.[6,25] However, pneumonia was found to be a risk factor for NIV failure in a prospective study.[6] NIV can be considered as initial mode of respiratory support in children with mild to moderate pneumonia with close monitoring till further evidence is available with larger RCTs. There is insufficient data regarding utility of CPAP and HHHFNC in pneumonia in children.

Immunocompromised Children

Immunocompromised children are mostly admitted with pneumonia leading to rapid progression to respiratory failure. Many of these patients require ETI and IMV which leads to complications associated with IMV such as ventilator associated pneumonia and ventilator induced lung injury contributing to increased mortality among these children. NIV helps these children by avoiding ETI and its associated complications besides decreasing work of breathing.[26,27] However, these children should be carefully monitored when on NIV and further interventions should be done as needed.

Postoperative and Postextubation

There is a paucity of literature to support the use of NIV in the postoperative period in children. However, NIV is often used in pediatric cardiac ICUs following cardiac surgery. In a retrospective study from the US Pediatric cardiac critical care consortium, NIV use across hospitals ranged from 32 to 65%.[28] The adjusted mean duration was 1-4 days. This data includes children given HHHFNC and positive airway pressure (CPAP and BiPAP). Similarly, in a retrospective study from a Spanish PICU, including all children following cardiac surgery from 2001 to 2012, NIV use (not including HHHFNC) increased from 13.2% in the first 6 years to 29.2% in the last 6 years, with a median duration of 3 days.[29] Similar results are available from post liver transplant patients in a small retrospective study for children below 12 years operated between 2001 and 2009.[30]

Some studies have categorized the use of NIV in the postextubation period as "prophylactic" if this was started soon after extubation (as planned) and compared the same in children in whom it was started after signs and symptoms of acute respiratory failure developed (called "nonprophylactic" or "rescue"). Children who received NIV prophylactically had shorter ICU and hospital stays. The authors opined that NIV can be safely applied to prevent extubation failure in the critically ill child with heart disease.[31]

CONCLUSION

Noninvasive ventilation has been used at a larger scale in recent years both in emergency and critical care areas and has shown promising results in acute respiratory failure. Although high quality evidence is still lacking regarding its use, there is progressive increase in research in this field which will provide answers in the near future. Judicious patient selection with early initiation of NIV may prevent progression to ETI and IMV. The patient needs to be closely monitored when on NIV, more than on IMV, to assess NIV failure or success. In case of non-improvement or worsening of clinical and laboratory parameters on NIV, respiratory support should be quickly escalated and the patient intubated tracheally and started on invasive mechanical ventilation. There are many ongoing RCTs involving the use of CPAP and HHHFNC which will provide concrete evidence regarding their use in future.

REFERENCES

1. Fedor KL. Noninvasive respiratory support in infants and children. Respir Care. 2017;62(6):699-717.
2. Cheifetz IM. Invasive and noninvasive pediatric mechanical ventilation. Respir Care. 2003;48(4): 442-53; discussion 453-8.

3. Viscusi CD, Pacheco GS. Pediatric Emergency Noninvasive Ventilation. Emerg Med Clin North Am. 2018;36(2):387-400.
4. Lee JH, Rehder KJ, Williford L, Cheifetz IM, Turner DA. Use of high flow nasal cannula in critically ill infants, children, and adults: a critical review of the literature. Intensive Care Med. 2013;39(2):247-57.
5. Mortamet G, Amaddeo A, Essouri S, Renolleau S, Emeriaud G, Fauroux B. Interfaces for noninvasive ventilation in the acute setting in children. Paediatr Respir Rev. 2017;23:84-8.
6. Bernet V, Hug MI, Frey B. Predictive factors for the success of noninvasive mask ventilation in infants and children with acute respiratory failure. Pediatr Crit Care Med J Soc Crit Care Med World Fed Pediatr Intensive Crit Care Soc. 2005;6(6):660-4.
7. James CS, Hallewell CPJ, James DPL, Wade A, Mok QQ. Predicting the success of non-invasive ventilation in preventing intubation and re-intubation in the paediatric intensive care unit. Intensive Care Med. 2011;37(12):1994-2001.
8. Mayordomo-Colunga J, Medina A, Rey C, Díaz JJ, Concha A, Los Arcos M, et al. Predictive factors of noninvasive ventilation failure in critically ill children: a prospective epidemiological study. Intensive Care Med. 2009;35(3):527-36.
9. Abboud PA, Roth PJ, Skiles CL, Stolfi A, Rowin ME. Predictors of failure in infants with viral bronchiolitis treated with high-flow, high-humidity nasal cannula therapy*. Pediatr Crit Care Med. 2012;13(6):e343-349.
10. Yañez LJ, Yunge M, Emilfork M, Lapadula M, Alcántara A, Fernández C, et al. A prospective, randomized, controlled trial of noninvasive ventilation in pediatric acute respiratory failure. Pediatr Crit Care Med. 2008;9(5):484-9.
11. Dohna-Schwake C, Stehling F, Tschiedel E, Wallot M, Mellies U. Non-invasive ventilation on a pediatric intensive care unit: feasibility, efficacy, and predictors of success. Pediatr Pulmonol. 2011;46(11):1114-20.
12. Wolfler A, Calderini E, Iannella E, Conti G, Biban P, Dolcini A, et al. Evolution of Noninvasive Mechanical Ventilation Use: A Cohort Study Among Italian PICUs. Pediatr Crit Care Med. 2015;16(5):418-27.
13. Essouri S, Carroll C, Pediatric Acute Lung Injury Consensus Conference Group. Noninvasive support and ventilation for pediatric acute respiratory distress syndrome: proceedings from the Pediatric Acute Lung Injury Consensus Conference. Pediatr Crit Care Med J Soc Crit Care Med World Fed Pediatr Intensive Crit Care Soc. 2015;16(5 Suppl 1):S102-110.
14. Basnet S, Mander G, Andoh J, Klaska H, Verhulst S, Koirala J. Safety, efficacy, and tolerability of early initiation of noninvasive positive pressure ventilation in pediatric patients admitted with status asthmaticus: a pilot study. Pediatr Crit Care Med J Soc Crit Care Med World Fed Pediatr Intensive Crit Care Soc. 2012;13(4):393-8.
15. Thill PJ, McGuire JK, Baden HP, Green TP, Checchia PA. Noninvasive positive-pressure ventilation in children with lower airway obstruction. Pediatr Crit Care Med J Soc Crit Care Med World Fed Pediatr Intensive Crit Care Soc. 2004;5(4):337-42.
16. Carroll CL, Schramm CM. Noninvasive positive pressure ventilation for the treatment of status asthmaticus in children. Ann Allergy Asthma Immunol Off Publ Am Coll Allergy Asthma Immunol. 2006;96(3):454-9.
17. Mayordomo-Colunga J, Medina A, Rey C, Concha A, Menéndez S, Arcos ML, et al. Non-invasive ventilation in pediatric status asthmaticus: a prospective observational study. Pediatr Pulmonol. 2011;46(10):949-55.
18. Korang SK, Feinberg J, Wetterslev J, Jakobsen JC. Non-invasive positive pressure ventilation for acute asthma in children. Cochrane Database Syst Rev. 2016;9:CD012067.
19. Baudin F, Buisson A, Vanel B, Massenavette B, Pouyau R, Javouhey E. Nasal high flow in management of children with status asthmaticus: a retrospective observational study. Ann Intensive Care. 2017;7(1):55.

20. Jat KR, Mathew JL. Continuous positive airway pressure (CPAP) for acute bronchiolitis in children. Cochrane Database Syst Rev. 2015;1:CD010473.
21. Beggs S, Wong ZH, Kaul S, Ogden KJ, Walters JAE. High-flow nasal cannula therapy for infants with bronchiolitis. Cochrane Database Syst Rev. 2014;(1):CD009609.
22. Ganu SS, Gautam A, Wilkins B, Egan J. Increase in use of non-invasive ventilation for infants with severe bronchiolitis is associated with decline in intubation rates over a decade. Intensive Care Med. 2012;38(7):1177-83.
23. Thia LP, McKenzie SA, Blyth TP, Minasian CC, Kozlowska WJ, Carr SB. Randomised controlled trial of nasal continuous positive airways pressure (CPAP) in bronchiolitis. Arch Dis Child. 2008;93(1):45-7.
24. Milési C, Matecki S, Jaber S, Mura T, Jacquot A, Pidoux O, et al. 6 cmH$_2$O continuous positive airway pressure versus conventional oxygen therapy in severe viral bronchiolitis: a randomized trial. Pediatr Pulmonol. 2013;48(1):45-51.
25. Abadesso C, Nunes P, Silvestre C, Matias E, Loureiro H, Almeida H. Non-invasive ventilation in acute respiratory failure in children. Pediatr Rep. 2012;4(2):e16.
26. Pancera CF, Hayashi M, Fregnani JH, Negri EM, Deheinzelin D, de Camargo B. Noninvasive ventilation in immunocompromised pediatric patients: eight years of experience in a pediatric oncology intensive care unit. J Pediatr Hematol Oncol. 2008;30(7):533-8.
27. Schiller O, Schonfeld T, Yaniv I, Stein J, Kadmon G, Nahum E. Bi-level positive airway pressure ventilation in pediatric oncology patients with acute respiratory failure. J Intensive Care Med. 2009;24(6):383-8.
28. Romans RA, Schwartz SM, Costello JM, Chanani NK, Prodhan P, Smith AH, et al. Epidemiology of noninvasive ventilation in pediatric cardiac intensive care units. Pediatr Crit Care Med. 2017;18:949-57.
29. Fernandez Lafever S, Toledo B, Leiva M, Padron M, Balseiro M, Carrillo A, et al. Non-invasive mechanical ventilation after heart surgery in children. BMC Pulmonary Med. 2016;16:167.
30. Murase K, Chihara Y, Takahashi K, Okamoto S, Segawa H, Fukuda K, et al. Use of noninvasive ventilation for pediatric patients after liver transplantation: decrease in the need for reintubation. Liver Transpl. 2012;18:1217-25.
31. Gupta P, Kuperstock JE, Hashmi S, Arnolde V, Gossett JM, Prodhan P, et al. Efficacy and predictors of success of noninvasive ventilation for prevention of extubation failure in critically ill children with heart disease. Pediatr Cardio. 2013;34:964-77.

Index

Page numbers followed by *b* refer to box, *f* refer to figure, *fc* refer to flowchart, and *t* refer to table.

A

Abrasions 85
Accessory muscle, use of 62, 67
Acidosis, severe 91
Acquired immunodeficiency
   syndrome 101, 149
Acute hypercapnic failure 78, 83
   contributors of 82
Acute hypercapnic respiratory
   failure 51, 63, 77, 262
   causes of 77
Acute hypoxemic respiratory failure
   101, 113, 172, 262, 266,
   269, 270, 276, 278, 280*fc*
   treatment of 260
Acute left ventricle dysfunction 105
Acute respiratory acidosis 51, 143
   prevention of 51
Acute respiratory distress syndrome
   53, 54, 73, 96, 99, 113,
   114, 116, 117*fc*, 176, 203,
   270, 317, 321
   de novo 115
   development of 82
   mild 63
   mild-to-moderate 197
   moderate-to-severe 183
   severity of 115
Acute respiratory failure 3, 11, 41,
   51-53, 62, 63, 63*b*, 67, 84,
   98, 109, 119, 120, 142, 143,
   149, 150, 153, 156, 159,
   163, 183, 197, 210, 264,
   269, 270, 317, 323
   pathophysiology of 78, 145
Adaptive servo ventilation 20, 26, 128
Adequate monitoring, requirements
   for 198
Adequate oxygenation and
   ventilation 320
Adjuvant therapies 40
Adrenaline 47
Advanced airways, use of 316
Aerophagia 68
Aerosol delivery
   device 46*f*
   factors influencing 191*f*
Aerosol deposition 44, 44*f*, 188, 189*f*

Aerosol generator 44
   types of 45, 192
Aerosol particles size 192
Aerosol system 188, 189
   components of 188
   factors determining efficiency of
      188
Aerosol therapy 40, 43, 186, 188
   common applications of 190, 190*t*
Agitation 79, 82
Air 275, 330
   leak 42, 67, 86
      compensation 15
      pressure 86
Airway 53, 73, 190
   clearance 311, 312
      techniques 311
   defects 307
   diseases 74
   dryness 57, 86
   inflammation 190
   injury 149
   obstruction, respiratory
      depression 184
   pressure 106*f*, 158
      continuous 246
   resistance 21
Alcohol intake 100
Allogeneic hematopoietic cell
   transplantations 101
Altitude compensation 132
Alveolar hypoventilation, primary 74
American thoracic society 11, 86,
   157, 306, 307
   clinical practice guidelines 216
Amikacin 190
Amphotericin B 190
Amyotrophic lateral sclerosis 74,
   239, 245, 251
Ancillary therapies 311
Anesthesia 53
Anterior horn cell 73
Antibiotics 190
Anxiety 242
Aortic blood pressure 106*f*
Apnea 124
   central 248, 254
   hypopnea index 125, 248, 249

Apneic oxygenation, preprocedure 262
Argyle nasal prongs 290*f*
Arm edema 85
Arrhythmia 56, 59, 79, 102, 158,
   167, 267
   cardiac 261
Arterial blood gas 62, 67, 199
   abnormalities 83
   analysis 204, 204*t*
Arterial blood pressure 165
Arterial carbon dioxide 51
   tension 78
Arterial oxygen partial pressure 40
Arterial pulse pressure 8
Aspergillus prevention 190
Asphyxia, less chances of 33
Aspiration 68, 167
   high risk of 102
   pneumonia 57, 85
   risk of 58
   worsening of 82
Asthma 73, 190, 322
   acute 51, 52, 74, 190
   severe 79
   chronic obstructive pulmonary
      disease overlap
      syndrome 53
   exacerbations 63
   pathophysiological feature of 52
Asynchrony 32
Atelectasis 54, 121, 140, 146
   bilateral lobar 121
   preventing 276
   treat postoperative 121
Atelectrauma 96
At-home ventilators 16*f*
Atrial natriuretic peptide synthesis 7
Automatic tube compensation 216
Auto-positive end-expiratory
      pressure 21
Auto-titrating continuous positive
      airway pressure 127, 129
Average volume assured pressure
   mode 210
   support 20, 23, 252
Awakening and breathing controlled
   trials 216

B

Backup respiratory rate 16, 251
Bag and mask, self-inflating 312
Bariatric surgery 120
Barotrauma 57, 59, 85, 96, 268
Becker's muscular dystrophy 134
Bernoulli's effect 289
Beta-agonists 190
Bilevel continuous positive airway pressure 297, 310
Bilevel noninvasive ventilation 51
Bilevel positive airway pressure 22, 23, 31, 40, 51, 64, 78, 101, 128, 129, 135, 241, 249, 317
  spontaneous mode 20
  therapy 302
  work 108
Biotrauma 96
Biphasic positive airway pressure 316, 319
Bite plates 32
Biventricular function 6fc, 7fc
Blood
  gas 70
    analysis 199
    worsening of 99
  pressure, reduction in 125
  products, large transfusion of 145
Blunt injury 99
Body mass index 83
Body weight, predicted 114
Borg dyspnea score 153
Borg scale, modified 153
Botulism 74
Boussignac continuous positive airway pressure 166f
  mask 166f
Bowel obstruction 79
Brain injury, traumatic 313
Brainstem 91fc
Breath
  enhanced jet nebulizer 46
  per minute 252
  stacking 140
Breathing
  glossopharyngeal 136
  measurement of 124
  patterns 16
  work of 21
British Thoracic Society 58
  Guidelines 198, 225
Bronchial asthma
  exacerbation of 85
  severe 3

Bronchiectasis 73, 74, 78, 245
Bronchiolitis 22, 322
Bronchitis 74
Bronchodilator 45, 190
Bronchopulmonary dysplasia 245, 286, 310
Bronchoscopy 171
  ultrasound guided 171
Bronchospasm 190
Bubble Continuous positive airway pressure system 288f
Bubble humidifier 43
Budesonide 47, 190
Bulbar involvement 253
Bulbar weakness 138
Burns 79

C

Capnography 203
  mainstream 206, 206f, 206t
  monitoring 203
  waveform 204, 204f
  understanding 204
Carbon dioxide 203, 205, 317
  arterial partial pressure of 216
  arterial pressure of 41
  cutaneous 206
  monitoring 247
  rebreathing 57
  transcutaneous measurement of 247
Cardiac arrest 56, 102
Cardiac disease 157
Cardiac failure 82
  chronic 242
Cardiac function 105
Cardiac origin, pulmonary edema of 113
Cardiac output 105
Cardiac parameters 200
Cardiac transmural pressure 105, 108
Cardiogenic pulmonary edema 51, 52, 63, 74, 98, 105, 109, 157, 197, 259, 260
  management of 10
  pathophysiology of 10, 105
Cardiopulmonary disease 154, 157
Cardiopulmonary interactions 11
Cardiopulmonary monitoring 312
Cardiorespiratory interaction 107f
Cardiovascular system, effects on 7
Care providers, training of 312
Ceftazidime 190

Central inspiratory drive, inadequate 307
Central nervous system
  abnormalities 74
  diseases 73
Central sleep apnea 254
Central venous pressure 9
Chemotherapy, receiving 149
Chest
  deformity, obese severe 27
  trauma 53, 99, 142
    non-flail 54
  wall 74, 236
    abnormalities 74
    deformity 51, 55, 63, 65, 77, 85, 142, 143, 144t, 235
    disease 74, 144
    disorders 142, 235
    trauma 74
  X-ray 295
Cheyne-Stokes
  breathing 26
  respiration 254
Child's inspiration 289
Chronic end-stage diseases 242
Chronic home respiratory support 313
Chronic hypercapnic respiratory failure 89
  management of 89
Chronic obstructive airway disease 74
Chronic obstructive pulmonary disease 3, 51, 63, 73, 77, 78, 89, 90, 96, 113, 138, 171, 179, 187, 190, 197, 210, 216, 218f, 233, 234, 236, 239, 240, 243, 245, 251, 259, 262, 267, 306
  acute exacerbation of 51, 63, 74, 86, 89, 163
  exacerbation 90f, 92fc, 190
  stable 90f
Chronic obstructive pulmonary disorder 50
Chronic respiratory
  conditions 233
  diseases 306
  failure 143, 179, 233, 235, 242, 306
  support 306
Claustrophobia 33, 34, 36, 57, 82, 86, 102, 131
Colistin 190
Collection bag 46
Coma 56
Concurrent infection 78

Index

Confusion 79
Consciousness
　altered 93
　impaired 56, 79, 102
Continuous capnography 208
　use of 208
Continuous cardiorespiratory
　　monitoring 320
Continuous flow devices 287, 288
Continuous positive airway pressure
　　3, 10, 13, 21, 40, 84, 97, 105,
　　108, 114, 119, 125, 127, 146,
　　150, 170, 186, 233, 241, 252,
　　259, 267, 285, 288f, 291,
　　292f, 295, 300, 317, 318
　components of 287
　delivery system, components of 287f
　device 289f
　failure of 293
　fixed 127, 129
　interfaces 291t
　machines 310
　principle of 286, 286f
　role of 146
　settings, adjustment of 292
　types of 287, 287t
　weaning from 293
Conventional bubble humidifier 264
Conventional invasive ventilation
　　113, 259
Conventional oxygen therapy 260,
　　261, 269, 270
Cor pulmonale 82
Corticosteroids 62, 149, 150
Cosmetic issues 131
Cough
　assist device 253, 311
　augmentation 253
　impaired 138
　reflex 146
Craniofacial anomalies 308
Critical care ventilator 66, 110
Cystic fibrosis 59, 245, 310-312

D

Daytime sleepiness, excessive 253
De Novo acute respiratory failure
　　51, 54
Dead space 31
　ventilation 92
Deep sedation 184
Deep vein thrombosis 85, 214, 241
Delirium 178
Delivery devices 318

Delivery room continuous positive
　　airway pressure during
　　resuscitation 286
Denitrogenation 169
Deoxyribonucleotidase 312
Desynchrony, state of 85
Device criteria 240
Dexmedetomidine 184
Diabetes mellitus 105, 124
Diaphragm 53
　movements of 5
Diaphragmatic dysfunction 96, 100, 119
　ventilator-induced 176
Diaphragmatic pacing 313
Diaphragmatic rupture 74
Disposable vapor transfer cartridge
　　264
Disuse atrophy 74
Domiciliary noninvasive ventilation
　　239
Downes score system, modified 296t
Draeger nasal prongs 290f
Drug
　class 190
　dose inhaler 45
Dry mouth 82
Dry powder inhaler 47, 189
Duchenne muscular dystrophy 134,
　　239, 251, 253
Dynamic transpulmonary pressure 158
Dyslipidemia 124
Dyspnea 143, 153, 158
　reduction of 153
　relieves 103
Dystrophinopathies 134

E

Early mobilization, cost-
　　effectiveness of 179
Early morning bifrontal headaches 253
Edema
　acute cardiogenic pulmonary 96
　fluid, leakage of 145
Effective aerosol drug delivery 189t
Ejection fraction, reduced 254
Electrocardiography, continuous 200
Electrolyte abnormalities 74
Emphysema 74
Encephalitis 73, 313
Encephalopathy
　hypercapnic 91
　persistent 82
End-expiratory lung volume 90,
　　125, 275

End-inspiratory transpulmonary
　　pressure 158
Endocrine disorders 74
Endoscopic retrograde Cholangio-
　　pancreatography 172
Endoscopy 63, 172
Endotracheal intubation 3, 51, 62,
　　96, 98, 146, 183, 259, 317
　preoxygenation before 267
　required 101
Endotracheal tube 290f, 316
End-tidal capnography 205
End-tidal carbon dioxide 199, 204f
　monitoring 204, 204t
Epoprostenol 190
Erectile dysfunction 125
Erythema 57, 85
Esophageal anastomosis, recent 56, 79
Esophageal balloon 158
European Pressure Ulcer Advisory
　　Panel 224
European Respiratory Society 11,
　　86, 157, 216
Exacerbation, acute 51
Excessive leaks around mask 68
Exhalation valve, position of 16
Expiratory positive airway pressure
　　3, 13, 16f, 21, 41, 64, 78,
　　97, 108, 128, 135, 240,
　　243, 319
Extubation failure 216
　high risk of 217

F

Face
　injury 34
　mask 96, 114, 234f, 254
　　simple 264
　　total 226, 237f
　pressure sores on 82
Facial
　burns 56
　hair 131
　skin lesions 85
　trauma 56, 79, 99, 102
Fat embolism syndrome 73
Fatty acids, hyperoxygenated 226
Fiberoptic bronchoscopy 171
First line respiratory support 149
Fisher and Paykel nasal prongs 290f
Flail chest 53, 73, 74, 146
　trauma 54
Flexible fiberoptic bronchoscope 171

Fluid
    flip 289f
    responsiveness, predicting 10
Fluticasone 190
Forced expiratory volume 53, 144
Forced vital capacity 144, 243
Free eyes 33
Free mouth 33
Full-face 32, 80, 109
    mask 35, 36, 101, 236, 308
Full-night studies 129
Functional residual capacity 8, 97, 144

G

Gas exchange 146, 158
    indices 144
    parameters 198
Gas flows 16
Gastric
    distension 33, 68, 200
    insufflation 57, 86, 223, 228
Gastroesophageal reflux, symptoms of 125
Gastrointestinal effects 297
Gastrointestinal procedures 173
Gastroscopy 172
Glasgow coma
    scale 50, 56, 83, 198, 239, 243
    score 200
Glucose tolerance, impaired 124
Greater respiratory impairment 158
Guillain-Barré syndrome 73, 74, 313

H

Haloperidol 184
Head
    and neck movements, restriction of 36
    injuries 99
Headgear placement 131
Health evaluation, acute physiology and chronic 50, 54, 84
Heart 106
    disease 323
    failure 7, 254, 260, 267
        acute decompensated 163, 262
        congestive 21, 64, 254, 266
        incidences 125
        programs for 254
    lung interaction 5, 11, 106, 108
        clinical applications of 9
    rate 295

Heat
    advantages of 187t
    and moisture exchanger 42t, 80, 186
        filter 187, 189
    disadvantages of 187t
Heated humidifier 41, 42t, 43, 187
    systems 187t
Helium 35, 35f, 80, 190, 236, 237f
Helmet mask 101
Hematopoietic stem cell transplant 149, 150
Hemodynamic effects 59
Hemodynamic instability 56, 57, 79, 102, 116, 178
    exclusion of 157
    severe 79
Hemothorax 53, 54, 146
High dependency unit 63, 197
High flow nasal cannula 84, 170, 257, 259, 264, 266t, 267, 271, 275, 280fc, 301, 303, 304, 317, 320
    administration of 303
    delivery 303f
    indications of 302
    infection 262
    oxygenation 259, 281
    therapy 268, 275, 279, 304
        heated humidified 300
High flow oxygen
    group 115
    therapy 264, 271
High oxygen requirement 255
Home bilevel positive airway pressure 245
Home care service 251
Home mechanical ventilation 252
    indications of 245
Home noninvasive ventilation 235, 237, 245
Home oxygen therapy 252, 313, 314
Home respiratory support 306, 307t, 314b
    indications of 307
    part of 310
    required 313
    weaning of 313
Home ventilation 231, 233, 238, 245, 251, 252, 254, 307t
    mainstay of 251
    major indications for 251
    require 307
Home ventilator 249
    and telemonitoring, monitoring accuracy of 245
    care 251

Hospital readmission, risk of 252
Hudson nasal prongs 290f
Humidification 40, 41, 131, 186, 188
    device 311
    types of 42
Humidified gas, warmed 266
Humidified oxygen, high flow 150
Humidity
    absolute 41, 187
    control of 227
Hybrid mask 237f
Hydration, adequate 235
Hydrogen peroxide 48
Hypercapnia 238, 252
    chronic daytime 241
    daytime 254
    persistent 252
    predominate 252
Hypercapnic failure 272
    acute on chronic 83
    moderate 272
Hypercapnic respiratory failure 113, 272
Hypercapnic subgroup 153
Hyperemia, local 247
Hypertension, chronic 105
Hypertonic saline therapy 312
Hypervolemia 9
Hypophosphatemia 215
Hypopnea 124, 248
Hypotension 57, 68, 85, 167
Hypoventilation 140, 172
    alveolar 72, 73
    central 245
    chronic 143
    congenital 313
    severe central 308
    syndrome 23
        congenital 308
Hypoxemia 54, 73, 105, 143, 167, 252, 270
    acute 100
    cycle of 105
    progressive 277
    severe 79, 261
    severity of 116
Hypoxemic acute respiratory failure 277
Hypoxemic respiratory failure 91, 96, 98, 101, 102fc, 103, 119, 146, 157, 235, 259, 260, 264, 267, 271
    post-traumatic 147
    preoxygenation in 271
Hypoxia 154, 172, 247
    severe chronic 307

Index

I

Ideal interface, characteristics of 30, 30*b*
Illness, acute 253
Iloprost 190
Infection
  acute 312
  control 48
Inflammatory cellular infiltrates 145
Influenza
  A 54
    H1N1 infection 158
  severe 266
Inhaled gas
  pressure of 42
  temperature of 42
In-home titration 130
  disadvantage of 130
Injury, diaphragmatic 100
Insomnia, severe 127
Inspiratory flow 15, 42
Inspiratory limb, single 278
Inspiratory oxygen fraction 40
Inspiratory positive airway pressure 3, 13, 16*f*, 21, 64, 78, 97, 108, 128, 145, 236, 240, 243, 251, 319
  titration of 135
Inspiratory time 23
Inspiratory trigger 15
Inspired oxygen 259
  ratio 115
  fraction of 17, 42, 79, 96, 97, 179, 187, 264, 288, 295, 295*f*
Insufflation-exsufflation devices 253
Intelligent volume assured pressure support 20
  ventilation 24
Intensive care unit 13, 17, 50, 63, 77, 96, 149, 159, 163, 177, 188, 197, 208, 216, 275, 300, 306
  acquired weakness, management of 177
  procedures 169
  ventilators 16*f*, 17, 17*t*
Interface
  change of 226
  choice of 79
  fit, proper 225
  material, proper 225
  types of 32, 190, 236
Interhospital transfer 163
Intermittent positive pressure ventilation 5

Internal flow sensors 294
Internal pneumatic stabilization 146
Intra-abdominal pressure 5
Intrahospital transfer 164
Intrathoracic pressure 5, 105
  effects of 7*fc*
Intubation bundle 170
Invasive artificial airway 169, 233
Invasive mechanical ventilation 3, 50, 56, 77, 96, 99, 102, 113, 151, 159, 176, 242, 276, 317
  complications of 149
  postextubation from 55
  weaning assist from 216
Invasive positive pressure ventilation 137
Invasive ventilation 13, 253, 259, 260, 306, 316
  elective 141
Ipratropium 190
  bromide 47
  nebulization 62
Ischemia 59
  cardiac 158
Isopropyl alcohol 48

J

Jacket ventilator 19
Jet nebulizer 45, 46
  correct use of 47
  types of 46
Jet reservoir 46
Jet turbine principle 166*f*

K

Kidney
  disease, chronic 124
  failure, chronic 105
Kussmaul's sign 9
Kyphoscoliosis 73, 74, 77, 85, 251
  early-onset 245
Kyphosis 142

L

Lacrimation 33
Lactate dehydrogenase 158
Leak test 246
Left ventricle 6, 7, 8*f*
  dysfunction development 105
Left ventricular
  dysfunction 82

  ejection fraction 261
  end-diastolic
    pressure 105
    volume 9
Lethargy 143
Levosalbutamol 47
Limb
  circuits, single 86, 251
  expiratory 291
  inspiratory 291
  number of 246
Low intensity ventilator strategy 234
Low ventilatory support 313
Lower motor neuron 138
Lung 74, 106, 136, 245
  abnormality 73
  capacity, total 90
  compliance 21
    reduced 318
  contusion 146
  disease
    acute interstitial 190
    chronic 252, 302, 310
    granulomatous 73
    interstitial 310
  failure 72
  inflation of 7
  injury 11
    acute 114, 152
    aggravating 114
    ventilator induced 96, 156, 285, 323
  parenchyma 53, 73, 145
    acute infection of 156
    severe infection of 156
  resection
    postoperative 120
    sequelae 245
  transplantation 121, 190
  volume 5, 7

M

Machine 246
  expiratory component 246
  inspiratory component 246
  unintentional leaks 246
Malignancy
  advanced 242
  hematologic 101, 266
Malnutrition 74
Mask
  comfort 67
  discomfort 68

intolerance 57
rotation 226
types of 101
Maximum expiratory pressure 144
Maximum inspiratory pressure 144, 243
Mean airway pressure 295
Mean blood oxygen 145
Mean systemic filling pressure 5, 6, 6f, 7
Mechanical ventilation 3, 98, 157, 214, 215f, 259, 260, 280, 295
  delivery of 285
  prolonged 215
Medicine, evolution of 245
Mental status 304
Metabolic acidosis 105
  presence of 116
Metabolic substances, accumulation of 224
Metastatic pain, severe 153
Metered dose inhaler 45, 45f
Midazolam 184
Molecular genetic testing 134
Monitoring and nursing care 295
Monitoring and weaning 195
Monitoring parameters 198
Morphine 153, 184
Motor functions, normal 139
Motor neuron disease 245
Mouth breathing 131
Mouthpiece 32, 79
Movement disorders 127
Mucociliary clearance 100
Multicenter randomized controlled trial 119
Multidrug resistant 190
  pneumonia 190
  tracheobronchitis 190
Multiorgan dysfunction syndrome 203
Multiorgan failure 116
Muscle
  abnormalities 74
  strength
    expiratory 253
    inspiratory 253
Muscular dystrophy 74, 142, 245, 313
Musculoskeletal self-injury, risk of 178
Myasthenia gravis 74
Myocardial infarction 11
Myocardium 108
Myopathy 134
Myotrauma 96

N

Narcolepsy 127
Nasal airway resistance 42
Nasal antihistamines 131
Nasal bridge 110, 223f
  ulceration 57
Nasal cannula 150, 264, 290, 300
  and masks, normal 261
  monitoring in high flow 275
  physiological effects of high flow 275
  role of high-flow 152
  settings of high flow 278
  set-up of high-flow 265f
  success, predictors of high flow 276
  therapy, newborn receiving high flow 303f
  treatment failure, predictors of high flow 276
  weaning from high flow 268, 275, 279
  wide-bore 275
Nasal congestion 57, 68, 86, 131
Nasal continuous positive airway pressure 285, 301
  contraindications 286
  failure 293
  indications 285
Nasal decongestants 235
Nasal dryness 68, 86
Nasal effects 297
Nasal glucocorticoids 131
Nasal high-frequency ventilation 285
Nasal interfaces 32, 33, 33f
  types of 290f
Nasal mask 32, 36, 79, 101, 137, 237f, 289
Nasal mucosa, keratinization of 42
Nasal neurally adjusted ventilator assist 285
Nasal oxygen, high flow 218, 262
Nasal pillows 32, 79, 101, 131, 236, 237f
Nasal prongs 289, 308
  secure fixation of 290f
Nasal sling 32
Nasal trauma 290f
  scoring chart 292f
Nasogastric tube 227
  insertion 57
Nasopharyngeal prong 290, 290f
  single 290f
Nebulization 40
  common drugs used for 47, 47t
Nebulizer 192

Negative pressure
  pulmonary edema 10
  ventilation 40
Neonatal intensive care unit 295
Neonates 285
Neonatology and pediatrics 283
Neuromuscular disease 33, 51, 55, 63, 65, 77, 85, 134, 235, 236, 240, 245, 249, 251, 253
  inherited 253
Neuromuscular disorders 59, 74, 242
  chronic 253
Neuromuscular junction 134, 136
Neuromuscular transmission 73
Neuromuscular weakness 149, 311, 312
Newborns, sample monitoring chart for 295f
Nocturnal arrhythmias 125
Nocturnal hypercapnia 134
Nocturnal hypoventilation 253
  reduce 239
Noncardiogenic pulmonary edema 74
Noninvasive approaches, novel 136
Noninvasive high-frequency ventilation 20, 26
Noninvasive home ventilators 13
Noninvasive interfaces 36
Noninvasive positive pressure ventilation 40, 50b, 62, 113, 115, 119, 171, 191f, 285, 293
  delivery 99
  devices 294
  failure of 295
  nasal interface 294
  settings, adjustment of 294
  types of 317
Noninvasive pressure support ventilation 294
Noninvasive respiratory support 316
Noninvasive ventilation 3 5, 11, 13, 17t, 19, 30, 37, 50, 51b, 56, 56t, 62, 63b, 64, 70, 77, 83, 89, 91fc, 96, 97, 102b, 105, 110, 113, 114b, 119, 140, 149, 156, 163, 167t, 169, 173, 176, 183, 184t, 187t, 188, 190, 197, 203, 210, 211t, 217, 223, 234, 245, 251, 254, 259, 262, 266, 285, 295f, 300, 308, 319, 323
  advantages of 4
  adverse effects of 200
  aerosol equipment for 44
  ambulation on 176

and tracheostomy 218
application of 62, 65, 66, 66f, 69fc, 98, 109, 217
classification of 20fc
complications of 50, 57t, 297
contraindications of 50, 143, 317
discontinuation of 68
disease specific 75
duration, stepwise reduction in 211
during transport 163
evidence for 150
failure 82, 91, 92, 93, 156, 320, 322
   higher risk of 151
   predictors of 116, 158
   reasons for 157
   strategies to reduce 92
fate of 82
favor humidification during 186
humidification in 187
immediate withdrawal of 212
in abdominal surgery, role of 119
in atelectasis, role of 121
in bariatric surgery, role of 120
in hypoxemic respiratory failure, role of 103
in postlung transplant, role of 121
in spinal surgery, role of 120
in thoracic surgery, role of 120
including newer modes, modes of ventilation for 19
indications for 50, 90, 210, 317
initiation of 64
interface 30, 237
   adopted 36
long-term 136, 233
management of 102fc, 318
mask 223f
mode 20fc, 210
   ventilators without 17
monitoring of 67b, 197, 200
nebulizer in 192f
outcome, predictors of 140
physiological benefits of 97b, 97fc
place of 142, 143
position of 44
potential benefits of 113b
practical aspects of 109
predictors of 116b, 138
pressure support, stepwise reduction in 211
protocol for application of 64
rationale of 3, 4, 89, 96
reasons for underfeeding on 227
rherapeutic benefits of 144t

role of 98, 99, 135, 137, 140
sedation during 183
settings 144
setup 101
skin damage during 37f
spacer in 192f
strategy 285
success 320
therapy, complications of 85
troubleshooting of 68t
use of 4, 50, 117fc, 134, 233, 321
utilization of 216
ventilation in 144, 236
ventilators for 13
weaning from 210
Noninvasive ventilator 19, 20, 101, 165
   understanding 14
Non-rebreathing reservoir mask 264
Normocapnic hypoxemia 143
Nosocomial infection, prevents 119, 316
Nosocomial pneumonia 85, 119
Novel techniques 140
Numeric rating scale 153
Nutrition 223, 227

O

Obesity 74, 77
   hypoventilation syndrome 63, 65, 83, 120, 210, 241, 245, 251, 252
   mild 252
Obstructive disorders
   of upper airways 317
   severe 247
Obstructive sleep apnea 22, 78, 82, 100, 120, 124, 125, 234, 235, 239, 241, 242, 245, 252, 269, 271
   classification 124
   goals of management 124
   indications of 125t
   modes of administration of 126, 126t
   signs of 124t
   symptoms of 124t
Onblanchable erythema 224
Ondine's curse 74
Opera trial 270
Operating room 163
Opioids 208
Oral airway 308
Oral dryness 68, 86

Oral interfaces 32, 32f, 131
Oral mask 236, 237f
Oral surgery especially soft palate 33
Organ dysfunction 83
   major 158
Organ failure 157
   extrapulmonary 114
   life-threatening 56
   presence of 270
Organ transplant 266
Organophosphate poisoning 74
Oronasal mask 34, 34f, 36, 101, 236, 237f, 318
Oropharyngeal airway 308
Orotracheal intubation 261
Orthopnea 254
Osserman classification, modified 137t
Osserman system, modified 136
Oximetry, continuous 67
Oxygen 40, 190, 208, 300
   abnormalities of delivery of 74
   administration of 157
   arterial
      partial pressure of 169
      pressure 157
   blender 275
   cannula, standard 290
   concentrator 233
   conserver device 311
   delivery devices 264
   delivery system 259
   flows 16
   group 151, 153
   heated humidified 275
   inspiratory 157
   saturation 154
   source 233, 310
   supplementation 269, 306, 310
   supply 15, 169
   therapy 10, 151, 300
      long-term 235, 240, 243, 251
   treatment, standard 280
   wastage of 311
Oxygenation 40, 105
   criteria 276

P

Pain, postoperative 53
Palliative care 51, 55, 153, 242
   settings 153, 154
Pancreatitis, acute 145
Pandemic viral illness 54

Paralysis 261
Parasomnia 127
Parenchymal defect 307
Partial pressure of oxygen 79
Passover humidifiers 43
Patent ductus arteriosus 73
Patient education and monitoring 237
Patient selection prior to transport 164
Patient's mental status 102
Patient-device interface 130
Patient-ventilator
   desynchrony 57, 86
   interfaces 3
   synchrony 67
Peak expiratory
   flow rate 43
   pressure 309
Peak inspiratory
   flow rate 264
   pressure 295f, 309
Pediatric acute lung injury consensus conference 321
Pediatric intensive care units 302
Pediatric settings, acute 317
Percutaneous gastrostomy 253
Perfusion inequality 72
Pericardial diseases 9
Phrenic nerve paralysis 245
Physical therapy 176
Physiological exchange parameters 198
Physiotherapy 223, 228
Pleural abnormalities 74
Pleural cavity abnormality 73
Pleural effusion 74
Pleural pressure 90, 106
Pneumatic jet nebulizer with reservoir tube 46
Pneumatic nebulizer 45
   types of 46
Pneumoconiosis 73
Pneumonia 22, 54, 59, 63, 73, 74, 82, 96, 98, 146, 149, 156, 157, 316, 322
   acute respiratory failure due to 157
   community acquired 91, 156, 158, 159
   incidence of 156, 261
   management of 98, 156
   mild-to-moderate 322
   ventilator-associated 51, 96, 156, 197, 214, 259, 323
   risk of 119
   venturi mask for 157
Pneumothorax 53, 54, 73, 79, 82, 268
   acute 56, 85
Poliomyelitis 74
Polymyositis 74
Poor cough 311
Poor nutritional status 100
Portable pressure ventilators 65
Portable ventilator 233
Positive airway pressure 125
   amount of 128
   modes of 126
   therapy 125
   initiation of 126
Positive end-expiratory pressure 3, 16, 16f, 58, 64, 67, 78, 96, 97, 108, 113, 149, 152, 156, 170, 184, 189, 191f, 259, 266, 286, 295
   adequacy of 67
Positive pressure ventilation 7fc, 13, 136, 233
   application of 89
Post-bariatric surgery 120
Post-brain injury sequelae 311, 313
Post-cardiac surgery 267
   postextubation hypoxemia 262
   respiratory failure 261
Post-cardiopulmonary resuscitation 267
Postextubation 51, 269, 270, 286, 293
   failure 214
   hypoxemia 262
   respiratory failure 55, 63, 77, 83, 214
   prevent 216
   support 267
Preintubation
   apneic oxygenation 261
   oxygenation 63, 262
Premature extubation 214
Prematurity 74
   apnea of 286, 293, 300, 302
Premorbid and comorbid state 83
Preoxygenation 169, 173, 269
Pressure
   alveolar 105, 106f
   areas, cushioning of 225
   control 78, 167
   expiratory 23
   generating device 288
   intrapleural 6, 7
   ramp 132
   relief 131
   settings, selecting 128
   sores 57, 68
   measures to prevent 224
   support 78, 97, 167
   adequacy of 67
   approach 66
   ventilation 80
   volume assured 20, 23
   ulcers 85, 214, 223, 223f, 226f
   stages of 224, 224f
   ventilation, volume-targeted 23
Pressure-based trigger 19
Pressure-targeted modes 27
Pressurized metered dose inhaler 45, 189, 190, 191f, 192, 192f
Primary pathology permits 301
Procedural sedation 173
Progressive illness 313
Propofol 184
Proportional-assisted ventilation 20, 24
Prostaglandin synthesis 7
Protein loss 234
Protocolized spontaneous breathing trial 215f
Pseudohypertrophic muscular paralysis 134
Pulmonary arterial hypertension 73
   pressure 92, 144
Pulmonary capillaries 73
Pulmonary compliance 100
Pulmonary contusions 53
Pulmonary edema 73, 105
Pulmonary effects 297
Pulmonary embolism 9, 73, 214
Pulmonary fibrosis 73, 82, 154, 245
Pulmonary hypertension 190, 310
Pulmonary infiltrate, severity of 158
Pulmonary interstitial edema, mechanical effect of 106
Pulmonary vascular resistance 8
   effects on 8
Pulmonary vasculature 53
   abnormality 73
Pulse
   oximeter 247, 312
   oximetry 198
   continuous 165
   lowest 271
   oxygen delivery system 311
   pressure variation 8, 10
Pulsus paradoxus 9
   reverse 9
Pump failure 72

Q
Quadriplegia 134, 138

R
Radiological atelectasis score 121
Randomized controlled trials 50, 52, 183, 216, 262, 270, 321
Rapid eye movement 127, 138, 247
Rapid shallow breathing index 199
Rebreathing 86
   promote 110
Recurrent atrial fibrillation 125
Relative humidity 187, 264
Remifentanil 184
Residual volume 90
Respiration through mouth 33
Respiratory acidosis 304
   acute on chronic 51
   and lethargy 145
   development of 52
Respiratory and cardiac muscles 134
Respiratory arrest 56, 79, 102, 267
Respiratory assist devices 251
Respiratory assistance 138
Respiratory comorbidities 137
Respiratory complications 139
Respiratory compromise 235
Respiratory disease 54, 87, 157, 304
Respiratory disorders 100
Respiratory distress 51, 67, 70, 153, 293, 301, 317
   causes of 322
   moderate-to-severe 62
   score 322
   severe 102
   syndrome 285, 300
      mild-moderate 304
Respiratory dysfunction 145
Respiratory effort
   absence of 248
   related arousal 125
Respiratory failure 51, 52, 54, 72, 73t, 74t, 96, 100, 134, 142, 217, 218f, 268, 276, 300, 370
   anticipated 300
   causes of 73t
   mechanism underlying 142
   perioperative 100
   physiology of
      type I 72
      type II 72
   postoperative 63, 119
   profound 134

   risk of severe 275
   severe 98
      acute 157
      type I 72
      type II 73, 234
Respiratory function 135, 259
Respiratory impairment
   signs of 253
   symptom of 253
Respiratory insufficiency,
   mechanism of 307
Respiratory mechanics 144
Respiratory muscle 52, 134
   diseases of 73
   dysfunction 234
   fatigue 4, 149
   mechanical failure, sign of 106
Respiratory pump, inadequate 307
Respiratory rate 62, 67, 83, 248, 269, 277, 278, 313
   analysis 248
   higher 270
   oxygenation index 277
   reduced 272
Respiratory secretions, excessive 79
Respiratory stimulation 247
Respiratory support
   adequacy of 312
   advancements in 134
   equipment for 309
   long-term 306
   mode of 134
Respiratory system, compliance of 91
Respironics BiPAP vision 15
Restrictive disease 27
Restrictive disorders 247
Restrictive thoracic disorders 85, 144
Rib fractures 53
Right atrial pressure 5, 6, 6f, 7, 9
Right ventricle 6, 7, 8f
Right ventricular
   dysfunction 82
   end-diastolic volume 8f
   failure 190
Rigid bronchoscope 171
Risperidone 184

S
Salbutamol 47, 62, 190
Salivation 33
Salmeterol 190
Salt and water retention 4 7
Scleroderma 74

Scoliosis 142
Second-generation systems 248
Secretion
   accumulation of 92
   clearance 200
   drying up of 82
Sedation 184, 261
   drugs used for 183, 184t
   indications for 183
   practices 183
   related issues 59
Seizures 184
Sensorium 67
   worsening of 70
Sepsis 74, 156
Series effect 8
Shock 145, 267
   circulatory 74
Shunt 146
Sickle cell disease 310
Sidestream capnography 206, 206f, 206t
   with nasal prongs, use of 207f
Silverman-Anderson scoring system 296t
Six-minute walk test 254
Skeletal muscle weakness 136
Skin
   damage 34
   lesions 223
   rash 57
   sores 223
Sleep
   architecture, impaired 249
   disordered breathing 254, 310
   hypoventilation 247
   sudden awakenings from 253
Sleepiness, daytime 125
Small volume nebulizer 43, 45, 46t
Sniff nasal
   inspiratory pressure 241
   pressure 236
Solid organ transplant 149, 150
Solid tumors 153
Spanish sleep network study 252
Spinal cord
   damage 245
   injury 139
      level of 139t
   trauma 73
Spinal injury, acute phase of 139
Split-night studies 130
Spontaneous awakening trials 216

Spontaneous breathing 43, 247
  effects of 6fc
  nebulization during 44f
  trials 215, 218f
Spontaneous respiration 106
  cardiovascular effects of 107
Status asthmaticus 9
Sterile water reservoir 264
Stress
  extramural 106f
  intramural 106f
Stroke 73
  volume variation 8, 10
Sudden heart failure 105
Supplemental oxygen 40, 261
Support staff, training of 301
Surgery, abdominal 53
Surrogate 158
Symptomatic sleep 254
Synchronicity 248
Synchronized noninvasive positive pressure ventilation 294
Systemic lupus erythematosus 74
Systemic vascular resistance 105
Systolic pressure variation 8, 10

T

Tachycardia 85
Tachypnea 70
Tank ventilators, development of 19
Telemonitoring 248
Temperature 279
Terbutaline 47
Tetanus 73
Tetraparesis, causes of 139t
Tetraplegia 36, 134, 138, 139, 140t
  causes of 139t
Therapy
  monitoring of 82
  titration of 81, 312
Third-generation systems 248
Thoracic cage abnormalities 245
Thoracoabdominal asynchrony 277
Thoracoabdominal dyssynchrony 304
Thoracoplasty 74, 142
Thoracotomy 140
Tidal breathing 90f
Tidal volume 20, 67, 90, 92
  monitoring 36
Tiotropium 190
Tissue ischemia 105
  local 224
Titration modality 129
Tobramycin 190
Tolerate oronasal masks 318

Tracheobronchomalacia 172
Tracheostomy 214, 308
  care 311
  tube 251, 254, 316
Traditional capnography 205
Traditional oxygen devices 264
Transcutaneous capnometry monitoring 208
Transcutaneous carbon dioxide 199
  monitoring 207
Transdiaphragmatic pressure 144
Transesophageal echocardiography 172
Translate sound 234
Transport, preparation for 165
Transverse myelitis 73
Trauma 51, 53, 63, 73, 145
  local 268
  management 146
Trigger 19
  sensitivity 319
Two finger rule 225f

U

Ultrasonic nebulizer 45, 47
Uncooperative patient (confused, agitated) 56
Upper airway 143, 311
  collapse 271
  obstruction 56, 74, 102
  fixed 79
  patency of 100
  surgery 79
Upper gastrointestinal tract surgery 143
Upper motor neuron 138
Upper respiratory tract 186

V

Vapor transfer cartridge 264
Variable flow devices 287, 288
Vascular problems defect 307
Vasoactive agents 190
Vena cava
  inferior 10
  superior 10
Venous return 5
Vented masks, use with 166
Ventilation 72, 92, 97, 251, 260, 308
  alveolar 4, 24
  effectiveness of 312
  homogenous distribution of 269
  intermittent mandatory 146
  mode of 64, 190
  volume-targeted 20

perfusion
  inequalities 97
  mismatch 234
  pressure-targeted 21
  strategy 235
  via tracheostomy 251
  volume-targeted 15
Ventilator 236, 288f, 309
  alarms 312
  and respiratory muscle pressure 158
  circuit, device in inspiratory limb of 45f
  dysfunction 312
  dyssynchrony 58
  failure 140
  free days, terms of 114
  interface 233
  mode of 43
    recent 24
    selection of 236
  parameters 67, 189
  pressures 45
  related factors 190
  settings 247
  tolerance of 67
  type of 42, 110
Ventilatory assist, neurally-adjusted 20, 25, 216, 294
Ventilatory control center 89, 91fc, 92
Ventilatory failure 253
Ventilatory parameters 199
Ventilatory settings 16
Ventilatory support 245
Ventilatory technique 36
Ventricular function 6
Ventricular interdependence 5, 8, 9f
Venturi mask 264
Vibrating mesh nebulizer 189, 190
Viral illness 51
Viral pneumonias 3
Vital capacity, waning 134
Vocal cords 259
Volume assist-control mode 20
Volutrauma 96
Vomiting 33, 34, 56
  severe 79

W

Weaning 63, 69
  failure 214
  noninvasive ventilation, strategies for 211
  pulmonary edema of 11

EU GSPR Authorised Reprsentative
Logos Europe, 9 rue Nicolas Poussin
1700, La Rochelle, France
Phone: +33 (0) 6 67 93 73 78
E-mail: contact@logoseurope.eu

www.ingramcontent.com/pod-product-compliance
Ingram Content Group UK Ltd.
Pitfield, Milton Keynes, MK11 3LW, UK
UKHW050454150426
5217IPUK00025B/1688